ADVANCED PHARMACEUTICS

Physicochemical Principles

Books are to be returned on or before
the last date below.

LIBREX-

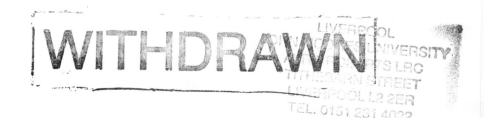

ADVANCED PHARMACEUTICS
Physicochemical Principles

Cherng-ju Kim

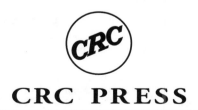

CRC PRESS

Boca Raton   London   New York   Washington, D.C.

Library of Congress Cataloging-in-Publication Data

Kim, Cherng-ju.
    Advanced pharmaceutics : physicochemical principles / Cherng-Ju Kim.
      p. cm.
    Includes bibliographical references and index.
    ISBN 0-8493-1729-0 (alk. paper)
      1. Drugs--Dosage forms. 2. Pharmacy. 3. Pharmaceutical technology. I. Title.

RS200.K54 2004
615'.4--dc22

2003066753

Visit the CRC Press Web site at www.crcpress.com

Preface

This book presents, in a mechanistic, quantitative manner, many of the necessary fundamentals required for pharmaceutics-related problems. It can be used to guide students and professionals until they understand the fundamentals well enough to focus their research areas and read articles in the literature. This book has evolved from several course notes at Temple University School of Pharmacy, particularly with the aid of books by J. R. Barrante (*Physical Chemistry for the Life Sciences*), R. Chang (*Physical Chemistry with Applications to Biological Systems*), A. T. Florence and D. Attwood (*Physicochemical Principles of Pharmacy*), A. Martin (*Physical Pharmacy*), O. Robbins, Jr. (*Ionic Reactions and Equilibria*), and Williams et al. (*Basic Physical Chemistry for the Life Sciences*). It is intended primarily for graduate students in pharmaceutics. This book can be taught in two semesters with supplemental material: Chapters 1 to 4 for the first semester and Chapters 5 to 7 for the second semester. I hope that this book will also be useful as a reference for pharmaceutical scientists engaged in drug product development.

I acknowledge Dean Peter H. Doukas at Temple University for his support and encouragement. I owe major debts to Professor Archie E. Hamielec and Dr. Ping I. Lee who introduced me to polymer engineering and pharmaceutics, respectively. I am grateful to graduate students who raised various questions and suggestions in diverse subject matters.

I am indebted to my wife and children for their patience, understanding, and assistance during the preparation of this book.

Cherng-ju Kim
Loma Linda, California

Author

Cherng-ju Kim, Ph.D., is an Associate Professor and Chair of Pharmaceutical Sciences, School of Pharmacy, Loma Linda University, Loma Linda, California. Before taking this position in 2002, Dr. Kim was Associate Professor and Director of Graduate Studies at the School of Pharmacy, Temple University, Philadelphia, Pennsylvania (1992–2002). Dr. Kim's primary research interests include the development of polymeric materials for controlled release drug delivery systems and the modulation of drug release kinetics. As the author of *Controlled Release Dosage Form Design* (Technomic Publishing, Lancaster, PA), Dr. Kim has published more than 50 papers and 3 patents in this field. Before becoming involved in drug delivery fields, Dr. Kim worked in the area of synthetic membranes (Zenon Environmental, Inc. and Advanced Membranes, Inc.). Dr. Kim received his B.S. in Chemical Engineering from Korea University, Seoul (1974), his M.E. in Environmental Engineering from Manhattan College, Riverside, New York (1979), and his Ph.D. in Chemical Engineering under the supervision of Prof. Archie Hamielec from McMaster University, Hamilton, Ontario, Canada (1984).

Contents

1 Thermodynamics

Thermodynamics is a branch of physical chemistry that deals quantitatively with the inter-exchange of heat and work evolved in physical and chemical processes. This subject is widely utilized to explain equilibrium systems in physical pharmacy. For example, a pharmaceutical scientist may use equilibrium thermodynamics to study isotonic solutions, solubility of drugs, distributions of drugs in different phases, or ionization of weak acids and weak bases. Even though the gas laws are not usually directly related to pharmaceutical science (with some exceptions such as aerosols), these concepts must be introduced when dealing with simple thermodynamic systems of gases and the universal gas constant, R.

1.1 IDEAL GASES

Robert Boyle discovered experimentally that the volume of a gas in a J–tube apparatus at a constant temperature varied in inverse proportion to the pressure. This is known as Boyle's law. Boyle's law may be expressed mathematically as:

$$V \propto \frac{1}{P} \quad \text{(constant temperature)} \tag{1.1}$$

where V and P are the volume and pressure of the gas, respectively.

In the early 19th century, Joseph Gay-Lussac, after following the work of Alexandre Charles, established that the volume of a gas increases linearly with temperature at constant pressure. Expressed mathematically, Charles's law states that:

$$V = V_o(1 + \alpha\, t) \quad \text{(constant pressure)} \tag{1.2}$$

where V_o is the volume of the gas at 0°C, α is the proportionality constant (or thermal expansion coefficient) for the gas, and t is the temperature (°C). It was found experimentally that α is independent of the nature of the gas and that it has the value of $\frac{1}{273.15}$ °C^{-1}. Substituting this value into Equation (1.2) yields:

$$V = V_o\left(\frac{273.15 + t}{273.15}\right) \tag{1.3}$$

In Equation (1.3), the volume of the gas becomes zero when the temperature is reduced to –273.15°C, which is the absolute zero temperature. The relation between the Celsius degree and the absolute scale (called Kelvin degree) is given by:

$$T(K) = 273.15 + t\ (°C) \tag{1.4}$$

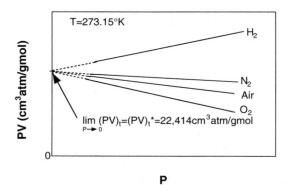

FIGURE 1.1 Variation of pressure–volume product with pressure.

The Kelvin degree scale was originally introduced by William Thomson. It is a thermodynamic temperature scale based on the second law of thermodynamics and is identical to the absolute temperature scale based on the above volume expansion arguments. Substituting Equation (1.4) into Equation (1.3) gives:

$$V = V_o \frac{T}{T_o} \quad \text{or} \quad \frac{V}{T} = \frac{V_o}{T_o} \tag{1.5}$$

where $T_o = 273.15$ K.

Volume is an extensive property, which is dependent on the quantity of substance (or substances) present in the system. Therefore, the volume of a gas at constant temperature and pressure is directly proportional to the number of moles of the gas, n (Avogadro principle). Unlike volume, temperature and pressure are intensive properties and are independent of the amount of material present in the system. Combining Equation (1.1) and Equation (1.5) with the Avogadro principle gives:

$$V \propto \frac{nT}{P} \quad \text{or} \quad PV = n\,RT \tag{1.6}$$

where R is the proportionality constant or gas constant. Equation (1.6) is known as the ideal gas law. The proportionality constant of Equation (1.6) is determined experimentally.

As the pressure approaches zero, all gases follow the ideal gas law. Experimentally, plotting PV against P and extrapolating to zero pressure gives the gas constant, R (see Figure 1.1). Since one mole of an ideal gas occupies 22.414 L at 0°C and 1 atmospheric pressure, then, R is:

$$R = \frac{PV}{nT} = \frac{1\,\text{atm} \times 22.414\,\text{L}}{1\,\text{mole} \times 273.15\,\text{K}} = 0.08206\,\text{L - atm / mole K} \tag{1.7}$$

TABLE 1.1

Values of the Ideal Gas Constant R

82.06	mL-atm K^{-1} mol^{-1}
1.987	cal K^{-1} mol^{-1}
8.314	J K^{-1} mol^{-1}
8.314×10^7	erg K^{-1} mol^{-1}
1.987	Btu (lb mol)$^{-1}$ R^{-1}

The value of R is dependent on the units used for each variable (i.e., P, V, T). The common values of R are listed in Table 1.1.

Example 1.1

Calculate the volume occupied by 23.6 g of a propellant, trifluorochloroethane, at 55°C and 720 mmHg pressure. Assume the gas follows the ideal gas law.

Solution

$$V = \frac{n\,RT}{P} = \frac{(23.6 \text{ g})(0.08206 \text{ L atm / mol K})(55° + 273.15°)}{(136 \text{ g / mole})(720 \text{ mmHg})(1 \text{ atm / 760 mmHg})} = 4.93 \text{ L}$$

In a mixture of gases in a container at constant temperature and pressure, each gas obeys the ideal gas law. The total pressure of the container is dependent on the total number of moles present in the container regardless of the nature of the gases. The individual pressures for each gas are called partial pressures (i.e., $P_1, P_2, P_3, \cdots$). The sum of these partial pressures is equal to the total pressure, P_T; this is known as Dalton's law of partial pressures. The mathematical expression for Dalton's law is as follows:

$$P_T = P_1 + P_2 + P_3 + \cdots\cdots\cdots + P_N \tag{1.8}$$

where N is the number of gases in the system.

Applying the ideal gas law gives:

$$P_T = \frac{(n_1 + n_2 + n_3 + \cdots\cdots)\,RT}{V} \tag{1.9}$$

where n_1, n_2, n_3, etc., represent the number of moles of each gas. Equation (1.8) and Equation (1.9) give the partial pressure of each gas *i* as:

$$P_i = \frac{n_i RT}{V} \tag{1.10}$$

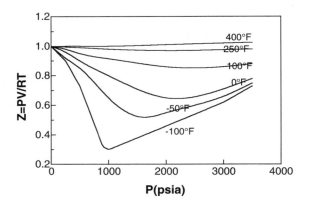

FIGURE 1.2 Compressibility factor diagram for methane.

From the ratio of Equation (1.9) to Equation (1.10), the mole fraction of the gas i, in the mixture, X_i, can be obtained by:

$$X_i = \frac{P_i}{P_T} = \frac{n_i}{n_1 + n_2 + n_3 + \cdots\cdots + n_T} \tag{1.11}$$

1.2 REAL GASES

As the pressure of a gas is increased and/or its temperature is lowered, the ideal gas law is not followed because the volume of the gas is not negligible and intermolecular forces do exist. If the ratio, $z = \frac{PV}{nRT}$, referred to as the *compressibility factor* for the gas, is plotted against P at constant temperature, then the values of Z deviate from ideal behavior, which is unity for an ideal gas (see Figure 1.2). This is attributed to the pressure build-up as gas molecules collide on the walls of a container. If the gas molecules adjacent to the walls exert intermolecularly attractive forces, the momentum of the gas molecules toward the wall will be decreased. Thus, the collisions of the gas molecules will be reduced, resulting in the pressure of the gas being less than that of an ideal gas. At high pressure, the gas molecules pack the container very closely together, causing the volume of the gas molecules to be a significant part of the total volume.

Van der Waals proposed the incorporation of two additional terms into the ideal gas law to account for the deviations from ideal behavior. The ideal gas law equation then becomes:

$$\left(P + \frac{a}{V^2}\right)(V - b) = RT \tag{1.12}$$

where a and b are constants and are determined experimentally. The constant a in Equation (1.12) accounts for the cohesive forces between the gas molecules, which

TABLE 1.2

Van der Waals Constants of Some Gases

Gas	a (L^2 atm/mol^2)	b (L/mol)
He	0.0353	0.0241
H_2	0.246	0.0267
N_2	1.35	0.0383
O_2	1.36	0.0319
CO_2	3.60	0.0427
CH_4	2.25	0.0428
H_2O	5.43	0.0303
NH_3	4.19	0.0373

drag other gas molecules around a single molecule, causing the pressure of the gas to be less than that of an ideal gas. The cohesive forces are dependent on the intermolecular distances and related to the density of the gas. The term a/V^2 is called the internal pressure per mole. This internal pressure will be used to describe the solubility of the molecules in liquids in Chapter 3. The constant b in Equation (1.12) accounts for the incompressibility of the gas molecules, known as the excluded volume occupied by the gas molecules. The excluded volume is approximately four times the volume of the gas molecules. The term $(V - b)$ represents the effective volume of the gas molecules that expand freely. The van der Waals constants for typical gases are listed in Table 1.2. At low pressure, the volume of the gas molecules is so large that the contribution of the excluded volume toward the total volume is very small and the term a/V^2 becomes negligible. Thus, under these conditions, Equation (1.12) is reduced to the ideal gas law expressed by Equation (1.6).

Example 1.2

Calculate the pressure produced by 75 g of ethanol in a 5.0 L container at 80°C by the ideal gas law and van der Waals equation. The van der Waals constants a and b are 12.02 L^2 atm/mol^2 and 0.08407 L/mol, respectively.

Solution

From the ideal gas law,

$$P = \frac{n\,RT}{V} = \frac{(75\text{ g})(0.08206\text{ Latm}/\text{mol K})(353.15\text{ K})}{(46\text{ g}/\text{mol})(5\text{ L})} = 9.45\text{ atm}$$

The van der Waals equation can be rewritten as:

$$P = \frac{n\,RT}{V - n\,b} - \frac{n^2 a}{V^2} = \frac{(75/46)(0.08206)(353.15)}{5 - (75/46)(0.08407)} - \frac{(75/46)^2(12.02)}{5^2}$$

$$= 8.44\text{ atm}$$

1.3 THERMODYNAMICS

It is common to observe in our daily life that different forms of energy may be interchanged. For example, electrical energy can be converted to heat. Thermodynamics is not only the study of the quantitative relationships of these energy changes but is also used as a tool to examine and predict the behaviors of physical, chemical, and biological processes in terms of energetics. The two principles of thermodynamics, the first and second laws, are extremely important to the understanding of energy. The first law, which pertains to the conservation of energy, states that energy may not be created or destroyed but may only change its form. The second law predicts the direction in which any given process will occur. Thermodynamics explains whether a process will proceed in a certain direction, but it does not reveal the time required or how many hurdles the system will go through to get there. In other words, it gives us the beginning and the end of a process even though it is independent of the pathways leading from the beginning to the end.

1.3.1 THE FIRST LAW OF THERMODYNAMICS

First, let us define a system and its surroundings. A system is a portion of the whole upon which one chooses to focus one's interest. A boundary separates the system from the rest of the whole. Mass and/or energy may enter or leave through the boundary. The surroundings of the system are anything outside the boundary of the system. In a closed system, energy may enter or leave during a particular process but no mass may be exchanged with the surroundings through the boundary. Systems in which both mass and energy can enter or leave during a process are called open systems.

The energy change in a system may occur through the absorption or loss of heat and by any work done on or by the system. No absolute energy value of the system is known, so one should consider the energy change from one state to another. Mathematically, the first law of thermodynamics states for both the system and its surroundings:

$$\int dE = 0 \tag{1.13}$$

where E is the internal energy of the system. The internal energy of a material should not be obtained from its position or movement as a whole. The internal energy is the motional energy retained by a molecule. In other words, it refers to the energy of the molecules making up the material. Equation (1.13) relates that a change in the energy of the surroundings is precisely compensated for by a change in the energy of the system. This leads to a total energy change of zero for the system and its surroundings when considered together. For the system alone, however, the first law states that:

$$\Delta E = q - w \tag{1.14a}$$

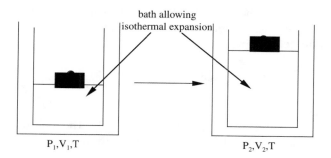

FIGURE 1.3 A cylinder with a frictionless piston holds a gas undergoing an isothermal expansion.

where ΔE is the energy change of the system and q and w are heat and work exchanged between the system and its surroundings, respectively. Heat absorbed by the system is assigned a positive value whereas a negative value corresponds to work done on the surroundings by the system. The change in internal energy is dependent only on the initial and final states, regardless of the pathways taken from the initial to final states. Such a system is referred to as a state function. For example, if a process starts at an initial state and travels many different paths and then comes back to the initial state, the change in internal energy for the system must be zero because $\Delta E = E_1 - E_2 = E_1 - E_1 = 0$. However, heat and work are always dependent on the pathways taken by the system from the initial to the final states. For example, when a person climbs the peak of a mountain, the internal change in energy level for the person is the height of the mountain climbed. The work the person does to reach the top of the mountain depends on the path taken to the peak (i.e., zigzag, straight-up walk, etc.). When applied to processes involving differential changes in the system, Equation (1.14a) may be written as:

$$dE = dq - dw \tag{1.14b}$$

Equation (1.14b) is advantageous when E, q, or w is expressed as a variable function, changing during a process. Some illustrations of the first law of thermodynamics are given as follows:

Isothermal expansion of an ideal gas: Let us consider that a cylinder fitted with a frictionless piston contains a gas and is heated to the system shown in Figure 1.3. Normally, the temperature of the system increases upon heating, but one wants to maintain a constant temperature for the system during this isothermal process. The piston exerts an external pressure on the system, and the gas expands. Since no temperature change takes place, the change in the internal energy is equal to zero ($\Delta E = 0$) because the internal energy is only a function of temperature. Then, Equation (1.14) becomes:

$$q - w = 0 \quad \text{or} \quad q = w \tag{1.15}$$

Because $\Delta E = 0$, the heat absorbed by the system must work on its surroundings by expanding against the external pressure. An infinitesimal increase of work, dw, done against the external pressure, P_{ext}, is given by:

$$dw = F \times dl = P_{ext} \times A \times dl = P_{ext}dV \qquad (1.16)$$

where dl is the infinitesimal distance and F and A are the force to move up the piston and the cross-sectional area of the piston, respectively. The total work done while moving the piston from the initial to final stage is given as:

$$w = \int P_{ext}dV \qquad (1.17)$$

It is important to point out that work is not a state function but is dependent on the pathway taken to reach the final state.

If a gas expands isothermally under a constant external pressure, Equation (1.17) becomes:

$$w = P_{ext}\int_{V_1}^{V_2} dV = P_{ext}(V_2 - V_1) \qquad (1.18)$$

where V_1 and V_2 are the initial and final volumes, respectively.

If a gas expands isothermally and the external pressure exerted on the gas varies, one must find a different relationship between P_{ext} and V. In other words, the value of external pressure must be known at every stage during the expansion or compression. If the gas expands or is compressed reversibly, the pressure difference between the internal gas pressure and external pressure is infinitesimally small, and thus the internal gas pressure (P_{gas}) is equal to the external pressure. Then P_{ext} in Equation (1.17) can be replaced with P_{gas} as:

$$w = \int P_{ext}dV = \int P_{gas}dV \qquad (1.19)$$

If the gas behaves ideally at a constant temperature, Equation (1.6) can be substituted into Equation (1.19), resulting in:

$$w = \int_{V_1}^{V_2} \frac{n\,RT}{V}dV = n\,RT\,\ln\!\left(\frac{V_2}{V_1}\right) = n\,RT\,\ln\!\left(\frac{P_1}{P_2}\right) \qquad (1.20)$$

If the gas obeys the van der Waals equation, the substitution of Equation (1.12) into Equation (1.19) yields:

$$w = \int_{V_1}^{V_2}\left(\frac{n\,RT}{V-n\,b} - \frac{n^2a}{V^2}\right)dV = n\,RT\,\ln\!\left(\frac{V_2-n\,b}{V_1-n\,b}\right) + n^2a\!\left(\frac{1}{V_2} - \frac{1}{V_1}\right) \quad (1.21)$$

Example 1.3
One mole of CO_2 gas at 25°C is allowed to expand reversibly and isothermally from a volume of 5 L to a volume of 15 L. Calculate the work done by the gas against the frictionless piston for an ideal gas and for a van der Waals gas. The van der Waals constants a and b are 1.94 L^2 atm/mol^2 and 0.0314 L/mol, respectively.

Solution
From Equation (1.21),

$$w = n\ RT\ \ln\left(\frac{V_2 - n\ b}{V_1 - n\ b}\right) + n^2 a\left(\frac{1}{V_2} - \frac{1}{V_1}\right)$$

$$= 1.987\ (298.15)\ \ln\left(\frac{15 - 0.0314}{5 - 0.0314}\right) + 1.94\left(\frac{1}{15} - \frac{1}{5}\right) = 653\ \text{cal}$$

From Equation (1.20),

$$w = n\ RT\ \ln\frac{V_2}{V_1} = 1.987\ (298.15)\ln\frac{15}{5} = 651\ \text{cal}$$

Isothermal vaporization of a liquid under a constant pressure: When a liquid in a frictionless piston is heated and its vapor pressure reaches the external pressure, the liquid vaporizes and therefore the system (liquid and its vapor) expands. Therefore, the system does work on the piston as $P_{ext}(V_{gas} - V_{liquid})$. However, the volume of vapor is much larger than that of the liquid, and thus the work done is $P_{ext}V_{gas}$. The heat absorbed is used to vaporize the liquid as the vapor does work on the surroundings (i.e., against the piston). The remaining energy is stored in the vapor state as internal energy according to the first law of thermodynamics.

Example 1.4
Calculate the energy change ΔE and w for the vaporization of one mole of ethanol at 78.3°C and 1 atmospheric pressure. The heat of vaporization of ethanol is 204 cal/g.

Solution
The heat required to vaporize is:

$$q = (1\ \text{mole})(204\ \text{cal}\ /\ \text{g})(46\ \text{g}\ /\ \text{mol}) = 9384\ \text{cal}$$

The work done by the vapor is:

$$w = P_{ext}\Delta V = P_{gas}V_{gas} = nRT = (1\ \text{mole})(1.987\ \text{cal}\ /\ \text{mol\ K})(351.45\ \text{K}) = 698\ \text{cal}$$

Then $\Delta E = q - w = 9384 - 698 = 8686\ \text{cal}$

1.3.2 ENTHALPY (HEAT CONTENT) AND HEAT CAPACITY

Let us consider that a system absorbs heat but is not allowed to expand. Under this condition no work is done on the system or by the system because dV is equal to zero. Thus, the heat absorbed is now the increase in internal energy of the system. The first law of thermodynamics is given by:

$$\Delta E = q_V - w = q_V - \int_{V_1}^{V_2} P_{ext} dV = q_V \tag{1.22a}$$

where q_V is the heat absorbed or lost by the system under constant volume. However, most physical, chemical, and biological processes are not carried out at constant volume, but rather at constant pressure (isobaric). For example, a chemical reaction in a round-bottom flask is done under a constant atmospheric pressure. If the process is isobaric and reversible, the first law of thermodynamics yields:

$$\Delta E = q_P - w = q_P - \int_{V_1}^{V_2} P_{ext} dV = q_P - P\Delta V \tag{1.22b}$$

where q_P is the heat absorbed or lost by the system at constant pressure and $P_{ext} = P$, the pressure of the system, because the process is reversible.

Equation (1.22b) may be rearranged to:

$$q_P = \Delta E + P\Delta V = E_2 - E_1 + PV_2 - PV_1 = \left(E_2 + PV_2\right) - \left(E_1 + PV_1\right) \tag{1.23}$$

Now a new thermodynamic term, enthalpy or heat content, is defined as:

$$H = E + PV \tag{1.24a}$$

In differential form, Equation (1.24a) becomes:

$$dH = dE + d(PV) \tag{1.24b}$$

Substituting Equation (1.24a) into Equation (1.23) yields:

$$q_P = H_2 - H_1 = \Delta H \tag{1.25}$$

It is important to point out that ΔH, like ΔE, is a state function. The change in enthalpy is independent of the path taken and dependent only on the initial and final states of the system. Equation (1.25) states that the amount of heat absorbed or lost during an isobaric process is equal to the change of enthalpy of the system. If the process is not isobaric but reversible, then from Equation (1.14b) and Equation (1.19),

$$dH = dE + d(PV) = q - PdV + PdV + VdP = q + VdP \qquad (1.26)$$

At constant pressure, Equation (1.26) becomes Equation (1.25).

When a system is heated, its temperature generally increases. This increase in temperature is dependent on the heat capacity of the system under constant volume or constant pressure. Therefore, the heat capacity is defined as the ratio of heat added to a system to its corresponding temperature change. If the system is under constant volume, the molar heat capacity is C_V, whereas the molar capacity is C_P for a system under constant pressure. Then,

$$C_V = \lim_{\Delta T \to 0} \frac{q_V}{\Delta T} = \left(\frac{\partial q}{\partial T}\right)_V = \left(\frac{\partial E}{\partial T}\right)_V \qquad (1.27a)$$

$$C_P = \lim_{\Delta T \to 0} \frac{q_P}{\Delta T} = \left(\frac{\partial q}{\partial T}\right)_P = \left(\frac{\partial H}{\partial T}\right)_P \qquad (1.27b)$$

Equation (1.27a) and Equation (1.27b) lead to:

$$dE = C_V dT \quad \text{and} \quad dH = C_P dT \qquad (1.28)$$

The changes in the internal energy and enthalpy during a temperature change due to the absorption of heat are given by:

$$\Delta E = \int_{T_1}^{T_2} C_V dT \quad \text{and} \quad \Delta H = \int_{T_1}^{T_2} C_P dT \qquad (1.29)$$

The heat capacity is a function of temperature. When the change in heat capacity is negligible over a small temperature change, the average value of heat capacity ($\overline{C}_V$ or $\overline{C}_P$) over the temperature range is used instead. Then Equation (1.29) is integrated to:

$$\Delta E = \overline{C}_V (T_2 - T_1) \quad \text{or} \quad \Delta H = \overline{C}_P (T_2 - T_1) \qquad (1.30)$$

If the temperature change varies broadly, the constant and average values of heat capacity cannot be used. Empirically, the heat capacity at constant pressure is expressed as a polynomial form of T as:

$$C_P = a + bT + cT^2 \qquad (1.31)$$

where a, b, and c are the constants determined experimentally.

Substituting Equation (1.31) into Equation (1.29) gives:

$$\Delta H = a(T_2 - T_1) + \frac{b}{2}(T_2^2 - T_1^2) + \frac{c}{3}(T_2^3 - T_1^3) \qquad (1.32)$$

The relationship between C_P and C_V is $C_P = C_V + R$. Differentiating Equation (1.24a) with respect to temperature yields:

$$\frac{dH}{dT} = \frac{dE}{dT} + \frac{d(PV)}{dT} \qquad (1.33)$$

Substituting Equation (1.28) and the ideal gas law into Equation (1.33) yields:

$$\frac{C_P dT}{dT} = \frac{C_V dT}{dT} + \frac{d(RT)}{dT} \quad \text{or} \quad C_P = C_V + R \qquad (1.34)$$

For solids and liquids, the change in volume is so small that C_P and C_V are almost the same.

Example 1.5

Calculate ΔE, ΔH, q, and w for the isobaric reversible expansion of one mole of an ideal gas from 25 to 75°C. The molar heat capacity of the gas is 8.96 cal/mol K.

Solution

From Equation (1.30),

$$\Delta H = \overline{C}_P(T_2 - T_1) = 8.96 \times (75 - 25) = 448 \text{ cal}$$

$$\Delta E = \overline{C}_V(T_2 - T_1) = 6.973 \times (75 - 25) = 348.65 \text{ cal}$$

Because the process is an isobaric expansion, $\Delta H = q = 448$ cal and w is given by:

$$w = q - \Delta E = 448 - 348.65 = 99.35 \text{ cal}$$

1.3.3 THERMOCHEMISTRY

Thermochemistry is a branch of thermodynamics that deals with the change of heat (enthalpy) in chemical reactions. The heat absorbed or lost in chemical reactions usually occurs at constant pressure rather than at constant volume. The change of heat is mostly expressed by ΔH, the enthalpy change of a process from reactants to products:

$$\Delta H = \sum H_{products} - \sum H_{reactants} \qquad (1.35)$$

If $\Delta H > 0$, heat must be supplied to the reaction (endothermic); if $\Delta H < 0$, heat is evolved during the reaction (exothermic). As mentioned before, if reactants or products are pure liquids or solids, as they are for most biochemical reactions, there is no volume change, so that $\Delta E = \Delta H$. However, if there are gas molecules in the reactants and/or products, the change of volume during the reactions is large and ΔV should be considered to calculate the enthalpy change.

To express the heat absorbed or evolved in any chemical reaction, the symbol ΔH°_{25} is used in which the superscript $^{\circ}$ indicates a standard state and the subscript specifies the temperature at which the reaction occurs. The standard state for a gas is 1 atm pressure and the standard state for liquids is the pure liquid under the same conditions. For solids, it refers customarily to a crystalline state at 1 atm. Unless otherwise denoted, 25°C is the standard state for temperature.

As discussed for a state function such as E, there is no absolute value of enthalpy of a chemical (reactant or product); it is determined experimentally. The enthalpy value of an individual compound is calculated based on the assigned base value. A value of zero corresponds to the enthalpy of the most stable form of an element in its standard state at 25°C. Heat of formation is defined as the heat absorbed or evolved in the formation of one mole of a compound from its elements in their standard states. The formation of ethanol involves the elements of solid carbon, hydrogen, and oxygen. However, even though these elements are put together and heated in a reaction vessel, ethanol is not formed. In this case, the heat of formation of ethanol is calculated based on Hess's law of constant heat summation. The law states that the heat absorbed or evolved during a chemical reaction under constant pressure is the same regardless of the pathways taken to get to the final state from the initial state. This is due to the fact that enthalpy or enthalpy change is a function of state. Let us apply this principle to the heat of formation of glucose from ethanol and carbon dioxide as given by:

$$2C_2H_5OH(l) + 2CO_2(g) \rightarrow C_6H_{12}O_6(s) \qquad \Delta H^{\circ}_{25} = 16.2 \text{ kcal / mol} \qquad (1.36)$$

where (l), (g), and (s) refer to the physical states of liquid, gas, and solid, respectively. The following reactions can be used to determine the heat of formation of glucose because their enthalpy changes can be determined experimentally:

$$C(s) + O_2(g) \rightarrow CO_2(g) \qquad \Delta H^{\circ}_{25} = -94.05 \text{ kcal / mol} \qquad (1.37)$$

$$H_2(g) + \tfrac{1}{2}O_2(g) \rightarrow H_2O(l) \qquad \Delta H^{\circ}_{25} = -68.32 \text{ kcal / mol} \qquad (1.38)$$

$$C_2H_5OH(l) + 3O_2(g) \rightarrow 2CO_2(g) + 3H_2O(l) \qquad \Delta H^{\circ}_{25} = -326.68 \text{ kcal / mol} \qquad (1.39)$$

Taking $2 \times (1.39) - 6 \times (1.38) - 6 \times (1.37)$ yields:

$$2C_2H_5OH(l) - 6H_2(g) - 6C(s) - 3O_2(g) \rightarrow -2CO_2(g) \qquad (1.40)$$

$$\Delta H^{\circ}_{25} = 2 \times (-326.68) - 6 \times (-68.32) - 6 \times (-94.05) = 320.86 \text{ kcal}$$

Rearranging Equation (1.40) yields:

$$2C_2H_5OH(1) + 2CO_2(g) \rightarrow 6H_2(g) + 6C(s) + 3O_2(g) \quad \Delta H^o_{25} = 320.86 \text{ kcal} \quad (1.41)$$

Turning Equation (1.41) around gives:

$$6H_2(g) + 6C(s) + 3O_2(g) \rightarrow 2C_2H_5OH(1) + 2CO_2(g) \quad \Delta H^o_{25} = -320.86 \text{ kcal} \quad (1.42)$$

When reactions are turned around, the sign for the enthalpy change must be changed. Adding Equation (1.36) and Equation (1.42) together yields:

$$6H_2(g) + 6C(s) + 3O_2(g) \rightarrow C_6H_{12}O_6(s) \quad \Delta H^o_{25} = -304.66 \text{ kcal / mol} \quad (1.43)$$

The heat of formation of one mole of glucose is −304.66 kcal.

Table 1.3 presents heats of formation for a number of substances determined by direct or indirect methods.

Example 1.6

Calculate ΔH^o_{25} for the esterification of oleic acid with methanol using the appropriate heats of formation for the compounds.

Solution

The esterification of oleic acid with methanol is:

$$C_{17}H_{34}COOH + CH_3OH \rightarrow C_{17}H_{34}COOCH_3$$

Applying Equation (1.35) to the data given in Table 1.3 yields:

$$\Delta H^o_{25} = (-174.2) - (-178.9) - (-57.04) = 61.74 \text{ kcal / mol}$$

A chemical reaction may be carried out at other temperatures rather than 25°C for the enthalpy change. The effect of temperature on ΔH at constant pressure can be given by differentiating Equation (1.35) with respect to temperature as:

$$\frac{d\Delta H}{dT} = \sum \frac{dH_{products}}{dT} - \sum \frac{dH_{reactants}}{dT} \quad (1.44)$$

The first and second terms on the right–hand side of Equation (1.44), (dH/dT), are the total heat capacities of all the products and reactants at constant pressure, respectively. Equation (1.44) then becomes:

$$\frac{d\Delta H}{dT} = C_{P,products} - C_{P,reactants} = \Delta C_P \quad (1.45)$$

TABLE 1.3
Standard Heats of Formation ΔH°_{25} for Selected Organic Compounds at 25°C (kcal/mol)

Substance	State	ΔH°_f	Substance	State	ΔH°_f
Acetic acid	l	−115.72	Glycine	s	−128.39
Acetaldehyde	g	−58.99	Glycinate ion	aq	−114.39
Acetone	l	-58.99	Glycylglycine	s	−178.29
L-Alanine	s	−134.49	Glycylglycinate	aq	−164.88
L-Alanine ion	aq	−133.34	L(+)-Lactic acid	s	−165.87
L-Alaninate ion	aq	−121.79	L(+)-Lactate ion	aq	−164.10
L-Arginine	s	−148.59	α-Lactose	s	−530.97
DL-Aspartic acid	s	−233.49	β-Lactose	s	−534.58
L-Aspartic acid	s	−232.43	DL-Leucine	s	−155.29
L-Aspartic acid ion	s	−228.28	L-Leucine	s	−154.59
L-Aspartate ion	aq	−216.49	L-Leucinate ion	aq	−143.54
Benzene	l	11.72	L-Malic acid	s	−263.69
Butyric acid	l	−127.89	L-Malate ion	aq	−201.39
Butyrate ion	aq	−127.99	α-Maltose	aq	−534.93
Carbon dioxide	g	−94.04	β-Maltose	aq	−534.81
Citric acid	s	−368.98	Methanol	l	−57.04
Citrate ion	aq	−362.10	L-Methionine	s	−181.89
Creatine	s	−128.21	Oxaloacetic acid	s	−235.29
L-Cysteine	s	−127.29	Oxaloacetate ion	aq	−189.59
L-Cystine	s	−249.59	Palmitic acid	s	−212.89
Ethanol	l	−66.20	Pyruvic acid	l	−139.99
Ethyl acetate	l	−115.19	Pyruvate ion	aq	−142.49
Formic acid	l	−97.80	2-Propanol	l	−75.97
Formate ion	aq	−97.99	Succinic acid	s	−224.85
Fumaric acid	s	−193.74	Succinate ion	aq	−217.17
Fumarate ion	aq	−185.79	Sucrose	s	−530.97
α-D-Glucose	s	−304.59	DL-Valine	s	−147.69
β-D-Glucose	s	−303.06	L-Valine	s	−147.69
Glycerol	l	−160.29	L-Valine ion	aq	−146.32
L-Glutamic acid	s	−241.19	L-Valinate ion	aq	−135.61
L-Glutamate ion	aq	−224.59	Water	l	−68.32

Source: Data from R. C. Wilhoit, Thermodynamic Properties of Biochemical Substances, in *Biochemical Microcalorimetry* (H. D. Brown, Ed.), Academic Press, New York, 1969.

where ΔC_p is the change in the heat capacity of the reaction. Equation (1.45) is called Kirchhoff's equation.

Integration of Equation (1.45) yields:

$$\int_{T_1}^{T_2} d\Delta H = \Delta H_{T_2} - \Delta H_{T_1} = \int_{T_1}^{T_2} \Delta C_p dT \qquad (1.46)$$

Example 1.7

Calculate ΔH°_{37} for the cellular respiration of glucose, at the physiological temperature of 37°C, based on the heat-of-formation data given in Table 1.3. Assume the heat capacities for all compounds are constant over low temperature and are 52.31, 7.02, 8.87, and 6.87 kcal/mol for glucose, oxygen, carbon dioxide, and water, respectively.

Solution

The cellular respiration of glucose is expressed by:

$$C_6H_{12}O_6(s) + 6O_2(g) \rightarrow 6CO_2(g) + 6H_2O(l)$$

Enthalpy change for this reaction is given by:

$$\Delta H^\circ_{25} = 6 \times (-94.05) + 6 \times (-68.32) - (-304.66) = 669.56 \text{ kcal / mol}$$

Integrating Equation (1.46) with the constant heat capacity change yields:

$$\Delta H_{T_2} = \Delta H_{T_1} + \Delta C_P(T_2 - T_1) \qquad (1.47)$$

ΔC_P is determined as:

$$\Delta C_P = 6 \times 8.87 + 6 \times 6.87 - 52.31 - 6 \times 7.02 = 0.01 \text{ cal / mol K}$$

The cellular respiration of glucose is then given by:

$$\Delta H^\circ_{37} = \Delta H^\circ_{25} + 0.01 \times 10^{-3} \times (310.15 - 298.15) = 669.56 \text{ kcal / mol}$$

Therefore, the effect of temperature on the enthalpy change is negligible.

1.3.4 HEAT ENGINE AND THE CARNOT CYCLE

In the previous sections, the energy changes in processes were discussed, and it was found that the total energy of a system and its surroundings is conserved. However, many processes obey the first law of thermodynamics but do not happen naturally. For example, ice never gets colder when in contact with warm water. Likewise, warm water does not get warmer when in contact with cold water. A homogeneous mixture of two gases cannot be separated into a high-pressure gas on one side and a low-pressure gas on the other side (Figure 1.4). If these processes were to occur and they did not violate the first law, they would be considered unnatural or not spontaneous due to the work done on the system. However, the opposite direction of these processes would occur spontaneously.

Consider a chemical reaction between hydrogen and nitrogen to form ammonia:

$$N_2 + 3H_2 \rightarrow 2NH_3$$

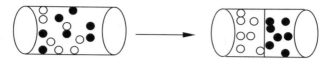

FIGURE 1.4 Separation of a homogeneous gas mixture.

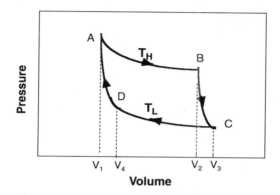

FIGURE 1.5 Pressure–volume relationship for the Carnot cycle.

When one part of nitrogen and three parts of hydrogen come into contact, the forward reaction goes to completion with the evolution of significant heat. In the reverse reaction, the evolved heat can be used with ammonia to regenerate nitrogen and hydrogen. This process does not violate the first law of thermodynamics since the forward reaction takes place naturally while the reverse reaction does not occur spontaneously. The first law of thermodynamics does not predict in which direction a particular physical, chemical, or biological process will happen spontaneously. Therefore another law of thermodynamics is needed to deal with the spontaneity of the process.

The reverse direction of a spontaneous process requires that some work must be done on the system. In 1824, Sadi Carnot, an engineer in Napoleon's army, presented an ideal engine in which the heat could not be completely converted into work. The engine had an ideal gas in a cylinder with a frictionless piston and employed a cyclic operation. In Figure 1.5, the pressure and volume are related to the four steps of the cycle. Initially, the engine contains an initial pressure of P_1, an initial volume of V_1, and an initial temperature of T_H as the initial state A.

The initial state undergoes an isothermal reversible expansion to the second state B at temperature T_H. Because the expansion is isothermal, $\Delta E = 0$ and from Equation (1.20), the work done on the system is given by:

$$q_{A \to B} = w_{A \to B} = RT_H \ln \frac{V_2}{V_1} \qquad (1.48)$$

The second operation is that the ideal gas at the second state B is further expanded adiabatically and reversibly to the third state C. Since the process is adiabatic, no heat is absorbed or lost (i.e., $q_{B \to C} = 0$), and the temperature drops from T_H to T_L. Then from Equation (1.14),

$$\Delta E = C_V (T_L - T_H) = -w_{B \to C} \tag{1.49}$$

The third operation involves the gas at the third state C at temperature T_L, which is compressed isothermally and reversibly to the fourth state D. Since the process is isothermal, $\Delta E = 0$ and the work done on the system is given by:

$$q_{C \to D} = w_{C \to D} = RT_L \ln \frac{V_4}{V_3} \tag{1.50}$$

Finally, the gas is further compressed adiabatically and reversibly to the initial state A. Therefore $q_{D \to A} = 0$ and

$$\Delta E = C_V (T_H - T_L) = -w_{D \to A} \tag{1.51}$$

The total work done on the system over the complete cycle is given by:

$$w_{total} = w_{A \to B} + w_{B \to C} + w_{C \to D} + w_{D \to A} \tag{1.52}$$

Since $w_{B \to C} = -w_{D \to A}$, Equation (1.52) becomes:

$$w_{total} = w_{A \to B} + w_{C \to D} = RT_H \ln \frac{V_2}{V_1} + RT_L \ln \frac{V_4}{V_3} \tag{1.53}$$

Because the second and fourth processes are adiabatic, the following relationship is applied to Equation (1.53):

$$\frac{V_3}{V_2} = \frac{V_4}{V_1} \quad \text{or} \quad \frac{V_4}{V_3} = \frac{V_1}{V_2} \tag{1.54}$$

Thus Equation (1.53) becomes:

$$w_{total} = R(T_H - T_L) \ln \frac{V_2}{V_1} \tag{1.55}$$

The total net work done by the system or the net heat absorbed by the system is illustrated by the inner area of ABCD in Figure 1.5. Because heat and work are not functions of state, net work should be done on the system or by the system even though the system returns to the initial state. The thermodynamic efficiency of the Carnot cycle is defined as the net work done by the system divided by the heat absorbed. Thus

$$\text{efficiency} = \frac{w}{q_{A \to B}} = \frac{R(T_H - T_L) \ln (V_2 / V_1)}{R T_H \ln (V_2 / V_1)} = \frac{T_H - T_L}{T_H} \qquad (1.56)$$

Equation (1.56) implies that the efficiency depends on the two operating temperatures of the engine. The smaller the numerator (temperature difference), the less heat absorbed is converted to work. If the lower temperature is at absolute zero, the efficiency becomes 100%. The engine described is not of interest to pharmaceutical scientists but important to engineers and others who deal with heat engines or refrigerators. However, this heat engine is of interest to all disciplines of science from the viewpoint of the development of absolute zero temperature.

Example 1.8

A heat engine operates between 130 and 30°C. How much heat must be taken from the high temperature to obtain 6 kcal of work? Assume there is no frictional loss of energy.

Solution

From Equation (1.56)

$$\frac{w}{q} = \frac{6}{q} = \frac{T_H - T_L}{T_H} = \frac{403.15 - 303.15}{403.15}$$

$$q = 6 \times \frac{403.15}{100} = 24.2 \text{ kcal}$$

1.3.5 THE SECOND LAW OF THERMODYNAMICS AND ENTROPY

From the discussion of heat engines, the second law of thermodynamics states that it is impossible to achieve heat, taken from a reservoir, and convert it into work without simultaneous delivery of heat from the higher temperature to the lower temperature (Lord Kelvin). It also states that some work should be converted to heat in order to make heat flow from a lower to a higher temperature (Principle of Clausius). These statements acknowledge that the efficiency of heat engines could never be 100% and that heat flow from high temperatures to low temperatures is not totally spontaneous. Simply, the second law states that natural processes occur spontaneously toward the direction in which less available work can be used.

Pharmaceutical scientists use the concept of spontaneity of heat flow for a chemical reaction or biological transformation of energy in an organism even though there is no heat engine or no high and low temperature reservoirs. According to the first law of thermodynamics (i.e., energy conservation), the net total work should be equal to $w_{total} = q_{A \to B} + q_{C \to D}$. Thus,

$$\text{efficiency} = \frac{q_{A\to B} + q_{C\to D}}{q_{A\to B}} = \frac{T_H - T_L}{T_H} \tag{1.57}$$

or
$$\frac{q_{A\to B}}{T_H} + \frac{q_{C\to D}}{T_L} = 0 \tag{1.58}$$

Equation (1.58) applies to any isothermal or adiabatic reversible cyclic processes. If there are many isothermal and adiabatic processes from high temperature T_H to low temperature T_L before the process goes back to its original state, any reversible cyclic process [Equation (1.58)] can be generalized as:

$$\sum_i \frac{dq_i}{T_i} = 0 \tag{1.59}$$

If each isothermal and adiabatic step is infinitesimal, Equation (1.59) for the entire cycle becomes:

$$\oint \frac{dq_{rev}}{T} = 0 \tag{1.60}$$

Equation (1.60) illustrates a very important thermodynamic property in which the quantity dq_{rev}/T becomes zero when the cyclic process is completed regardless of the paths taken from the initial to final states. Such a property is known as a state function, as are P, V, T, E, and H. Clausius suggested defining a new thermodynamic state function, called "entropy" and denoted as S, where $dq_{rev}/T = dS$, so that

$$\oint \frac{dq_{rev}}{T} \equiv \oint dS = 0 \tag{1.61}$$

Therefore, any finite change in entropy can be given by:

$$\int_1^2 dS = S_2 - S_1 = \Delta S = \int \frac{dq_{rev}}{T} \tag{1.62}$$

For an irreversible cyclic process, the summation of dq/T is less than 0, so the efficiency of an irreversible process is lower than that of a reversible one (Clausius):

$$\text{(irreversible process)} \quad \frac{q_H^{irrev} + q_L^{irrev}}{q_H^{irrev}} < \frac{T_H - T_L}{T_H} \quad \text{(reversible process)} \tag{1.63}$$

Therefore,

$$\oint \frac{dq_{irrev}}{T} < 0 \qquad (1.64)$$

The second law of thermodynamics can be restated in terms of entropy regardless of heat engines, chemical reactions, or biological transformations of energy in living organisms, as follows:

1. The change in entropy of the system and the surrounding for any reversible processes is equal to zero.
2. The system and the surrounding react spontaneously in the direction in which the entropy of an irreversible process increases.

Therefore, unlike internal energy and enthalpy, entropy is easily used to predict the direction of a spontaneous process. Thus

$$\Delta S_{system} + \Delta S_{surroundings} = 0, \quad \text{the system is at equilibrium}$$

$$\Delta S_{system} + \Delta S_{surroundings} > 0, \quad \text{spontaneously occurs}$$

$$\Delta S_{system} + \Delta S_{surroundings} < 0, \quad \text{does not spontaneously occur}$$

However, it is very difficult to measure the entropy change of a system and its surroundings in a biological process (i.e., processes occurring in plants and animals). Later in this chapter, a new thermodynamic term, "free energy," will be used to describe the spontaneity of a process.

Example 1.9

One mole of an ideal gas expands reversibly from 5 to 15 L while the temperature drops from 65 to 25°C. Calculate the entropy change of the gas.

Solution

From Equation (1.14b), Equation (1.16), and Equation (1.28),

$$dq_{rev} = dE + dw = dE + PdV$$

$$= C_V dT + \frac{RT}{V} dV \qquad (1.65)$$

Then

$$dS = \frac{dq_{rev}}{T} = C_V \frac{dT}{T} + R \frac{dV}{V} \qquad (1.66)$$

Integrating Equation (1.66) yields:

$$\Delta S_{system} = S_2 - S_1 = C_V \int_{T_1}^{T_2} \frac{dT}{T} + R \int_{V_1}^{V_2} \frac{dV}{V} = C_V \ln \frac{T_2}{T_1} + R \ln \frac{V_2}{V_1} \quad (1.67)$$

Assume C_V $(= \frac{3}{2}R)$ to be constant. The entropy change of the system during the expansion is given by:

$$\Delta S_{system} = \left(\frac{3}{2}\right)(1.987) \ln \frac{298.15}{338.15} + (1.987) \ln \frac{15}{5} = -0.375 + 2.183 = 1.81 \text{ kcal}$$

Equation (1.67) can be rearranged to incorporate a pressure term:

$$\Delta S_{system} = C_V \ln \frac{T_2}{T_1} + R \ln \frac{P_1 T_2}{P_2 T_1} = (C_V + R) \ln \frac{T_2}{T_1} + R \ln \frac{P_1}{P_2}$$

$$= C_P \ln \frac{T_2}{T_1} + R \ln \frac{P_1}{P_2} \quad (1.68)$$

1.3.6 THE THIRD LAW OF THERMODYNAMICS

Equation (1.62) can be rewritten for $T_1 = 0 \text{ K}$ as:

$$\int_0^T dS = S_T - S_0 = \int_0^T \frac{dq_{rev}}{T} = \int_0^T \frac{\Delta H}{T} = \int_0^T \frac{C_P}{T} dT \quad (1.69)$$

where S_0 and S_T are the entropy of the system at absolute zero temperature and at temperature T, respectively. The heat capacity of a crystalline material approaches zero as the temperature nears absolute zero. The third law of thermodynamics states that the entropy of a pure crystalline substance is equal to zero at absolute zero temperature. As a result, one can calculate the absolute entropy of each element at any temperature with the knowledge of its heat capacity as:

$$S_T = \int_0^T \frac{C_P}{T} dT \quad (1.70)$$

If the heat capacity is not constant, it must be used as a function of temperature for Equation (1.70), for which the integration must then be carried out. When the temperature nears the absolute zero temperature, $C_P = aT^3$ where $a = 2.27 \times 10^{-4} \text{ cal} \cdot \text{mol}^{-1} \text{ K}^{-4}$. If there are some phase changes before reaching the temperature T, the entropy of phase transitions must be incorporated into the calculation for the absolute entropy:

$$S_T = \int_0^T \frac{C_P}{T} dT = \int_0^{T_m} \frac{C_{P,1}}{T} dT + \frac{\Delta H_m}{T_m} + \int_{T_m}^{T_b} \frac{C_{P,2}}{T} dT + \frac{\Delta H_b}{T_b} + \int_{T_b}^{T} \frac{C_{P,3}}{T} dT \quad (1.71)$$

TABLE 1.4
Absolute Entropies of Various Substances at 25°C in cal/mol K

Substance	State	ΔS^o	Substance	State	ΔS^o
Acetic acid	l	38.20	Fumarate ion	aq	25.20
Acetaldehyde	g	63.15	α-D-Glucose	s	50.70
Acetone	l	47.50	β-D-Glucose	s	54.50
L-Alanine	s	30.88	Glycerol	l	48.90
L-Alanine ion	aq	45.90	L-Glutamic acid	s	44.98
L-Alaninate ion	aq	29.10	L-Glutamate	aq	30.50
L-Arginine	s	59.90	Glycine	s	24.74
l-Aspartic acid	s	40.66	Glycylglycine	s	45.40
L-Aspartic acid ion	aq	54.80	L(+)-Lactic acid	s	34.30
L-Aspartate ion	aq	21.50	α-Lactose	s	92.30
Benzene	l	29.76	DL-Leucine	s	49.50
Butyric acid	l	54.10	L-Leucine	s	50.10
Carbon dioxide	g	51.05	L-Leucinate ion	aq	39.30
Citrate ion	aq	22.00	α-Maltose	s	96.40
Creatine	s	45.30	β-Maltose	s	95.70
L-Cysteine	s	40.60	Methanol	l	30.30
L-Cystine	s	67.06	L-Methionine	s	55.32
Ethanol	l	38.49	2-Propanol	l	43.16
Ethyl acetate	l	62.80	Succinic acid	s	42.00
Formic acid	s	30.82	Sucrose	s	86.10
Formate ion	l	21.90	L-Valine	s	42.72
Fumaric acid	s	39.70	Water	l	16.70

Source: Data from R. C. Wilhoit, Thermodynamic Properties of Biochemical Substances, in *Biochemical Microcalorimetry* (H. D. Brown, Ed.), Academic Press, New York, 1969.

where the subscripts m and b denote the melting and boiling temperatures, respectively. Based on the absolute entropy value of a substance, one is able to calculate the change in entropies for the formation of other compounds:

$$\Delta S_f^o = \sum S_{products}^o - \sum S_{reactants}^o \tag{1.72}$$

The absolute entropies of various substances are listed in Table 1.4.

1.4 FREE ENERGY

In Section 1.3.6, it was shown that the entropy of a system and its surroundings dictates the direction of the spontaneity of a process. This spontaneity proceeds until the maximum entropy occurs. When the maximum entropy takes place, the system and its surroundings are at equilibrium. However, it is not always easy to measure or calculate the entropy or entropy changes for the surroundings. A new criterion of spontaneity and equilibrium may be developed based only on changes in the state function of the system. In this way, one is able to determine the spontaneity of chemical or biological processes in living organisms carried out isothermally, isobarically, or isochorically even though there is no work and conversion of heat to work such as in a heat engine. A new thermodynamic state function, "free energy," is now introduced.

1.4.1 FREE ENERGY FUNCTIONS

Helmholtz and Gibbs introduced two independent free energy functions. They are represented by Helmholtz free energy A and Gibbs free energy G as follows:

$$A = E - TS \tag{1.73a}$$

$$G = H - TS \tag{1.73b}$$

A, E, G, H, T, and S are thermodynamic state functions, independent of the path of a process. Changes in A and G from one state to another at constant temperature can be written by:

$$\Delta A = \Delta E - T\Delta S \tag{1.74a}$$

$$\Delta G = \Delta H - T\Delta S \tag{1.74b}$$

If the process is reversible, the system will do maximum work given by:

$$\Delta E = q_{rev} - w_{max} \tag{1.75}$$

At constant temperature, Equation (1.61) is substituted into Equation (1.75) by

$$\Delta E = T\Delta S - w_{max} \tag{1.76}$$

Combining Equation (1.74a) with Equation (1.76) yields:

$$-w_{max} = \Delta A \tag{1.77}$$

Equation (1.77) implies that the maximum work done by the system under isothermal conditions can be carried out by the change of Helmholtz free energy. The state function A is known as the work function. The Helmholtz free energy is not useful for most chemical and biological processes since these processes occur at constant pressure rather than at constant volume.

At constant pressure, Equation (1.24) becomes:

$$\Delta H = \Delta E + P\Delta V \tag{1.78}$$

Substituting Equation (1.78) and Equation (1.74a) into Equation (1.74b) gives:

$$\Delta G = \Delta A + P\Delta V \qquad (1.79)$$

Substituting Equation (1.77) into Equation (1.79) yields:

$$-\Delta G = w_{max} - P\Delta V \qquad (1.80)$$

The $-\Delta G$ in Equation (1.80) is the useful work or net work at constant temperature and pressure to carry out the process; not the work done by the expansion of volume. If a volume of the solution during the chemical or biological processes of liquids or solids does not increase, the work $P\Delta V$ is not useful for the process.

For an irreversible spontaneous process, $TdS > dq_{irrev}$ combined with $dE = dq - dw$ yields:

$$TdS > dE + PdV \qquad (1.81)$$

Substituting Equation (1.80) into Equation (1.81) along with the first law ($dE = dq - dw$) and the second law ($dq = TdS$) gives:

$$dG < VdP - SdT \qquad (1.82)$$

At constant temperature and pressure ($dT = 0$ and $dP = 0$), Equation (1.82) becomes:

$$(dG)_{T,P} < 0 \qquad (1.83)$$

For a thermodynamically reversible process under the same conditions, $T\Delta S = q_{rev}$ so that:

$$(dG)_{T,P} = 0 \qquad (1.84)$$

If $(dG)_{T,P} > 0$, the system cannot occur spontaneously. As mentioned before, one determination of a spontaneous process is the increase in entropy of a system and its surroundings, but the more practical criterion is the decrease in free energy of the system alone, excluding its surroundings. The change in free energy can be determined easily for chemical and biological processes at constant temperature and pressure. Once equilibrium is established, the system does not depart spontaneously from equilibrium, and the free energy of the system is a minimum so that a small change in the equilibrium system does not alter the free energy much (i.e., $\Delta G = 0$).

Pharmaceutical scientists deal with many cases of equilibrium systems, as will be described in the following chapters. The equilibrium of two phases of a pure substance — vapor–liquid, vapor–solid, or liquid–solid — will be discussed here. When phase 1 and phase 2 are in equilibrium:

$$M(\text{phase } 1) \rightleftharpoons M(\text{phase } 2) \qquad (1.85)$$

Any changes in the free energies of the substance M in phase 1 and phase 2 are equivalent, and Equation (1.82) then becomes:

$$dG_1 = -S_1 dT + V_1 dP = dG_2 = -S_2 dT + V_2 dP \qquad (1.86)$$

Equation (1.86) can be rearranged to:

$$\frac{dP}{dT} = \frac{S_2 - S_1}{V_2 - V_1} = \frac{\Delta S}{\Delta V} \qquad (1.87)$$

Since the entropy change during the phase transition at temperature T is $\Delta S = \Delta H / T$, then Equation (1.87) gives:

$$\frac{dP}{dT} = \frac{\Delta H}{T \Delta V} \qquad (1.88)$$

For a liquid–vapor system, a vapor–solid system, and a liquid–solid system, $\Delta V = V_v - V_l \cong V_v$, $\Delta V = V_v - V_s \cong V_v$, and $\Delta V = V_l - V_s \cong M(\rho_l^{-1} - \rho_s^{-1})$, respectively, where M and ρ are the molecular weight and density of the substance, respectively. Substituting these relationships into Equation (1.88) along with the ideal gas law and integrating the resulting equation yields:

$$\int_{P_1}^{P_2} \frac{dP}{P} = \ln \frac{P_2}{P_1} = \int_{T_1}^{T_2} \frac{\Delta H}{RT^2} dT = \frac{\Delta H}{R} \left(\frac{1}{T_1} - \frac{1}{T_2} \right) \qquad (1.89)$$

where ΔH is the enthalpy change during the phase change (i.e., the heat of vaporization for vapor–liquid systems and the heat of sublimation for vapor–solid systems). This equation is known as the Clausius–Clapeyron equation for vapor–liquid and vapor–solid systems. For a liquid–solid system, Equation (1.88) becomes:

$$\frac{dP}{dT} = \frac{\Delta H}{TM(\rho_l^{-1} - \rho_s^{-1})} \qquad (1.90)$$

Integration of Equation (1.90) yields:

$$\int_{P_1}^{P_2} dP = P_2 - P_1 = \int_{T_1}^{T_2} \frac{\Delta H}{TM(\rho_l^{-1} - \rho_s^{-1})} dT = \frac{\Delta H}{M(\rho_l^{-1} - \rho_s^{-1})} \ln \frac{T_2}{T_1} \qquad (1.91)$$

where ΔH is the heat of fusion of the solid.

Example 1.10

The vapor pressure of water at 25°C is 24 mmHg. What is the vapor pressure at 85°C? The heat of vaporization of water is 9.8 kcal/mol.

Solution

From Equation (1.89)

$$\ln\frac{P_2}{24} = \frac{9800}{1.987}\left(\frac{1}{298} - \frac{1}{358}\right) = 2.77 \quad P_2 = 384 \text{ mmHg}$$

1.4.2 FUNDAMENTAL EQUATIONS OF THERMODYNAMICS AND THEIR USES

The first and second laws of thermodynamics and the Helmholtz and Gibbs free energies are rearranged to obtain the relationships between the state functions (i.e., E, H, A, and G) and temperature, pressure, and volume. For an infinitesimal process the first law is given by:

$$dE = dq - dw \tag{1.92}$$

If one considers $dw = PdV$ or $w = PV$ and Equation (1.62), then Equation (1.92) yields:

$$dE = TdS - PdV \tag{1.93}$$

Analogously, the enthalpy change is given by:

$$dH = dE + d(PV) = TdS - PdV + PdV + VdP = TdS + VdP \tag{1.94}$$

The Helmholtz and Gibbs free energies can thus be written by:

$$dA = dE - d(TS) = dE - TdS - SdT$$
$$= TdS - PdV - TdS - SdT = -PdV - SdT \tag{1.95}$$

and

$$dG = dH - d(TS) = dH - TdS - SdT$$
$$= TdS + VdP - TdS - SdT = VdP - SdT \tag{1.96}$$

Equation (1.93), Equation (1.94), Equation (1.95), and Equation (1.96) are the four basic equations of thermodynamics from which partial derivatives can be derived in terms of the temperature, pressure, and volume. For example, if the process runs reversibly at constant volume ($PdV = 0$) or at constant entropy ($TdS = 0$), then Equation (1.93) gives:

$$dE = TdS \quad \text{or} \quad \left(\frac{\partial E}{\partial S} \right)_V = T \qquad (1.97)$$

$$dE = -PdV \quad \text{or} \quad \left(\frac{\partial E}{\partial V} \right)_S = -P \qquad (1.98)$$

Therefore, Equation (1.93) can be written by:

$$dE = TdS - PdV = \left(\frac{\partial E}{\partial S} \right)_V dS + \left(\frac{\partial E}{\partial V} \right)_S dV \qquad (1.99)$$

Similarly, Equation (1.94), Equation (1.95), and Equation (1.96) can be written by:

$$dH = TdS + VdP = \left(\frac{\partial H}{\partial S} \right)_P dS + \left(\frac{\partial H}{\partial P} \right)_S dP \qquad (1.100)$$

$$dA = -SdT - PdV = \left(\frac{\partial A}{\partial T} \right)_V dT + \left(\frac{\partial A}{\partial V} \right)_T dV \qquad (1.101)$$

$$dG = -SdT + VdP = \left(\frac{\partial G}{\partial T} \right)_P dT + \left(\frac{\partial G}{\partial P} \right)_T dP \qquad (1.102)$$

The following additional six partial derivatives can be obtained from equations from Equation (1.100) to Equation (1.102):

$$\left(\frac{\partial H}{\partial S} \right)_P = T \quad \left(\frac{\partial H}{\partial P} \right)_S = V \qquad (1.103)$$

$$\left(\frac{\partial A}{\partial T} \right)_V = -S \quad \left(\frac{\partial A}{\partial V} \right)_T = -P \qquad (1.104)$$

$$\left(\frac{\partial G}{\partial T} \right)_P = -S \quad \left(\frac{\partial G}{\partial P} \right)_T = V \qquad (1.105)$$

Equation (1.97), Equation (1.98), Equation (1.103), Equation (1.104), and Equation (1.105) are the Maxwell relations, which with the aid of the Euler theorem are very useful in obtaining quantities not easily determined by other methods. Readers interested in this subject should consult the physical chemistry books listed at the end of this chapter. However, two important applications of the thermodynamic relationships are discussed here: internal pressure and the Gibbs–Helmholtz equation.

The internal pressure of a gas can be derived from the Helmholtz free energy. The internal pressure is the change in internal energy with respect to volume at constant temperature [i.e., $(\partial E / \partial V)_T$]. Taking the derivative of Equation (1.73a) with respect to volume at constant temperature gives:

$$\left(\frac{\partial A}{\partial V}\right)_T = \left(\frac{\partial E}{\partial V}\right)_T - T\left(\frac{\partial S}{\partial V}\right)_T \qquad (1.106)$$

Substituting Equation (1.104) into Equation (1.106) yields:

$$\left(\frac{\partial E}{\partial V}\right)_T = -P + T\left(\frac{\partial S}{\partial V}\right)_T \qquad (1.107)$$

Applying the Euler theorem to the second term on the right–hand side of Equation (1.107) gives:

$$\frac{\partial}{\partial V}\left(\frac{\partial A}{\partial T}\right)_V = -\left(\frac{\partial S}{\partial V}\right)_T = \frac{\partial}{\partial T}\left(\frac{\partial A}{\partial V}\right)_T = -\left(\frac{\partial P}{\partial T}\right)_V \qquad (1.108)$$

Substituting Equation (1.108) into Equation (1.107) yields:

$$\left(\frac{\partial E}{\partial V}\right)_T = -P + T\left(\frac{\partial P}{\partial T}\right)_V \qquad (1.109)$$

If a gas obeys the van der Waals equation, Equation (1.12) can be written as:

$$P = \frac{RT}{V - b} - \frac{a}{V^2} \qquad (1.110)$$

Taking the derivative of P with respect to T at constant volume V gives:

$$\left(\frac{\partial P}{\partial T}\right)_V = \frac{R}{V - b} = \frac{1}{T}\left(P + \frac{a}{V^2}\right) \qquad (1.111)$$

Substituting Equation (1.111) into Equation (1.109) gives:

$$\left(\frac{\partial E}{\partial V}\right)_T = \frac{a}{V^2} \qquad (1.112)$$

where a/V^2 is the internal pressure of a gas as mentioned in Section 1.2 and will be used to determine the solubility of a nonelectrolyte in Section 3.1.2.

Another important equation, the Gibbs–Helmholtz equation, is derived from the Maxwell relations. A chemist may use this equation to determine the enthalpy change in a reaction, and a pharmaceutical scientist may use it to calculate colligative properties (i.e., freezing point depression and boiling point elevation). The expression for free energy with respect to temperature at constant pressure is given by Equation (1.105):

$$\left(\frac{\partial G}{\partial T}\right)_P = -S \tag{1.105}$$

According to the Kirchhoff equation and Equation (1.73b), Equation (1.105) gives:

$$\left(\frac{\partial \Delta G}{\partial T}\right)_P = \frac{\Delta G - \Delta H}{T} \tag{1.113}$$

Differentiation of $\Delta G/T$ with respect to temperature at constant pressure gives:

$$\frac{\partial}{\partial T}\left(\frac{\Delta G}{T}\right) = -\frac{\Delta G}{T^2} + \frac{1}{T}\left(\frac{\partial \Delta G}{\partial T}\right)_P \tag{1.114}$$

Substituting Equation (1.114) into Equation (1.113) yields:

$$\left[\frac{\partial}{\partial T}\left(\frac{\Delta G}{T}\right)\right]_P = -\frac{\Delta H}{T^2} \tag{1.115}$$

which can be rearranged to:

$$\left[\frac{\partial(\Delta G/T)}{\partial(1/T)}\right]_P = \Delta H \tag{1.116}$$

By taking the slope of the plot of $\Delta G/T$ vs. $1/T$, one can determine the enthalpy change for a reaction. The equilibrium constants at different temperatures under constant pressure, freezing point depression, and boiling point elevation may be calculated from Equation (1.116), as will be discussed in Chapter 3.

1.4.3 FREE ENERGY OF FORMATION AND STANDARD FREE ENERGY CHANGE

Free energy and its change are state functions. As is the case with enthalpy, the absolute value of free energy cannot be calculated. The free energy of an element

TABLE 1.5
Standard Free Energies of Formation of Selected Substances at 25°C in kcal/mol

Substance	State	ΔG_f°	Substance	State	ΔG_f°
Acetic acid	l	−93.08	Glycerol	l	−114.60
Acetaldehyde	g	−33.24	L-Glutamic acid	s	−174.69
Acetone	l	−36.70	L-Glutamate ion	aq	−153.79
L-Alanine	s	−88.48	Glycine	s	−90.27
L-Alanine ion	aq	−91.91	Glycinate ion	aq	−77.46
L-Alaninate ion	aq	-75.25	Glycylglycine	s	-117.47
L-Arginine	s	−156.99	Glycylglycinate	aq	−106.53
DL-Aspartic acid	s	−174.29	L(+)-Lactic acid	s	−125.05
L-Aspartic acid	s	−174.31	L(+)-Lactate ion	aq	−123.49
L-Aspartic acid ion	s	−175.39	α-Lactose	s	−374.48
L-Aspartate ion	aq	−152.64	DL-Leucine	s	−85.70
Benzene	l	−41.30	L-Leucine	s	−85.20
Butyric acid	l	−90.60	L-Leucinate ion	aq	−70.89
Butyrate ion	aq	−88.92	α-Maltose	aq	−376.08
Carbon dioxide	g	−94.26	β-Maltose	aq	−375.74
Citrate ion	aq	−277.88	Methanol	l	−39.75
Creatine	s	−63.10	L-Methionine	s	−121.50
L-Cysteine	s	−81.90	Palmitic acid	s	−108.80
L-Cystine	s	−163.89	Pyruvate ion	aq	−41.00
Ethanol	l	−41.63	2-Propanol	l	−43.16
Ethyl acetate	l	−80.70	Succinic acid	s	−42.00
Formic acid	l	−82.70	Succinate ion	aq	−22.20
Formate ion	aq	−80.00	Sucrose	s	−86.10
Fumaric acid	s	−156.12	DL-Valine	s	−43.30
Fumarate ion	aq	−143.84	L-Valine	s	−42.72
α-D-Glucose	s	−217.62	L-Valine ion	aq	−57.40
β-D-Glucose	s	−217.22	Water	l	−56.69

Source: Data from R. C. Wilhoit, Thermodynamic Properties of Biochemical Substances, in *Biochemical Microcalorimetry* (H. D. Brown, Ed.), Academic Press, New York, 1969.

in its standard state (1 atmospheric pressure and 25°C) is zero. The standard free energy of formation of a compound is obtained from Equation (1.74b):

$$\Delta G_f^\circ = \Delta H_f^\circ - T\Delta S_f^\circ \qquad (1.117)$$

where the superscript ° again denotes the standard state. The standard free energies of formation for selected compounds at 25°C are presented in Table 1.5.

Example 1.11

Calculate the free energy of formation of L-alanine at 25°C for the reaction:

$$3C(\text{graphite}) + \tfrac{7}{2}H_2(g) + O_2(g) + \tfrac{1}{2}N_2(g) \rightarrow C_3H_7O_2N(s)$$

Solution

From Table 1.3,

$$\Delta H_f^{\circ}[C_3H_7O_2N(s)] = -134.50 \text{ kcal}$$

From Table 1.4,

$$\Delta S_{298}^{\circ} = \sum S_{\text{products}}^{\circ} - \sum S_{\text{reactants}}^{\circ} = 30.88 - 3\times1.36 - \tfrac{7}{2}\times31.21 - 49.00 - \tfrac{1}{2}\times45.77$$

$$= -154.33 \text{ cal / mol K}$$

$$\Delta G_f^{\circ} = \Delta H_f^{\circ} - T\Delta S_{298}^{\circ} = -134,500 - 298\times(-154.33) = -88.51 \text{ kcal / mol}$$

Analogous to the enthalpy change of a reaction, the free energy change of a reaction can be calculated by:

$$\Delta G_T^{\circ} = \sum \Delta G_{f,\text{products}}^{\circ} - \sum \Delta G_{f,\text{reactants}}^{\circ} \tag{1.118}$$

Using the free energy of formation and Equation (1.118), one is able to tell whether chemical or biological reactions are spontaneous and calculate the change in free energy for the reaction. Let us examine the synthesis of glucose:

$$6CO_2(g) + 6H_2O(l) \rightarrow C_6H_{12}O_6(s) + 6O_2(g)$$

The change in free energy for the reaction is given by:

$$\Delta G_{298}^{\circ} = (-217.63 + 0) - (6\times(-94.26) + 6\times(-54.64)) = 676.77 \text{ kcal}$$

The above synthetic reaction does not occur spontaneously due to the positive sign in the change in free energy for the reaction. However, in plants, photons or light quanta supply the excess amount of free energy, and then the following photosynthetic reaction can occur:

$$6CO_2(g) + 6H_2O(l) + n\,h\nu \rightarrow C_6H_{12}O_6(s) + 6O_2(g)$$

The free energy change for the above photosynthetic reaction is negative. The cellular respiration of glucose (see Example 1.7) will take place spontaneously because its change in free energy is −676.77 kcal.

Another example of using free energy is the conversion of chemical energy into chemical work, light, and electrical energy production in living systems. The chemical bond energy of adenosine triphosphate (ATP) is used to do chemical work. The formation of glutamine from glutamic acid and ammonia is not a favorable reaction pathway because the free energy change for the reaction based on 1 M concentrations of products and reactants gives a positive value.

$$\text{L-glutamic acid} + NH_3 \rightarrow \text{L-glutamine} + H_2O \qquad \Delta G^{\circ}_{298} = 3.4 \text{ kcal}$$

Living cells produce L-glutamine by a different reaction pathway using the chemical energy of ATP. ATP undergoes enzymatic hydrolysis to form adenosine diphosphate (ADP) and phosphate (P_i). During the hydrolysis of a 1 M concentration of ATP, the standard free energy at pH 7.0 and 25°C is measured:

$$ATP + H_2O \rightarrow ADP + \text{phosphate } (P_i) \qquad \Delta G^{\circ}_{298} = -7.3 \text{ kcal}$$

These reactions are not independent but are coupled to other reactions:

$$ATP + \text{L-glutamic acid} + NH_3 \rightarrow \text{L-glutamine} + ADP + \text{phosphate} \qquad \Delta G^{\circ}_{298} = -3.9 \text{ kcal}$$

Therefore the free energy change for the above reaction occurring in living cells is a negative value. The chemical energy generated from the breakdown of ATP to ADP is used for the formation of the amide bond in L-glutamine.

1.4.4 FREE ENERGY AND CHEMICAL EQUILIBRIUM

The free energy of a system composed of various substances is dependent on the quantities of individual species present, as well as temperature and pressure. However, the free energy of the system as a whole is not the summation of the free energies of each species in the pure state because species may behave differently in the mixture as compared to the pure state. Thus, the free energy of the mixture is given by:

$$G = \sum \overline{G}_i n_i \qquad (1.119)$$

where $\overline{G}_i$ and n_i are the partial molar free energy and the number of moles of the species i in the mixture, respectively. The partial free energy is known as the chemical potential and is denoted by μ, for which Equation (1.119) then becomes:

$$G = \sum \mu_i n_i \qquad (1.120)$$

$$\mu_i = \left(\frac{\partial G}{\partial n_i} \right)_{T,P,n_j} \qquad (1.121)$$

Equation (1.121) states that the chemical potential of the species i is the change in free energy with respect to the change in number of moles of the species i while the compositions of other species are held constant. Partial molar quantities also follow the same thermodynamic rules.

The variation of the free energy of a system (gas) with respect to pressure at constant temperature is given by:

$$dG = VdP \quad \text{[from Equation (1.105)]} \tag{1.122}$$

When we assume that the gas behaves ideally, then $V = RT / P$, and Equation (1.122) becomes:

$$dG = \frac{RT}{P} dp \tag{1.123}$$

Integrating Equation (1.123) yields:

$$\int_{G_1}^{G_2} dG = G_2 - G_1 = RT \int_{P_1}^{P_2} \frac{dP}{P} = RT \ln \frac{P_2}{P_1} \tag{1.124}$$

If the gas is initially in its standard state (i.e., P_1^o and G^o), then Equation (1.124) yields:

$$G = G^o + RT \ln \frac{P_2}{P_1^o} \tag{1.125}$$

where G is the free energy of the ideal gas at pressure P_2.

Therefore the chemical potential of species i can be given by:

$$\mu_i = \mu_i^o + RT \ln \frac{P_i}{P_i^o} \tag{1.126}$$

where μ_i^o is the chemical potential of species i in standard state and commonly chosen as its pure state. If the mixture behaves ideally, $P_i / P_i^o = X_i$, where X_i is the mole fraction of species i. Equation (1.126) then yields:

$$\mu_i = \mu_i^o + RT \ln X_i \tag{1.127}$$

If the behavior of the gas is far from its standard state, the activity, designated "a," is related to the chemical potential as:

$$\mu_i = \mu_i^o + RT \ln a_i \tag{1.128}$$

The activity of the species i in the mixture is the product of concentration and activity coefficient, γ_i, determined experimentally as:

$$a_i = \gamma_i C_i \tag{1.129}$$

Let us consider the general chemical reaction of two reactants and two products at constant temperature and pressure expressed by:

$$aA + bB \;\rightleftharpoons\; cC + dD \tag{1.130}$$

The free energy change for the above reaction is given by:

$$\Delta G = \sum_{products} n_i\mu_i - \sum_{reactants} n_i\mu_i = c\mu_C + d\mu_D - a\mu_A - b\mu_B \tag{1.131}$$

Substituting Equation (1.128) into Equation (1.131) yields:

$$\Delta G = \Delta G^\circ + RT \ln \frac{a_C^c a_D^d}{a_A^a a_B^b} \tag{1.132}$$

where $\Delta G^\circ = c\mu_C^\circ + d\mu_D^\circ - a\mu_A^\circ - b\mu_B^\circ$ and is defined as the free energy change for the reaction when all chemical compounds are in their standard states. When all the compounds are in their standard states, the natural log term of Equation (1.132) becomes zero and the ratio of products to reactants approaches unity. Therefore, $\Delta G = \Delta G^\circ$. If the concentrations of all the compounds are very dilute and each compound behaves ideally, the activity coefficient becomes unity and the concentration term can be used.

The natural logarithm term of Equation (1.132) is called the reaction quotient and is designated by the letter Q. Equation (1.132) then becomes:

$$\Delta G = \Delta G^\circ + RT \ln Q \tag{1.133}$$

When the reaction quotient furnishes the minimum value of the free energy change for the reaction, which is zero (i.e., $\Delta G = 0$), the reaction is in equilibrium and $Q = K$, where K is the equilibrium constant. Equation (1.133) becomes:

$$\Delta G = 0 = \Delta G^\circ + RT \ln K \tag{1.134}$$

If $K = 1$, the standard free energy change is zero and the reaction is at equilibrium. If $K > 1$, the reaction will proceed forward because ΔG° becomes negative and the products have more free energy than the reactants. The equilibrium thus lies to the right. If $K < 1$, ΔG° is positive and the reaction will proceed in reverse. The equilibrium then lies to the left.

Example 1.12

The free energy of the hydrolysis of ATP in its standard state is -7.3 kcal/mol based on a standard 1 M concentration of each substance. Calculate the free energy change when the concentrations of ATP, ADP, and phosphate (P_i) in human erythrocytes at pH 7.0 are 2.25, 0.25, and 1.65 mM, respectively. Assume that the solution behaves ideally.

Solution

The hydrolysis of ATP occurs in the following manner:

$$ATP + H_2O \;\rightleftharpoons\; ADP + phosphate\ (P_i)$$

$$\Delta G = \Delta G^\circ + RT \ln \frac{C_{ADP} C_{phosphate}}{C_{ATP}}$$

$$\Delta G = -7300 + 1.987 \times 298.15 \times \ln \frac{(2.50 \times 10^{-4})(1.65 \times 10^{-3})}{2.25 \times 10^{-3}} = -12.4 \text{ kcal / mol}$$

If the equilibrium concentrations of the substances are known, one can calculate the standard free energy for the reaction. For example, 0.0200 M glucose 1-phosphate changes to glucose 6-phosphate in the presence of phosphoglucomutase. The final equilibrium concentrations of glucose 1-phosphate and glucose 6-phosphate are 0.00100 and 0.0190 M, respectively. The equilibrium constant is then given by:

$$K = \frac{[\text{glucose 6 - phosphate}]}{[\text{glucose 1 - phosphate}]} = \frac{0.0190}{0.00100} = 19.0$$

Then, the standard free energy change for the reaction is:

$$\Delta G^\circ = -RT \ln K = -1.987 \times 298.15 \times \ln 19.0 = -1.74 \text{ kcal / mol}$$

The effect of temperature on the equilibrium constant can be related to the Gibbs–Helmholtz equation:

$$\left[\frac{\partial}{\partial T} \left(\frac{\Delta G^\circ}{T} \right) \right]_P = -\frac{\Delta H^\circ}{T^2} \qquad (1.115)$$

From Equation (1.134),

$$\ln K = -\frac{\Delta G^\circ}{RT} \qquad (1.135)$$

Substituting Equation (1.135) into Equation (1.115) yields:

$$\frac{d}{dT}(\ln K) = \frac{\Delta H^{\circ}}{RT^2} \tag{1.136}$$

Integrating Equation (1.136) from the temperature limits T_1 to T_2 gives:

$$\ln \frac{K_2}{K_1} = -\frac{\Delta H^{\circ}}{R}\left(\frac{1}{T_2} - \frac{1}{T_1}\right) = \frac{\Delta H^{\circ}}{R}\left(\frac{T_2 - T_1}{T_1 T_2}\right) \tag{1.137}$$

Assume ΔH° is constant. Equation (1.137) is known as the van't Hoff equation. The van't Hoff equation allows the determination of ΔH° when two equilibrium constants are measured at two temperatures.

When the heat capacity of reactants and products (i.e., ΔC_p°) is independent of temperature,

$$\Delta H_2^{\circ} = \Delta H_1^{\circ} + \Delta C_p^{\circ}(T_2 - T_1) \tag{1.138}$$

Integrating Equation (1.136) with Equation (1.138) then gives:

$$\ln\left(\frac{K_2}{K_1}\right) = \frac{\Delta H_1^{\circ}}{R}\left(\frac{T_2 - T_1}{T_1 T_2}\right) + \frac{\Delta C_p^{\circ}}{R}\left(\frac{T_1}{T_2} - \ln\frac{T_1}{T_2} - 1\right) \tag{1.139}$$

If the heat capacity of reactants and products at constant pressure is expressed as the second polynomial form of T as shown in Equation (1.31), the heat capacity of the reaction is given by:

$$d\Delta H^{\circ}/dT = \Delta C_p^{\circ} = \Delta a + \Delta bT + \Delta cT^2 \tag{1.140}$$

Integrating Equation (1.136) along with Equation (1.140) yields:

$$\ln\left(\frac{K_2}{K_1}\right) = \frac{\Delta H_o}{R}\left(\frac{1}{T_1} - \frac{1}{T_2}\right) + \frac{\Delta a}{R}\ln\left(\frac{T_2}{T_1}\right) + \frac{\Delta b}{2R}(T_2 - T_1) + \frac{\Delta c}{6}(T_2^2 - T_1^2) \tag{1.141}$$

where ΔH_o is the constant and $\Delta a = \sum_i v_i a_i$, and so on.

Figure 1.6 shows the effect of temperature on the equilibrium constants for CO_2 solubility in water and vaporization of water.

Example 1.13

L-Aspartate converts enzymatically to fumarate and ammonium ion as follows:

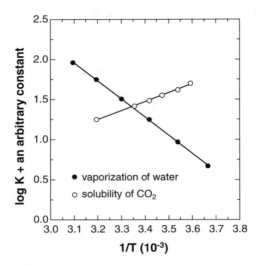

FIGURE 1.6 The effect of temperature on the equilibrium constants. [Graph reconstructed from data by W. Stumm and J. J. Morgan, *Aquatic Chemistry: An Introduction Emphasizing Chemical Equilibria in Natural Waters*, Wiley Interscience, New York, 1981, p. 71.]

$$\text{L-aspartate (aq)} \rightleftharpoons \text{fumarate (aq)} + NH_4^+ \text{ (aq)}$$

It was found that $\Delta H°$ is 14.5 kcal/mol and the equilibrium constant at 29°C is 7.4×10^{-3} mol/L. Calculate the equilibrium constant and entropy change at 37°C.

Solution
From the van't Hoff equation,

$$\ln \frac{K_{310}}{7.4 \times 10^{-3}} = \frac{14,500}{1.987} \left(\frac{310.15 - 302.15}{302.15 \times 310.15} \right) = 0.623$$

$$K_{310} = 0.0138 \text{ mol / L}$$

$$\Delta G_{310}^° = -RT \ln K = 1.987 \times 310.15 \times \ln 0.0138 = 2640 \text{ cal / mol}$$

$$\Delta G_{310}^° = 2640 = \Delta H_{310}^° - T\Delta S_{310}^° = 14500 - 310.15 \times \Delta S_{310}^°$$

$$\Delta S_{310}^° = 38.2 \text{ cal / mol K}$$

When considering the effect of temperature on equilibrium constant, the sign and magnitude of $\Delta H°$ are the determining factors. However, the spontaneity of a reaction is determined by the sign and magnitude of $\Delta S°$, which determines the effect of temperature.

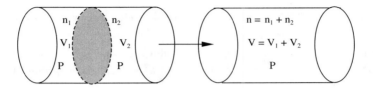

FIGURE 1.7 The mixing of two ideal gases at constant temperature and pressure.

1.4.5 THE THERMODYNAMICS OF MIXING

Consider a mixture of two ideal gases or two ideal solutions separated by a trans-
forming partition as shown in Figure 1.7. When the partition is removed, the gases
mix. The mixing is assumed to be reversible, and no changes in volume and temperature occur. The entropy changes for gases 1 and 2 are given by Equation (1.67):

$$\Delta S_1 = n_1 R \ln \frac{V_1 + V_2}{V_1} \quad \text{and} \quad \Delta S_2 = n_2 R \ln \frac{V_1 + V_2}{V_1} \tag{1.142}$$

Under the same temperature and pressure, the mole fractions of the two gases
in the final mixture, x_1 and x_2, are:

$$x_1 = \frac{n_1}{n_1 + n_2} = \frac{V_1}{V_1 + V_2} = 1 - x_2 \tag{1.143}$$

The total entropy change of the two gases is:

$$\Delta S_{mixing} = \Delta S_1 + \Delta S_2 = -\left(n_1 + n_2\right) R \left(x_1 \ln x_1 + x_2 \ln x_2\right) \tag{1.144}$$

The free energy change of the gas mixture is given by Equation (1.121):

$$dG = \mu_1 d n_1 + \mu_2 d n_2 \tag{1.145}$$

The free energy change of mixing is the free energy change of forming the
solution from the pure components at the same temperature and pressure:

$$\Delta G_{mixing} = G_{solution} - G_{pure\ components} \tag{1.146}$$

Substituting Equation (1.127) and Equation (1.145) into Equation (1.146) yields:

$$\Delta G_{mixing} = \int_0^{n_1} (\mu_1^o + RT \ln x_1)\, dn_1 + \int_0^{n_2} (\mu_2^o + RT \ln x_2)\, dn_2$$
$$\tag{1.147}$$
$$- \int_0^{n_1} \mu_1^o\, dn_1 - \int_0^{n_2} \mu_2^o\, dn_2$$

$$\Delta G_{mixing} = n_1 RT \ln x_1 + n_2 RT \ln x_2 = (n_1 + n_2) RT \left(x_1 \ln x_1 + x_2 \ln x_2 \right) \quad (1.148)$$

The value of x ranges from 0 to 1 and thus the value of $\ln x$ is negative. The free energy change of mixing will be negative for all possible compositions of an ideal solution.

The enthalpy change of mixing can be calculated from Equation (1.74b):

$$\Delta H_{mixing} = \Delta G_{mixing} + T\Delta S_{mixing}$$

$$= (n_1 + n_2) RT \left(x_1 \ln x_1 - x_1 \ln x_1 + x_2 \ln x_2 - x_2 \ln x_2 \right) = 0 \quad (1.149)$$

Suppose the chemical reaction:

$$2A(g, \ \Delta H_f^\circ = 7.93 \text{ kcal / mol}, \ \Delta S_f^\circ = 57.4 \text{ cal / K }) \ \rightleftharpoons$$

$$B(g, \ \Delta H_f^\circ = 2.19 \text{ kcal / mol}, \ \Delta S_f^\circ = 72.7 \text{ cal / K })$$

Let us define δ to be the extent of reaction. When only A is present, $\delta = 0.0$ and when only B is present, $\delta = 1$. Assume that initially only 1 mole of A is present. As the reaction progresses, $(1-\delta)$ moles of A and δ moles of B coexist. Then, enthalpy change as a function of the extent of reaction is:

$$\Delta H_{reaction} = 2 \times (1 - \delta) \times 7.93 + 2.19 \ \delta$$

And $\Delta H_{mixing} = 0$. Entropy change without mixing is a linear function of the extent of reaction like enthalpy:

$$\Delta S_{no \ mixing} = 2 \times (1 - \delta) \times 0.0574 + 0.0727 \ \delta$$

Entropy of mixing as a function of the extent of reaction is calculated by Equation (1.144):

$$\text{total number of moles} \ n = n_A + n_B$$

$$n_B = \delta \quad n_A = 2 \times (1 - \delta) \quad n = 2 - \delta$$

$$\Delta S_{mixing} = -(2 - \delta) \ R \left[\left(\frac{2 - 2\delta}{2 - \delta} \right) \ln \left(\frac{2 - 2\delta}{2 - \delta} \right) + \left(\frac{\delta}{2 - \delta} \right) \ln \left(\frac{\delta}{2 - \delta} \right) \right] \quad (1.150)$$

The free energy change as a function of the extent of reaction at 25°C is then calculated:

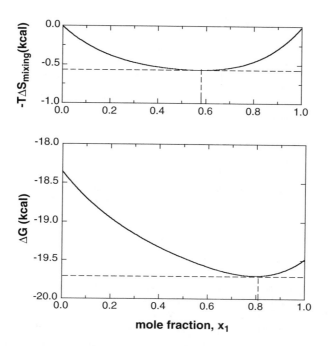

FIGURE 1.8 The enthalpy change of mixing and free energy change as a function of the extent of reaction at 25°C.

$$\Delta G = \Delta G_{no\ mixing} + \Delta G_{mixing} = \Delta G_{no\ mixing} - T\Delta S_{mixing}$$

$$= 2 \times (1 - \delta) \times (7.93 - 298 \times 0.0574) + \delta(2.19 - 298 \times 0.0727)$$

$$+ (2 - \delta) \times 298 \times 1.987 \times 10^{-3} \tag{1.151}$$

$$\times \left[\left(\frac{2 - 2\delta}{2 - \delta} \right) \ln \left(\frac{2 - 2\delta}{2 - \delta} \right) + \left(\frac{\delta}{2 - \delta} \right) \ln \left(\frac{\delta}{2 - \delta} \right) \right]$$

ΔS_{mixing} and $\Delta G_{reaction}$ as functions of the extent of reaction are plotted in Figure 1.8. The minimum value of $-T\,\Delta S_{mixing}$ is positioned at about $\delta = 0.57$. The position of the minimum depends on the ratio of the number of moles of reactants and products. The greater the number of moles of reactants, the closer the position is toward the product side. However, the minimum in free energy change is located at about $\delta = 0.81$ (i.e., $\partial \Delta G / \partial \delta = 0$). The equilibrium constant is then calculated:

$$K = \frac{\delta}{(2 - 2\delta)^2} = \frac{0.81}{0.38^2} = 5.61$$

SUGGESTED READINGS

1. J. R. Barrante, *Physical Chemistry for the Life Sciences*, Prentice-Hall, Englewood Cliffs, NJ, 1977, Chapters 1–4.
2. R. Chang, *Physical Chemistry with Applications to Biological Systems*, 2nd Ed., Macmillan, New York, 1981, Chapters 2, 6, and 7.
3. S. Glasstone and D. Lewis, *Elements of Physical Chemistry*, Van Nostrand Co., Maruzen Asian Ed., Tokyo, 1960, Chapters 2–4.
4. H. Kuhn and H.-D. Forsterling, *Principles of Physical Chemistry*, John Wiley & Sons, New York, 2000, Chapters 13–16.
5. K. J. Laidler and J. H. Meiser, *Physical Chemistry*, Benjamin/Cummings, Menlo Park, CA, 1982, Chapters 1–4.
6. A. L. Lehninger, *Bioenergetics*, W. A. Benjamin, Inc., Menlo Park, CA, 1971.
7. A. Martin, *Physical Pharmacy*, 4th Ed., Lea and Febiger, Philadelphia, 1993, Chapter 3.
8. C. K. Mathews and K. E. van Holde, *Biochemistry*, Benjamin/Cummings, Redwood City, CA, 1990, Chapter 3.
9. O. Robbins, Jr., *Ionic Reactions and Equilibria*, MacMillan, New York, 1967, Chapters 5 and 6.
10. J. M. Smith and H. C. van Ness, *Introduction to Chemical Engineering Thermodynamics*, 3rd Ed., McGraw-Hill, New York, 1975, Chapters 2–5.
11. I. Tinoco, Jr., K. Sauer, and J. C. Wang, *Physical Chemistry: Principles and Applications in Biological Sciences*, 3rd Ed., Prentice Hall, NJ, 1995, Chapters 1–5.
12. V. R. Williams, W. L. Mattrice, and H. B. Williams, *Basic Physical Chemistry for the Life Sciences*, 3rd Ed., W. H. Freeman and Co., San Francisco, 1978, Chapters 1–3.

PROBLEMS

1. Calculate the work done when a drop of ice (1 μm) evaporates to water at 0°C and 1 atm. The density of water and ice are 1.0 g/cm³ and 0.915 g/cm³, respectively.

2. Hot air at 50°C is blown through 50 kg of a cold metal solid that has been cooled to −10°C. The air leaves at 20°C and enters into a house for cooling. Calculate the volume of air at 20°C that is obtained by this operation. The density of air at 20°C and 1 atm is 1.20×10^{-3} g/cm³; the density of the metal is 2.5 g/cm³. The heat capacity of the metal and air at constant pressure are 500 J/K/kg and 1000 J/K/kg, respectively.

3. Calculate the heat absorbed or released by the system when 100 g of water is frozen at 0°C and 1 atm.

4. Calculate the enthalpy change of the oxidation of glycine to produce urea:

$$2NH_2CH_2COOH(s) + 3O_2 \longrightarrow NH_2CONH_2(s) + 3CO_2(1\ atm) + 3H_2O(l)$$

5. Calculate the entropy change at the standard condition for the formation of 1 mole of water from H_2 and O_2 gases:

$$H_2(g) + O_2(g) \longrightarrow H_2O(l)$$

6. Calculate the entropy change for the conversion of pyruvic acid ($CH_3COCOOH$) into acetaldehyde and CO_2 by the enzyme pyruvate decarboxylase at 25°C and 100 atm.

7. Calculate the entropy change when hot water (80°C) comes in contact with cold water (5°C). The heat capacity of water at constant pressure is 75 J/K/mol. Heat is not lost to the surroundings during this operation.

8. Calculate the free energy change of hydrolysis of glycylglycine at 25°C and 1 atm in a dilute aqueous solution at 37°C and 1 atm:

$$H_3N^+CH_2CONHCH_2COO^-(aq) + H_2O(l) \longrightarrow 2H_3N^+CH_2COO^-(aq)$$

9. Derive the equation

$$\left(\frac{\partial S}{\partial P}\right)_T = -\left(\frac{\partial V}{\partial T}\right)_P$$

10. Calculate the equilibrium constant for the following reaction at 25°C:

$$CH_3COCOOH(l) \longrightarrow CH_3COH(g) + CO_2(g)$$

11. Calculate the free energy, enthalpy, and entropy changes at 0°C and 50°C for ionization of 4-aminopyridine. The ionization constants at 0 and 50°C are 1.35×10^{-10} and 3.33×10^{-9}, respectively.

12. Calculate the hydrogen ion concentration of water at 37°C. The enthalpy change at 1 atm is 55.84 kJ. The equilibrium constant of water at 25°C is 1.0×10^{-14}.

13. Calculate the ionization constant and free energy change at standard condition for the conversion of glycerol to glycerol-1-phosphate by ATP:

$$glycerol + ATP \longrightarrow glycerol\text{-}1\text{-}phosphate + ADP$$

The steady-state concentrations of ATP and ADP in the living cell are 10^{-3} M and 10^{-4} M, respectively. The equilibrium ratio of glycerol-1-phosphate to glycerol is 770 at 25°C and pH 7.

14. How much heat is absorbed or evolved during the conversion of L-aspartic acid to L-alanine and $CO_2(g)$ at 25°C and 1 atm?

$$H_2NCH(CH_2COOH)COOH \rightleftharpoons H_2NCH(CH_3)COOH + CO_2$$

15. For an ideal gas, evaluate

$$\left(\frac{\partial T}{\partial P}\right)_S, \left(\frac{\partial T}{\partial S}\right)_P, \text{ and } \left(\frac{\partial T}{\partial S}\right)_V$$

2 Ionic Equilibrium

Many commercially available and investigational drugs are anionic or cationic salt forms of weak acids or weak bases (undissociated). Their properties (solubility, partition coefficient, bioavailability, etc.) are strongly dependent upon the degree of ionization, the pH of the solution, and other constituents in the solutions of the drugs. In this chapter, ionic equilibrium calculations will be demonstrated in order to facilitate study of their properties.

2.1 STRONG ACIDS AND STRONG BASES

2.1.1 pH OF THE SOLUTION OF A STRONG ACID OR STRONG BASE

When a strong acid (e.g., HCl) is placed in water, the acid ionizes completely as:

$$HCl + H_2O \rightarrow H^+ + Cl^- \tag{2.1}$$

Three species are present in the aqueous solution of the strong acid: H^+, OH^-, and Cl^-. H^+, generated from HCl, suppresses the ionization of H_2O. This leads to the lower concentration of H^+ in water than the theoretical concentration of H^+ coming from both HCl and H_2O. To calculate the concentration of H^+ and other species in the aqueous solution, three equations are required:

1. Equilibrium: Since HCl is fully ionized, there is no reverse reaction (only forward reaction). However, water is dissociated into H^+ and OH^- at equilibrium with the following relationship:

$$K_w = [H^+][OH^-] = 1 \times 10^{-14} \qquad \text{at } 25°C \tag{2.2}$$

   where K_w is the ionization constant of water.
2. Material Balance: The concentration of Cl^- is produced only from HCl and is equal to the concentration of HCl initially present in the solution, C_a.

$$C_a = [Cl^-] \tag{2.3}$$

3. Electroneutrality: The solution containing the ionic species must be electrically neutral in order for the ionic species to be separated from each other so that there is no net charge accumulation. The total concentration of the positive charges in the solution should be equal to the total concentration of negative charges in the solution:

$$[H^+] = [OH^-] + [Cl^-] \tag{2.4}$$

There are three unknown concentration terms and three independent equations. Substituting Equation (2.1) and Equation (2.3) into Equation (2.4) yields:

$$[H^+] = C_a + \frac{K_w}{[H^+]} \tag{2.5}$$

Equation (2.5) becomes a quadratic equation by transposing and the concentration of H$^+$ is given by:

$$[H^+] = \frac{C_a + \sqrt{C_a^2 + 4K_w}}{2} \tag{2.6a}$$

One can follow the same procedure described above for calculating the concentration of OH$^-$ in a solution of a strong base (e.g., NaOH). The resulting equation is:

$$[OH^-] = \frac{C_b + \sqrt{C_b^2 + 4K_w}}{2} \tag{2.6b}$$

where C_b is the concentration of the strong base initially present.

If the concentration of a strong acid or strong base is equal to or greater than 10^{-6} M, the second term of the right-hand side of Equation (2.5) is negligible compared to the initial concentration of the strong acid or strong base:

$$[H^+] \cong C_a \quad \text{and} \quad [OH^-] \cong C_b \tag{2.7}$$

When the concentration of the strong acid or strong base is less than 10^{-6} M, Equation (2.6a) or Equation (2.6b) must be used, respectively. For example, the pH of 10^{-7} M HCl is not 7 but 6.79, as calculated from Equation (2.6a):

$$[H^+] = \frac{10^{-7} + \sqrt{10^{-14} + 4 \times 10^{-14}}}{2} = 1.62 \times 10^{-7} M$$

or
$$pH = -\log\ (1.62 \times 10^{-7}) = 6.79$$

2.1.2 TITRATION CURVE OF A STRONG BASE WITH A STRONG ACID

As a strong acid mixes with a strong base (i.e., titration), the pH of the solution changes with increasing amounts of a strong acid added to an initial volume of a strong base. The units for the mass balance equation should be moles, not moles/liter (i.e., concentration unit). Suppose a volume V_b of NaOH with concentration C_b is titrated with a volume V_a of HCl with concentration C_a. Then,

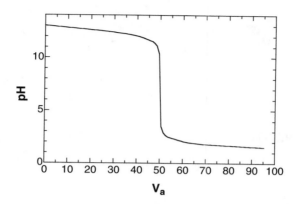

FIGURE 2.1 Titration curve for 50 mL of 0.1 M NaOH with 0.1 M HCl.

Equilibrium: $$[H^+][OH^-] = K_w \qquad (2.2)$$

Mass balance: $$[Na^+](V_a + V_b) = C_b V_b, \quad [Cl^-](V_a + V_b) = C_a V_a \qquad (2.7a)$$

Electroneutrality: $$[H^+] + [Na^+] = [Cl^-] + [OH^-] \qquad (2.7b)$$

Substitution of [Cl⁻] and [Na⁺] from Equation (2.7a) and [OH⁻] from Equation (2.2) into Equation (2.7b) yields:

$$[H^+] + \frac{C_b V_b}{V_a + V_b} = \frac{C_a V_a}{V_a + V_b} + \frac{K_w}{[H^+]} \qquad (2.7c)$$

Rearranging Equation (2.7c) gives:

$$V_a = V_b \left(\frac{C_b + [H^+] - K_w / [H^+]}{C_a - [H^+] + K_w / [H^+]} \right) \qquad (2.7d)$$

This gives the titration curve of pH vs. volume added as illustrated in Figure 2.1 for titrating 50 mL of 0.1 M NaOH with 0.1 M HCl. At the equivalence point (i.e., $C_b V_b = C_a V_a$), pH = 7.

Equation (2.7d) can be written in terms of the degree of completion of the titration, φ_{ab}:

$$\varphi_{ab} = \frac{C_a V_a}{C_b V_b} \qquad (2.7e)$$

$$\varphi_{ab} = \frac{1 + \dfrac{[H^+] - K_w / [H^+]}{C_b}}{1 - \dfrac{[H^+] - K_w / [H^+]}{C_a}} \tag{2.7f}$$

For titration of a strong acid with a strong base, Equation (2.7d) and Equation (2.7f) can be used by switching a to b and $[H^+]$ to $[OH^-]$.

2.2 MONOPROTIC WEAK ACIDS AND WEAK BASES

2.2.1 pH of the Solution of a Monoprotic Weak Acid or Weak Base

When a weak acid is dissolved in water, the acid will undergo ionization. The ionization of a weak acid, HA, in water can be expressed as:

$$HA + H_2O \; \rightleftharpoons \; H^+ + A^- \tag{2.8}$$

Four species are present in the solution of the weak acid at equilibrium: HA, A^-, H^+, and OH^-. To calculate the concentrations of the four species in the solution, four equations are needed:

1. Equilibrium: Since the forward and backward reactions are reversible, the equilibrium equation for HA and A^- is given by:

$$K_a = \frac{[H^+][A^-]}{[HA]} \tag{2.9}$$

   where K_a is the ionization constant.
   The water equilibrium is given by:

$$K_w = [H^+][OH^-] \tag{2.2}$$

2. Material Balance: Since HA and A^- coexist in equilibrium, the sum of the concentration of HA and A^- in equilibrium must equal the total concentration of the weak acid initially added to the solution, C_a.

$$C_a = [HA] + [A^-] \tag{2.10}$$

3. Electroneutrality: The three ionic species are composed of one positive charge (H^+) and two negative charges (OH^- and A^-). The sum of $[H^+]$ must equal the sum of $[OH^-]$ and $[A^-]$ as:

$$[H^+] = [OH^-] + [A^-] \tag{2.11}$$

Substituting Equation (2.10) for [HA] and Equation (2.11) for [A⁻] into Equation (2.9) yields:

$$K_a = \frac{[H^+][H^+ - OH^-]}{C_a - [H^+ - OH^-]} \tag{2.12a}$$

One can calculate the concentration of H^+ or OH^- in equilibrium by the substitution of Equation (2.2) into Equation (2.12a). The resulting equation becomes a troublesome cubic one, which cannot be solved easily:

$$[H^+]^3 + [H^+]^2 K_a - [H^+](C_a K_a + K_w) - K_w K_a = 0 \tag{2.12b}$$

One can simplify Equation (2.12a) under certain conditions because some concentration terms are assumed to be negligible in comparison to others:

1. $[H^+] >> [OH^-]$. The concentration of H^+ is much greater than that of OH^- because the ionization of HA produces H^+. However, this assumption is dependent on how strong or weak the weak acid is. The stronger the acid, the more justifiable the assumption will be. Applying the assumption ($[H^+] >> [OH^-]$) to Equation (2.12a) yields:

$$K_a = \frac{[H^+]^2}{C_a - [H^+]} \tag{2.13}$$

Substituting Equation (2.2) into Equation (2.13) yields a quadratic equation:

$$[H^+]^2 + K_a[H^+] - K_a C_a = 0 \tag{2.14}$$

and the concentration of H^+ in equilibrium is given by:

$$[H^+] = \frac{-K_a + \sqrt{K_a^2 + 4K_a C_a}}{2} \tag{2.15}$$

2. $C_a >> [H^+]$. Equation (2.13) can be further simplified under the assumption that the concentration of H^+ produced is very small compared to the total concentration of the acid initially added to the solution. When $C_a >> [H^+]$ is applied, Equation (2.13) becomes:

$$K_a = \frac{[H^+]^2}{C_a} \tag{2.16}$$

or
$$[H^+] = \sqrt{K_a C_a} \tag{2.17}$$

3. $C_a \gg [H^+] - [OH^-]$. When a diluted concentration of the weak acid is used, the concentration of H^+ produced is very small compared to that of water. In this case, the concentration of the acid is much greater than the concentration difference between H^+ and OH^- (i.e., $C_a \gg [H^+] - [OH^-]$). Thus Equation (2.12a) becomes:

$$K_a = \frac{[H^+][H^+ - OH^-]}{C_a} \qquad (2.18)$$

or $$[H^+] = \sqrt{K_a C_a + K_w} \qquad (2.19)$$

One may decide which equations should be used to calculate the concentration of H^+. In general, one should proceed with the calculation from the simplest one to the most difficult one.

Example 2.1

Calculate the pH of a 0.01 *M* solution of salicylic acid whose $K_a = 1.06 \times 10^{-3}$ at 25°C.

Solution

First, assume $C_a \gg [H^+]$. Using Equation (2.17),

$$[H^+] = \sqrt{K_a C_a} = \sqrt{1.06 \times 10^{-3} \times 0.01} = 3.26 \times 10^{-3} M$$

Now, check the assumption of $C_a \gg [H^+]$. How do we define $\gg$ (or "much greater than")? Generally speaking, if the concentration of H^+ is smaller than 5% of C_a, one can use $\gg$. The percentage of $[H^+]$ with respect to C_a is given by:

$$[H^+]/C_a = 3.26 \times 10^{-3} / 0.01 = 0.326$$

The assumption ($C_a \gg [H^+]$) is not a valid one. Use Equation (2.15) to calculate $[H^+]$ under the assumption that $[H^+] \gg [OH^-]$:

$$[H^+] = \frac{-1.06 \times 10^{-3} + \sqrt{(1.06 \times 10^{-3})^2 + 4 \times 1.06 \times 10^{-3} \times 0.01}}{2} = 2.77 \times 10^{-3} M$$

It is shown that $[H^+] \gg [OH^-]$. Therefore, the pH of the solution of the acid is given by:

$$pH = -\log (2.77 \times 10^{-3}) = 2.56$$

This same basic approach (equilibrium, material balance, and electroneutrality equations) applies to the calculation of the concentration of OH^- in a solution of a weak base at equilibrium. The resulting equation is:

$$K_b = \frac{[OH^-][OH^- - H^+]}{C_b - [OH^- - H^+]} \qquad (2.20)$$

where K_b is the ionization constant of the weak base. One can simplify Equation (2.20) under certain assumptions analogous to the cases of weak acids, as follows:

Assumption	Equation	
$[OH^-] \gg [H^+]$	$[OH^-] = \dfrac{-K_b + \sqrt{K_b^2 + 4K_bC_b}}{2}$	(2.21a)
$C_b \gg [OH^-]$	$[OH^-] = \sqrt{K_bC_b}$	(2.21b)
$C_b \gg [OH^- - H^+]$	$[OH^-] = \sqrt{K_bC_b + K_w}$	(2.21c)

Example 2.2

What is the pH of a 0.0033 M solution of cocaine base, which has an alkalinity constant (K_b) of 2.6×10^{-6}?

Solution

First, assume that $C_b \gg [OH^-]$. Using Equation (2.21b),

$$[OH^-] = \sqrt{K_bC_b} = \sqrt{2.6 \times 10^{-6} \times 0.0033} = 9.3 \times 10^{-5} M$$

Check that $[OH^-]/C_b = 9.3 \times 10^{-5} / 0.0033 = 0.028$, which is smaller than 0.05. The assumption is valid. The pH of the cocaine solution is given by:

$$pH = 14 - pOH = 14 + \log(9.3 \times 10^{-5}) = 9.97$$

Once the concentration of H+ is known, one can determine the concentrations of the other species in terms of [H+] based on Equation (2.9) and Equation (2.10).

$$[HA] = \alpha_0 C_a, \quad \alpha_0 = \frac{[H^+]}{[H^+] + K_a}, \qquad (2.22a)$$

$$[A^-] = \alpha_1 C_a, \quad \alpha_1 = \frac{K_a}{[H^+] + K_a}, \qquad (2.22b)$$

$$[B] = \beta_0 C_b, \quad \beta_0 = \frac{K_a}{[H^+] + K_a} \qquad (2.22c)$$

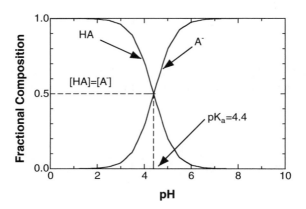

FIGURE 2.2 Equilibrium composition curve of ibuprofen ($pK_a = 4.4$).

$$[BH^+] = \beta_1 C_b, \quad \beta_1 = \frac{[H^+]}{[H^+] + K_a} \qquad (2.22d)$$

Equilibrium fractional mole compositions of ibuprofen ($pK_a = 4.4$) are shown in Figure 2.2.

Example 2.3

Calculate the concentration of un-ionized salicylic acid and ionized salicylate of a 0.01 M solution of salicylic acid as shown in Example 2.1.

Solution

The concentration of $[H^+]$ of 2.77×10^{-3} M was calculated in Example 2.1. The concentrations of the un-ionized salicylic acid and ionized salicylate can be calculated as:

$$\alpha_o = \frac{[H^+]}{[H^+] + K_a} = \frac{2.77 \times 10^{-3}}{2.77 \times 10^{-3} + 1.06 \times 10^{-3}} = 0.723$$

$$\alpha_1 = 1 - \alpha_o = 1 - 0.723 = 0.277$$

Therefore, the concentrations of the un-ionized salicylic acid and ionized salicylate are 7.23×10^{-3} M and 2.77×10^{-3} M, respectively.

Example 2.4

Calculate the pH of a mixture of 0.01 M acetic acid, HAc, ($pK_a = 4.8$) and 0.001 M benzoic acid, HBa, ($pK_a = 4.2$).

Solution

The electroneutrality equation is given by:

$$[H^+] = [Ac^-] + [Ba^-] + [OH^-]$$

Substituting Equation (2.9) for acetic acid and benzoic acid into the above equation yields:

$$[H^+] = \frac{C_{AA}K_{AA}}{[H^+]+K_{AA}} + \frac{C_{BA}K_{BA}}{[H^+]+K_{BA}} + \frac{K_w}{[H^+]}$$

where the subscripts AA and BA denote acetic acid and benzoic acid, respectively. The above equation is solved by iteration (trial and error). However, $[OH^-]$ is very small compared to other terms and can be neglected. Start with $[H^+]=10^{-3.7}$.

$$[H^+] = \frac{0.01 \times 10^{-4.8}}{10^{-3.7}+10^{-4.8}} + \frac{0.001 \times 10^{-4.2}}{10^{-3.7}+10^{-4.2}} = 7.36 \times 10^{-4} + 2.40 \times 10^{-4} = 9.76 \times 10^{-4}$$

A second iteration with $[H^+]=10^{-3.3}$ gives $[H^+]=10^{-3.38}$, and a third iteration with $[H^+]=10^{-3.34}$ yields the same $[H^+]$. Therefore, $pH = 3.34$.

2.2.2 TITRATION CURVE OF A WEAK ACID WITH A STRONG BASE

As illustrated in Section 2.1.2, the titration curve of a weak acid with a strong base can be constructed in terms of pH versus volume of the strong base. Consider a weak acid (e.g., HA) of volume V_a; its concentration C_a is titrated with a strong base (e.g., NaOH) of volume V_b and concentration C_b. The mass balances and electroneutrality equation can be given by:

$$[HA]+[A^-] = \frac{C_a V_a}{V_a + V_b}, \quad [Na^+] = \frac{C_b V_b}{V_a + V_b} \qquad (2.23)$$

$$[H^+] + [Na^+] = [A^-] + [OH^-] \qquad (2.24)$$

Substituting Equation (2.9) into Equation (2.23) yields:

$$[A^-] = \frac{C_a V_a}{V_a + V_b} \frac{K_a}{[H^+]+K_a} \qquad (2.25)$$

Substituting Equation (2.25) and $[Na^+]$ of Equation (2.23) into Equation (2.24) gives:

$$[H^+] + \frac{C_b V_b}{V_a + V_b} = \frac{C_a V_a}{V_a + V_b} \frac{K_a}{[H^+]+K_a} + \frac{K_w}{[H^+]} \qquad (2.26)$$

Rearranging Equation (2.26) for V_b versus $[H^+]$ yields:

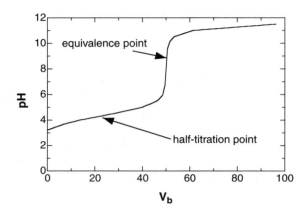

FIGURE 2.3 Titration curve of 50 mL of 0.01 M ibuprofen ($pK_a = 4.4$) with 0.01 M NaOH.

$$V_b = V_a \frac{\dfrac{K_a C_a}{[H^+] + K_a} + \dfrac{K_w}{[H^+]} - [H^+]}{C_b - \dfrac{K_w}{[H^+]} + [H^+]} \quad \text{or} \quad \varphi_{ab} = \frac{\alpha_1 - \dfrac{[H^+] - K_w[H^+]}{C_a}}{1 + \dfrac{[H^+] - K_w/[H^+]}{C_b}} \quad (2.27)$$

Figure 2.3 shows the titration curve of 50 mL of 0.01 M ibuprofen with 0.01 M NaOH.

When a volume V_a of the mixture of a strong acid (e.g., HCl) with a concentration C_{a1} and a monoprotic weak acid (HA) with a concentration C_{a2} is titrated with a strong base (e.g., NaOH) with a concentration C_b and a volume V_b, the charge balance and mass balance can be written:

$$[H^+] + [Na^+] = [Cl^-] + [A^-] + [OH^-] \tag{2.28a}$$

$$[HA] + [A^-] = \frac{C_{a2} V_a}{V_a + V_b} \qquad [Cl^-] = \frac{C_{a1} V_a}{V_a + V_b} \tag{2.28b}$$

Substituting Equation (2.9) into Equation (2.28b) yields:

$$[A^-] = \frac{C_{a2} V_a}{V_a + V_b} \frac{K_a}{[H^+] + K_a} \tag{2.28c}$$

Substituting Equation (2.23), Equation (2.28b), and Equation (2.28c) into Equation (2.28a) gives:

$$\left(C_b + [H^+] - [OH^-]\right) V_b = \left(C_{a1} + C_{a2} \frac{K_a}{[H^+] + K_a} + [H^+] - [OH^-]\right) V_a \tag{2.28d}$$

Rearranging Equation (2.28d) for V_b versus $[H^+]$ gives:

$$V_b = V_a \frac{C_{a1} + \dfrac{C_{a2}K_a}{[H^+] + K_a} + \dfrac{K_w}{[H^+]} - [H^+]}{C_b - \dfrac{K_w}{[H^+]} + [H^+]}$$

or

$$\varphi_{ab} = \frac{1 + \alpha_{A^-}\left(\dfrac{C_{a2}}{C_{a1}}\right) - \dfrac{[H^+] - K_w / [H^+]}{C_{a1}}}{1 + \dfrac{[H^+] - K_w / [H^+]}{C_b}} \qquad (2.28e)$$

where

$$\varphi_{ab} = \frac{C_b V_b}{C_{a1} V_a}$$

Equation (2.7d) and Equation (2.27) can be generalized for four possible different types of titration of strong/weak acids with strong/weak bases as:

$$V_b = V_a \frac{\left\{ bK_w + [H^+] \right\} \left\{ \left(1 + a[H^+]\right)\left(K_w - [H^+]^2 + C_a[H^+]\right) \right\}}{\left\{ 1 + a[H^+] \right\} \left\{ C_b[H^+]^2 + \left(bK_w + [H^+]\right)\left([H^+]^2 - K_w\right) \right\}} \qquad (2.29)$$

where $a = 1 / K_a$ for a weak acid and $b = 1 / K_b$ or $a = b = 0$ for a strong acid or base.

2.2.3 pH of the Solution of Salts of Weak Acids or Weak Bases

Section 2.2.1 discussed the ionic equilibria of undissociated acids or bases. The majority of commercial (or investigational) drugs are the salt forms of weak acids or weak bases. Let us examine the ionic equilibria when the salt formed between a weak base and a strong acid (HBX) is placed into solution. When the salt is placed into a solution, it completely dissociates into HB^+ and X^-. The ionic weak acid (HB^+) is further hydrolyzed as:

$$HBX \longrightarrow HB^+ + X^- \qquad (2.30a)$$

$$HB^+ + H_2O \rightleftharpoons H^+ + B \qquad (2.30b)$$

where B is the undissociated weak base. Five species are present in the solution of the salt: HB^+, X^-, H^+, OH^-, and B. Five equations are required to solve the concentration of the five species. The same approach used in the case of the undissociated acid can be applied as follows:

1. Equilibrium:

$$K_w = [H^+][OH^-] \qquad (2.2)$$

$$K_a = \frac{[H^+][B]}{[HB^+]} \qquad (2.31a)$$

2. Mass balance: According to Equation (2.30a) and Equation (2.30b), one can derive two material balance equations as follows:

$$C_a = [X^-] \qquad (2.31b)$$

$$C_a = [HB^+] + [B] \qquad (2.31c)$$

3. Electroneutrality:

$$[H^+] + [HB^+] = [OH^-] + [X^-] \qquad (2.32)$$

Substituting Equation (2.31b), Equation (2.31c), and Equation (2.32) into Equation (2.31a) yields:

$$K_a = \frac{[H^+][H^+ - OH^-]}{C_a - [H^+ - OH^-]} \qquad (2.33)$$

This shows that the ionic equilibrium calculation for the salt formed between the weak base and the strong acid is identical for the undissociated acid. Therefore, one may use Equation (2.15), Equation (2.17), and Equation (2.19) for the calculation of H^+ in the solution of a salt between a weak base and a strong acid. Equation (2.21a), Equation (2.21b), and Equation (2.21c) may be used for the calculation of OH^- in the solution of the salt between a weak acid and a strong base along with Equation (2.20).

Example 2.5

Calculate the pH of a 0.165 *M* solution of sodium sulfathiazole. The acidity constant for sulfathiazole is 7.6×10^{-8}.

Solution

The chemical drug is the salt of a weak acid. Therefore, one can use the equations derived for an undissociated base. First, we assume that $C_b \gg [OH^-]$,

$$[OH^-] = \sqrt{K_b C_b} = \sqrt{\frac{K_w C_b}{K_a}} = \sqrt{\frac{10^{-14} \times 0.165}{7.6 \times 10^{-8}}} = 1.47 \times 10^{-4} M$$

$[OH^-]/C_b = (1.47 \times 10^{-4})/0.165 = 8.9 \times 10^{-4}$, which is smaller than 0.05. This shows that the assumption is valid. The pH of the solution is then given by:

$$pH = 14 - pOH = 14 + \log (1.47 \times 10^{-4}) = 10.2$$

Example 2.6

Find the pH of a mixture of 10^{-4} M NaOH and 10^{-5} M of sodium benzoate, NaBa, ($pK_a = 4.2$).

Solution

The mass balance equations are given by:

$$[Na^+] = C_{NaOH} + C_{NaBa}$$

$$[HBa] + [Ba^-] = C_{NaBa}$$

The electroneutrality equation is given by:

$$[H^+] + [Na^+] = [OH^-] + [Ba^-]$$

Substituting $[Na^+]$ and $[Ba^-]$ from the mass balance equation into the electroneutrality equation yields:

$$[H^+] + [HBa] + C_{NaOH} = [OH^-]$$

Substitution of Equation (2.9) for benzoic acid into the above equation gives:

$$[H^+] + \frac{C_{NaB}[H^+]}{[H^+] + K_{NaB}} + C_{NaOH} = [OH^-]$$

A first approximation of $[H^+] = 10^{-10}$ gives:

$$[OH^-] = 10^{-10} + \frac{10^{-5} \times 10^{-10}}{10^{-10} + 10^{-4.2}} + 10^{-4} = 10^{-4}$$

The pH of the solution is 4.

2.2.4 pH OF THE SOLUTION OF A MIXTURE OF CONJUGATE ACIDS AND BASES: HENDERSON–HASSELBALCH EQUATION

The cases described in the previous sections are ones that deal only with undissociated weak acids or weak bases, or when the ionized weak acids or bases are present in a solution. However, there are many cases in which both undissociated acids and their conjugate bases are present in a solution; this situation can be created by adding the conjugate base into the solution of a weak acid or by partially neutralizing the weak acid with a strong base. Mixtures of an undissociated weak acid and its conjugate base or an undissociated weak base and its conjugate acid are known as *buffers*. Let us examine the equilibrium calculations of the known amount of HA (C_a) and the known amount of its conjugate base as a salt (NaA) (C_b) in a solution. Again, five species are present in the solution. The same approach as previously discussed will be applied:

1. Equilibrium:

$$K_a = \frac{[H^+][A^-]}{[HA]} \qquad (2.9)$$

$$K_w = [H^+][OH^-] \qquad (2.2)$$

2. Material balance: The total amount of the weak acid and its conjugate base at equilibrium should be the amount of the weak acid and its conjugate base initially present as:

$$C_a + C_b = [HA] + [A^-] \qquad (2.34)$$

From the complete dissociation of NaA, one can obtain:

$$C_b = [Na^+] \qquad (2.35)$$

3. Electroneutrality: There should be no net charge among the four ionic species as follows:

$$[Na^+] + [H^+] = [OH^-] + [A^-] \qquad (2.36)$$

Substituting Equation (2.35) into Equation (2.36) and solving the resulting equation for [A⁻] followed by substituting it into Equation (2.34) yields:

$$[A^-] = C_b + [H^+] - [OH^-] \qquad (2.37)$$

$$[HA] = C_a - [H^+ - OH^-] \tag{2.38}$$

Substituting Equation (2.37) and Equation (2.38) into Equation (2.9) yields:

$$K_a = \frac{[H^+][C_b + H^+ - OH^-]}{C_a - [H^+ - OH^-]} \tag{2.39}$$

If there is no conjugate base in the solution, Equation (2.39) becomes Equation (2.12a). Equation (2.39) is cubic and so is not easy to solve. Let us simplify it under certain assumptions.

If we assume $[H^+]$ is much greater than $[OH^-]$, Equation (2.39) becomes:

$$K_a = \frac{[H^+][C_b + H^+]}{C_a - [H^+]} \tag{2.40}$$

Assuming $C_a \gg [H^+]$ and $C_b \gg [H^+]$, Equation (2.40) further reduces to:

$$[H^+] = K_a \frac{C_a}{C_b} \tag{2.41}$$

Equation (2.41) is identical to Equation (2.9) if one considers that C_a and C_b are the equilibrium concentrations of HA and A^-, respectively. Taking the logarithm of Equation (2.41) for the mixture of a weak acid and its conjugate base gives:

$$pH = pK_a + \log\left(\frac{[salt]}{[acid]}\right) \tag{2.42}$$

For the ionization of a weak acid by a strong base, Equation (2.42) can be rewritten as:

$$pH = pK_a + \log\left(\frac{[ionized]}{[un\text{-}ionized]}\right) = pK_a + \log\left(\frac{\alpha}{1-\alpha}\right) \tag{2.43}$$

where α is the degree of ionization. Equation (2.41), Equation (2.42), and Equation (2.43) are the Henderson–Hasselbalch equations for a weak acid.

Example 2.7

Calculate the pH change when 0.005 *M* of sodium salicylate is added to a 0.01 *M* solution of salicylic acid.

Solution

The concentration of H^+ of a 0.01 M solution of salicylic acid has been calculated in Example 2.1 and given as:

$$[H^+] = 2.77 \times 10^{-3} M$$

The pH of the solution after adding 0.005 M sodium salicylate under the assumptions of $C_a \gg [H^+]$ and $C_b \gg [OH^-]$ is given by:

$$[H^+] = K_a \frac{C_a}{C_b} = (1.06 \times 10^{-3}) \frac{0.01}{0.005} = 2.12 \times 10^{-3} M$$

Checking the assumption: $[H^+]/C_a = (2.12 \times 10^{-3})/0.01 = 0.212$, which is larger than 0.05. Therefore, the assumption is not a valid one, so Equation (2.40) should be used:

$$K_a = \frac{[H^+][C_b + H^+]}{C_a - [H^+]} = \frac{[H^+][0.005 + H^+]}{0.01 - [H^+]} = 1.06 \times 10^{-3}$$

$$[H^+]^2 + (0.005 + 1.06 \times 10^{-3})[H^+] - 0.01 \times 1.06 \times 10^{-3} = 0$$

$$[H^+] = \frac{-0.00606 + \sqrt{(0.00606)^2 + 4 \times 0.01 \times 1.06 \times 10^{-3}}}{2} = 0.00142 M$$

The concentration of H^+ decreases from 2.77×10^{-3} to 1.42×10^{-3} (51.3% of the initial value). The pH changes from 2.56 to 2.85.

For a mixture of a weak base and its conjugate acid, the equivalent equation to Equation (2.39) is given by:

$$K_b = \frac{[OH^-][C_a + OH^- - H^+]}{C_b - [OH^- - H^+]} \tag{2.44}$$

Equation (2.44) can be simplified as follows:

Assumption	*Equation*	
$[OH^-] \gg [H^+]$	$K_b = \dfrac{[OH^-][C_a + OH^-]}{C_b - [OH^-]}$	(2.45a)
$C_a \gg [H^+]$ and $C_b \gg [OH^-]$	$[OH^-] = K_a \dfrac{C_b}{C_a}$	(2.45b)

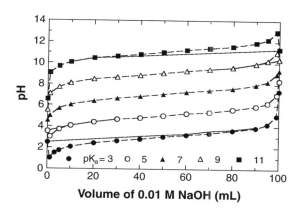

FIGURE 2.4 Exact and Henderson–Hasselbalch pH as a function of base volume during titration of 100 mL of 0.01 M weak acid. Solid lines without symbols represent the exact pH; symbols represent the Henderson–Hasselbalch pH. [Graph reconstructed from data by Po and Senozon, *J. Chem. Ed.*, 78, 1499 (2001).]

The Henderson–Hasselbalch equation for a weak base can be written as:

$$pH = pK_a + log\left(\frac{[base]}{[salt]}\right) = pK_a + log\frac{[un\text{-}ionized]}{[ionized]} = pK_a + log\frac{1-\alpha}{\alpha} \quad (2.46)$$

The discrepancy of the values of $[H^+]$ determined by Equation (2.39) and Equation (2.41), which are called the exact and approximate equations, respectively, can be very high even at moderate concentrations (e.g., 0.01 M) and at pH values close to the pK_a (e.g., 3). This occurs because the Henderson–Hasselbalch equation uses the initial molarities of [HA] and $[A^-]$. The error is dependent on the pK_a and concentrations of acid and conjugate base. For acids with a pK_a close to 7 (i.e., 5–9), the Henderson–Hasselbalch equation is suitable to determine $[H^+]$ as long as the ratio of acid to conjugate base is not too small or too large. However, when the pK_a departs by more than two units, the Henderson–Hasselbalch equation is not suitable to calculate $[H^+]$. As shown in Example 2.7, the percent error between Equation (2.39) and Equation (2.41) is 49.3%. If the ratio of the acid to the conjugate base is larger than 10, the percent error becomes more than 350%. In addition, when the concentration of the acid decreases to 0.001 M and the ratio is 10, the percent error becomes more than 1500%. In this case, the dissociation of the acid and unionization (or hydrolysis) of conjugate salt should be taken into account for calculating $[H^+]$ [i.e., Equation (2.39)]. Figure 2.4 displays the comparison of the exact and Henderson–Hasselbalch equations for an acid with a concentration of 0.01 M.

The Henderson–Hasselbalch equation shows the same pH as long as the ratio of weak acid to conjugate base is constant. As pointed out before, the pH of buffers is dependent on the total concentration of buffer agents. Equation (2.39) can be transformed to:

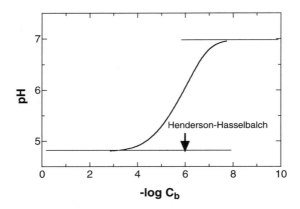

FIGURE 2.5 The effect of the total concentration of weak acid ($pK_a = 4.8$)–conjugate buffer on the pH of the buffer.

$$C_b = \frac{\left(1 + \dfrac{K_a}{[H^+]}\right)\left([H^+] - \dfrac{K_w}{[H^+]}\right)}{\left(\dfrac{C_a}{C_b}\dfrac{K_a}{[H^+]} - 1\right)} \qquad (2.47)$$

Figure 2.5 shows the effect of total concentration of buffer on the pH of equimolar weak acid–conjugate buffer. The Henderson–Hasselbalch equation fails to predict the pH of the buffer at concentrations of 10^{-3} M or less.

Example 2.8

As shown in Example 2.5, the pH of the solution of 0.165 M sodium sulfathiazole is 10.17, which is high. HCl is added to lower the pH. How much can one lower the pH without precipitating the weak acid (sulfathiazole)? The molar solubility of the weak acid is 0.002 M.

Solution

When HCl is added to the solution of sodium sulfathiazole, anionic sulfathiazole (Sulf⁻) will convert to the weak acid sulfathiazole (SulfH) as follows:

$$Sulf^- + H^+ \rightleftarrows SulfH + H_2O$$

If one keeps adding HCl, the amount of SulfH produced will exceed the solubility of SulfH in water, thus causing precipitation. Therefore, one can add HCl up to the saturated concentration of SulfH. Only 0.002 M of SulfH can be produced from 0.165 M sodium sulfathiazole without precipitation. The remaining concentration of Sulf⁻ is equal to 0.163 M (0.165 − 0.002 M). The pH at which the saturated concentration of SulfH is produced is given by:

$$pH = pK_a + \log \frac{[\text{salt}]}{[\text{un-ionized}]} = 7.12 + \log\left(\frac{0.165 - 0.002}{0.002}\right) = 9.03$$

The ionization constants for selected pharmaceutical drugs and reference weak acids and weak bases are listed in Table 2.1.

It is interesting to find the pH of a solution containing the salt of a weak acid (HA) and a weak base (B) where they have the same concentration. The equilibrium, mass balance, and electroneutrality equations can be given as:

1. Equilibrium:

$$K_{a1} = \frac{[H^+][A^-]}{[HA]} \tag{2.9}$$

$$K_{b1} = \frac{[H^+][B]}{[BH^+]} \tag{2.48}$$

$$K_w = [H^+][OH^-] \tag{2.2}$$

2. Mass balance:

$$C_a = [HA] + [A^-] = C_b = [BH^+] + [B] = C \tag{2.49}$$

3. Electroneutrality:

$$[H^+] + [BH^+] = [A^-] + [OH^-] \tag{2.50}$$

Substituting Equation (2.9) for [HA] and Equation (2.48) for [B] into Equation (2.49), solving for [A$^-$] and [BH$^+$], and then substituting the resulting equations into Equation (2.50) yields:

$$[H^+] + \frac{C[H^+]}{[H^+] + K_{b1}} = \frac{CK_{a1}}{[H^+] + K_{a1}} + [OH^-] \tag{2.51}$$

Instead of having a cubic equation in [H$^+$], Equation (2.51) is rearranged to:

$$C = \frac{K_w / [H^+] - [H^+]}{\dfrac{[H^+]}{[H^+] + K_{b1}} - \dfrac{K_{a1}}{[H^+] + K_{a1}}} \tag{2.52}$$

If [H$^+$] and [OH$^-$] are small, Equation (2.51) or Equation (2.52) becomes:

TABLE 2.1
Ionization Constants for Drugs and Weak Acids and Bases

Chemical	pK$_a$	Chemical	pK$_a$
Acetaminophen	9.9 (phenol)	Lidocaine	7.9
Acetic acid	4.8	Lorazepam	11.5, 1.3
Adriamycin	8.2	Malonic acid	2.8
Albuterol	9.3, 10.3	Mefenamic acid	4.3
Allyamine	10.7	Methotrexate	4.8, 5.5, 3.8
p-Aminobenzoic acid	2.4 (amine), 4.9	Metoprolol	9.7
Aminophylline	5.0	Metronidazole	2.6
Amoxicillin	2.4 (carboxyl)	Morphine	8.0, 9.6 (phenol)
	7.4 (amine)	Naproxen	4.2
	9.6 (phenol)	Nicotine	3.1, 8.0
Ampicillin	2.7, 7.3 (amine)	Nicotinic acid	4.8
Ascorbic acid	4.2, 11.6	o-Nitrophenol	7.2
Aspirin	3.5	Oxazepam	1.8, 11.1
Atropine	9.7	Oxytetracycline	3.3, 7.3, 9.1
Barbital	7.8	Penicillin G	2.8
Benzoic acid	4.2	Phenacetin	2.2
p-Bromophenol	9.2	Phenobarbital	7.5
Caffeine	14.0, 0.6 (amine)	Pilocarpine	1.6, 7.1
Camphoric acid	4.7	Prazosin	6.5
Chlorothiazide	6.7, 9.5	Procaine	9.0
Cimetidine	6.8	Propranolol	9.5
Cocaine	8.4	Propylparaben	8.4
Codeine	7.9	Pseudoephedrine	9.9
o-Cresol	10.3	Quinidine	4.2, 8.3
Dextromethorphan	8.3	Quinine	4.2, 8.8
Dextrose	12.1	Resorcinol	6.2
Doxorubicin	8.2, 10.2	Riboflavin	1.7, 10.2
Ephedrine	9.6	Saccharin	1.6
Erythromycin	8.8	Salicylic acid	3.0, 13.4 (phenol)
17α-Estradiol	10.7	Scopolamine	7.6
Ethanolamine	9.5	Succinic acid	4.2 (1st), 5.6 (2nd)
Fluorouracil	8.0, 13.0	Sulfadiazine	6.5, 2.0
Formic acid	3.7	Sulfisoxazole	5.0
Gentamicin	8.2	Tetracycline	3.3, 7.7, 9.5
Glutamic acid	4.3	Theophylline	8.8, 0.7(amine), 3.5
Glycolic acid	3.8	Thiamine	4.8, 9.0
Homatropine	9.7	Triethanolamine	7.8
p-Hydroxybenzoic acid	4.1	Urea	0.2
Indomethacin	4.5	Viomycin	8.2, 10.3, 12.0
Isoproterenol	8.7 (amine), 9.9 (phenol)	Warfarin	5.1
Lactic acid	3.9		

Source: The data are taken from J. E. Thompson, *A Practical Guide to Contemporary Pharmacy Practice,* Williams and Wilkins, Baltimore, 1998.

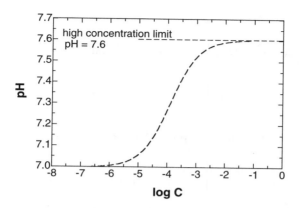

FIGURE 2.6 Dependence of pH for the salt of a weak acid ($pK_{a1} = 4.5$) and weak base ($pK_{a2} = 10.7$) on concentration.

$$\frac{[H^+]}{[H^+]+K_{b1}} = \frac{K_{a1}}{[H^+]+K_{a1}} \quad \text{or} \quad [H^+] = \sqrt{K_{a1}K_{b1}} \qquad (2.53)$$

Figure 2.6 shows a plot of concentration versus pH with $pK_{a1} = 4.5$ and $pK_{b1} = 10.7$. As the concentration decreases, the pH of the solution approaches 7.00, whereas the pH of the solution is either higher or lower than 7 as the concentration increases, depending on pK_{a1} and pK_{b1}. In this case the upper limit is

$$\tfrac{1}{2}(4.5+10.7) = 7.6$$

2.2.5 Buffer Solutions and Buffer Capacity

As mentioned before, a buffer solution contains a mixture of a weak acid and its conjugate base or of a weak base and its conjugate acid. The important aspect of the buffer solution is that the pH of the solution is minimally changed when small amounts of acid or base are added or when the solution is slightly diluted. Let us now examine a buffer solution made of a weak acid HA (0.3 M), whose pK_a is 4.90, and its conjugate base NaA (0.3 M). A small quantity of HCl (0.05 M) is accidentally added to the solution. The conjugate base (A^-) will react with H^+ as follows:

$$A^- + H^+ \rightleftharpoons HA + H_2O$$

Therefore, the amount of A^- will be reduced and the amount of HA will be increased as:

$$[A^-] = [\text{ionized}] = 0.3 - 0.05 = 0.25 \; M$$

$$[HA] = [\text{un-ionized}] = 0.3 + 0.05 = 0.35 \ M$$

After the addition of HCl, the pH of the solution is given by Equation (2.41) as:

$$pH = pK_a + \log\frac{[\text{ionized}]}{[\text{un-ionized}]} = 4.90 + \log\frac{0.25}{0.35} = 4.75$$

Before the addition of HCl, $pH = pK_a = 4.90$ because equal amounts of the acid and its conjugate base are initially present. This demonstrates that a 0.15 difference in pH was caused by the addition of HCl.

However, the degree of pH change executed by adding a strong acid or a strong base depends on the concentration of the buffer. A low buffer concentration (e.g., 0.05 M) will not be effective for buffering a similar or higher concentration of a strong acid or a strong base (0.05 M or higher). One should know the capacity of the buffer for a given buffer concentration at a given pH. The buffer capacity, β, is defined as:

$$\beta = -\frac{dC_A}{dpH} = \frac{dC_B}{dpH} \tag{2.54}$$

where C_A and C_B are the concentrations of a strong acid and a strong base added to a buffer, respectively. When a strong base (NaOH) is added to a buffer solution consisting of a weak acid and its conjugate base, Equation (2.11) will be changed to:

$$[Na^+] + [H^+] = C_B + [H^+] = [OH^-] + [A^-] \tag{2.55a}$$

or

$$C_B = [OH^-] + [A^-] - [H^+] \tag{2.55b}$$

Differentiating C_B with pH yields:

$$\beta = \frac{dC_B}{dpH} = \frac{d[A^-]}{dpH} + \frac{d[OH^-]}{dpH} - \frac{d[H^+]}{dpH} \tag{2.56}$$

The terms on the right-hand side of Equation (2.56) can be rewritten as follows:

$$\frac{d[A^-]}{dpH} = (C_a + C_b)\frac{d[H^+]}{dpH}\frac{d\alpha_1}{d[H^+]} = 2.303(C_a + C_b)\frac{K_a[H^+]}{(K_a + [H^+])^2} \tag{2.57a}$$

$$\frac{d[H^+]}{dpH} = -\frac{2.303d[H^+]}{d\ln[H^+]} = -2.303[H^+] = -\beta_{H^+} \tag{2.57b}$$

$$\frac{d[OH^-]}{dpH} = \frac{2.303d[OH^-]}{d\ln[OH^-]} = 2.303[OH^-] = \beta_{OH^-} \tag{2.57c}$$

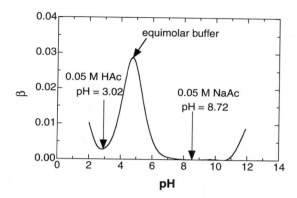

FIGURE 2.7 Buffer capacity of acetate buffer with respect to pH (C = 0.05M).

where C_a and C_b are the concentrations of the weak acid and its conjugate base initially present, respectively. Substituting Equation (2.57a) through Equation (2.57c) into Equation (2.56) yields:

$$\beta = \frac{dC_B}{dpH} = 2.303\left([OH^-]+[H^+]+\frac{(C_a+C_b)K_a[H^+]}{(K_a+[H^+])^2}\right) \quad (2.58)$$

Substituting Equation (2.9) into Equation (2.58) yields:

$$\beta = \frac{dC_B}{dpH} = 2.303\left([OH^-]+[H^+]+\frac{(C_a+C_b)[HA][A^-]}{[HA]+[A^-]}\right) \quad (2.59)$$

Now, if we assume $[H^+] \gg [OH^-]$,

$$\beta = \frac{dC_B}{dpH} = 2.303\left([H^+]+\frac{(C_a+C_b)[HA][A^-]}{[HA]+[A^-]}\right) = 2.303\left([H^+]+\frac{(C_a+C_b)K_a[H^+]}{(K_a+[H^+])^2}\right) \quad (2.60)$$

If we assume $C_a \gg [H^+]$ and $C_b \gg [H^+]$,

$$\beta = \frac{dC_B}{dpH} = 2.303\left(\frac{(C_a+C_b)[HA][A^-]}{[HA]+[A^-]}\right) = 2.303\left(\frac{(C_a+C_b)K_a[H^+]}{(K_a+[H^+])^2}\right) \quad (2.61)$$

The variation of buffer capacity of the acetate buffer with respect to pH is shown in Figure 2.7 for the total concentration of 0.05 *M*.

Example 2.9

Calculate the pH and buffer capacity of a buffer prepared with 100 mL of 0.10 *M* NaOH and 135 mL of 0.30 *M* CH_3COOH. The pK_a of CH_3COOH is 4.74. Calculate the change in pH when 0.001 *M* of HCl is added to the solution.

Solution

When the two solutions are mixed, the actual concentration of NaOH and CH_3COOH in $(100 + 135)$ mL will be:

$$0.10\ M \times \frac{100\ \text{mL}}{(100+135)\ \text{mL}} = 0.043\ M\ \text{NaOH}$$

$$0.30\ M \times \frac{135\ \text{mL}}{(100+135)\ \text{mL}} = 0.172\ M\ CH_3COOH$$

Therefore, $0.043\ M$ of CH_3COOH will be ionized and $0.129\ M$ of CH_3COOH will remain in the solution. The pH of the buffer is:

$$pH = pK_a + \log\left(\frac{0.043}{0.129}\right) = 4.26$$

The buffer capacity is given by:

$$\beta = 2.303\frac{(0.043+0.129)\times 10^{-4.74}\times 10^{-4.26}}{(10^{-4.26}+10^{-4.74})^2} = 0.0636\ M$$

The buffer capacity of the above buffer is $0.0636\ M$ per pH. The addition of HCl gives $\Delta C_a = 0.001$ and then,

$$\Delta pH = -\Delta C_a / \beta = 0.001 / 0.0792 = 0.013$$

Equation (2.61) is a parabolic one and has a maximum. The maximum buffer capacity can be derived at $d\beta / dpH = 0$:

$$\frac{d\beta}{dpH} = \frac{2.303(C_a + C_b)K_a(K_a - [H^+])}{(K_a + [H^+])^3} = 0 \qquad (2.62)$$

Therefore, the maximum buffer capacity occurs at $pH = pK_a$. The maximum buffer capacity is given by:

$$\beta = 0.576(C_a + C_b) \qquad (2.63)$$

The maximum buffer capacity of the buffer in Example 2-9 is equal to $0.576(0.172 + 0.043) = 0.124$. Therefore, it is recommended that a weak acid whose pK_a is close to the required pH should be chosen for a buffer solution.

If there is a weak acid and a weak base in a solution, the buffer capacity of the solution can be determined by the same approach as in the case of a weak acid alone. When a strong base, C_B, is added to the solution containing HA, A$^-$, B, and BH$^+$, the electroneutrality balance can be written as:

$$[Na^+]+[H^+]+[BH^+] = C_B +[H^+]+[BH^+] = [OH^-]+[A^-] \qquad (2.64a)$$

or

$$C_B = [OH^-]+[A^-]-[BH^+]-[H^+] \qquad (2.64b)$$

Differentiating C_B with pH yields:

$$\beta = \frac{dC_B}{dpH} = \frac{d[OH^-]}{dpH} + \frac{d[A^-]}{dpH} - \frac{d[H^+]}{dpH} - \frac{d[BH^+]}{dpH} \qquad (2.65)$$

The last term on the right-hand side of Equation (2.65) can be expressed as:

$$\frac{d[BH^+]}{dpH} = (C_a' + C_b')\frac{d[OH^-]}{dpH}\frac{d\beta_1}{d[OH^-]} = 2.303(C_a' + C_b')\frac{K_a[OH^-]}{(K_b +[OH^-])^2} \qquad (2.66)$$

where C_b' and C_a' are the concentrations of the weak base and its conjugate acid in the solution, respectively, and β_1 is given by:

$$\beta_1 = \frac{K_b}{K_b +[OH^-]} \qquad (2.22b)$$

Substituting Equation (2.57a) through Equation (2.57c) and Equation (2.66) into Equation (2.65) yields:

$$\beta = \frac{dC_B}{dpH} = 2.303\left([OH^-]+[H^+]+\frac{(C_a +C_b)K_a[H^+]}{(K_a +[H^+])^2} + \frac{(C_a' +C_b')K_b[OH^-]}{(K_b +[OH^-])^2}\right)$$

$$= 2.303\left([OH^-]+[H^+]+\frac{[HA][A^-]}{[HA]+[A^-]} + \frac{[B][BH^+]}{[B]+[BH^+]}\right) \qquad (2.67)$$

Buffer solutions commonly used in pharmaceutical applications are listed in Table 2.2.

2.2.6 EFFECT OF IONIC STRENGTH ON BUFFERS

The solutions are considered so dilute that the effect of ionic strength can be neglected (ideal solution). Mathematical expressions derived so far in this chapter use a molar concentration term. If the chemical activity deviates from ideal solution behavior, the ionization of a weak acid or weak base may be given in terms of activity rather than molar concentration to account for interactions in the real solution as follows:

TABLE 2.2
Buffer Solutions

Name	pH Range	Stock Solutions	
		A	B
KCl/HCl	1.0–2.2	KCl 0.2 N	HCl 0.2 N
Glycine/HCl	1.2–3.4	Glycine 0.1M in NaCl 0.1 N	HCl 0.1 N
Na citrate/HCl	1.2–5.0	Disodium citrate 0.1 M	HCl 0.1 N
K biphthalate/HCl	2.4–4.0	K biphthalate 0.1 M	HCl 0.1 N
K biphthalate/NaOH	4.2–6.2	K biphthalate 0.1 M	NaOH 0.1 N
Na citrate/NaOH	5.2–6.6	Disodium citrate 0.1 M	NaOH 0.1 N
Phosphate	5.0–8.0	KH_2PO_4 1/15 M	Na_2HPO_4 1/15 M
Na barbital/HCl	7.0–9.0	Na barbital 0.1 M	HCl 0.1 N
Na borate/HCl	7.8–9.2	Half-neutralized boric acid 0.2 M	HCl 0.1 N
Glycine/NaOH	8.6–12.8	Glycine 0.1 M in NaCl 0.1 N	NaOH 0.1 N
Na borate/NaOH	9.4–10.6	Half-neutralized boric acid 0.2 M	NaOH 0.1 N
Citric acid/phosphate	2.2–7.8	Citric acid 0.1 M	Na_2HPO_4 0.2 M
Citrate/phosphate/borate/HCl	2.0–12.0	To citric acid and phosphoric acid (ca. 100 ml), each equivalent to 100 ml NaOH 1 N, add 3.54 g cryst. boric acid and 343 ml NaOH 1 N and make up the mixture to 1 L	HCl 0.1 N
Acetate	3.8–5.6	Na acetate 0.1 N	Acetic acid 0.1 N
Dimethylglutaric acid/NaOH	3.2–7.6	β,β-dimethylglutaric acid 0.1 M	NaOH 0.2 N
Piperazine/HCl	8.8–10.6	Piperazine 1 M	HCl 0.1 N
Tetraethylethylenediamine	5.0–6.8 8.2–10.6	Tetraethylethylenediamine 0.1 M	HCl 0.1 N
Trismaleate	5.2–8.6	Tris acid maleate 0.2 M	NaOH 0.2 N
Dimethylaminoethylamine	5.6–7.4 8.6–10.4	Dimethylaminoethylamine 1 M	HCl 0.1 N
Tris/HCl	7.2–9.0	Tris 0.2 M	HCl 0.1 N
Carbonate	9.2–10.8	Na carbonate anhydrous 0.1 M	$NaHCO_3$ 0.1M

$$K_a = \frac{a_{H+}\, a_{A^-}}{a_{HA}} = \frac{(\gamma_{H+}[H^+])(\gamma_{A^-}[A^-])}{\gamma_{HA}[HA]} \qquad (2.68)$$

where γ is the activity coefficient. The pH based on the hydrogen ion activity $(-\log a_{H^+})$ is given by:

$$pH = pK_a + \log\left(\frac{[A^-]}{[HA]}\right) + \log \gamma_{A^-} - \log \gamma_o \qquad (2.69)$$

where γ_o is the activity coefficient for the un-ionized species.

Debye–Hückel developed a theory for the activity coefficients of an ionic solution at a molecular level. A selected ion in the ideally diluted solution is statistically well distributed and there are no interactions between ions present in the solution. In contrast, the ion in the concentrated solution is surrounded by the excess of counter ions in the vicinity of the ion, as the counter ions are attracted by Coulombic forces, while ions of the same charge are repelled. Thus, "ion atmosphere" is created. As a result, there is a difference in reversible work between the concentrated w_{rev} and dilute solutions $w_{rev, ideal}$:

$$w_{rev} - w_{rev, ideal} = -\frac{1}{2} \frac{e^2}{4\pi\varepsilon\varepsilon_o r_D} N \tag{2.70}$$

where e is the charge, ε is the dielectric constant of the solvent, ε_o is the permittivity of the vacuum, N is the number of ions, and r_D is the average distance of the counter ions from the selected ion.

If a small amount n of the selected ion from an ideally dilute solution $(\gamma = 1, c_o)$ is transferred to a solution of the same ion (γ, c), then Equation (2.70) becomes:

$$w_{rev} - w_{rev, ideal} = n\,RT\left(\ln\frac{\gamma c}{c_o} - \ln\frac{c}{c_o} \right) = -\frac{1}{2} \frac{e^2}{4\,\pi\varepsilon\varepsilon_o r_D} N \tag{2.71}$$

Rearranging Equation (2.71) for ions with arbitrary charge, ze, gives:

$$\ln\gamma = -\frac{1}{2kT}\left(\frac{(ze)^2}{4\,\pi\varepsilon\varepsilon_o r_D} \right) \tag{2.72}$$

where $nR = k$, k is the Boltzman constant, and T is the absolute temperature (K). According to the theory of Gouy and Chapman, the average distance r_D is given by:

$$\frac{1}{r_D} = \frac{\kappa}{1 + \kappa R_{min}} \tag{2.73}$$

$$\kappa = \sqrt{\frac{2e^2 N_A}{\varepsilon\varepsilon_o kT}}\,\sqrt{\mu} \tag{2.74}$$

where $1/\kappa$ is the thickness of the electrical double layer, R_{min} is the minimum distance between the ion and the counterion, N_A is Avogadro's number, and μ is the ionic strength given by:

$$\mu = \frac{1}{2}\sum_i c_i z_i^2 \tag{2.75}$$

where c_i and z_i are the concentration and the charge of ion i, respectively.
Substituting Equation (2.73) and Equation (2.74) into Equation (2.72) yields:

$$\ln \gamma = \frac{Az_i^2 \sqrt{\mu}}{1 + BR_{min}} \tag{2.76}$$

where

$$A = \left(\frac{e^3}{(4\,\pi\varepsilon_o)^{3/2}} \right) \sqrt{\frac{2\pi N_A}{k^3}} \frac{1}{(\varepsilon T)^{3/2}} \tag{2.77a}$$

$$B = \left(\frac{2e}{(4\,\pi\varepsilon_o)^{1/2}} \right) \sqrt{\frac{2\pi N_A}{k}} \frac{1}{(\varepsilon T)^{1/2}} \tag{2.77b}$$

For very weak ionic strength, Equation (2.76) is further simplified to:

$$\ln \gamma = -Az_i^2 \sqrt{\mu} \tag{2.78}$$

which is known as Debye–Hückel's limiting law.

Activity coefficients of anions and cations in an electrolyte solution cannot be determined independently. Thus, the mean activity coefficient, $\gamma_\pm$ is defined by:

$$\gamma_\pm = \left(\gamma_+^{z_+} \gamma_-^{z_-} \right)^{1/(z_+ + z_-)} \tag{2.79}$$

Guntelberg proposed a simple equation for the hydrated ion size by assuming $BR_{min} = 1$, since ions are approximately 1 Å and B is on the order of 10^8 cm^{-1}.

$$\log \gamma_\pm = -\frac{Az_+z_-\sqrt{\mu}}{1 + \sqrt{\mu}} \tag{2.80}$$

However, Equation (2.76) does not fit the experimental data, especially for $\mu > 0.1$. Empirical polynomial terms are then introduced to Equation (2.80). The Davies equation is proposed for the equation of the first polynomial term for water:

$$\log \gamma_\pm = -(0.51)\, z_+z_-\left(\frac{\sqrt{\mu}}{1 + \sqrt{\mu}} - 0.2\mu \right) \tag{2.81}$$

This equation is useful for an ionic strength up to 0.5 M. Table 2.3 lists the various activity coefficient equations.

TABLE 2.3
Individual Ion Activity Coefficient

	Approximation Equation	Ionic Strength (M)
Debye–Hückel	$\log \gamma_{\pm} = -A z_{+} z_{-} \sqrt{\mu}$	< 0.005
Extended Debye–Hückel	$= -A z_{+} z_{-} \dfrac{\sqrt{\mu}}{1 + aB\sqrt{\mu}}$	<0.1
Guntelberg	$= -A z_{+} z_{-} \dfrac{\sqrt{\mu}}{1 + \sqrt{\mu}}$	<0.1, for mixed ions
Davies	$= -A z_{+} z_{-} \left(\dfrac{\sqrt{\mu}}{1 + \sqrt{\mu}} - 0.2\mu \right)$	<0.5

Note: $A = 1.82 \times 10^{6} (\varepsilon T)^{-3/2}$ and $B = 56.3(\varepsilon T)^{-1/2}$ (where ε is a dielectric constant); and $z_{\pm}$ is the charge of the ion; A and B $\approx$ 0.51 and 0.33 for water at 25°C, respectively; a is an adjustable parameter.

Source: Taken from Stumm and Morgan, *Aquatic Chemistry*, Wiley Interscience, New York, 1981.

The activity coefficient of un-ionized molecules follows a simple "salting out" model of the ionic strength:

$$\log \gamma_{o} = b \mu \qquad (2.82)$$

where b ≈ 0.1 and depends on the species.
Equation (2.69) becomes:

$$pH = pK_{a} + \log\left(\frac{[A^{-}]}{[HA]}\right) - 0.51\left(\frac{\sqrt{\mu}}{1 + \sqrt{\mu}} - 0.2\,\mu\right) - 0.1\,\mu \qquad (2.83)$$

It is interesting to see that Equation (2.69) becomes the equation in which the activity coefficient of the un-ionized weak acid is assumed to be unity when Equation (2.80) is used as follows:

$$pH = pK_{a} + \log\left(\frac{[A^{-}]}{[HA]}\right) - \frac{0.51\sqrt{\mu}}{1 + \sqrt{\mu}} \qquad (2.84)$$

Example 2.10
Calculate the pH of a buffer solution containing 0.05 M acetic acid and 0.1 M sodium acetate. The pK_{a} of acetic acid is 4.74. The ionic strength of the solution is 0.10 M.

Solution

$$pH = 4.74 + \log\left(\frac{0.1}{0.05}\right) - \frac{0.51\sqrt{0.10}}{1 + \sqrt{0.10}} = 4.92$$

If the activity coefficient correction is not considered, the pH of the solution is given by:

$$pH = 4.74 + \log\left(\frac{0.1}{0.05}\right) = 5.04$$

There are many measurement techniques for activity coefficients. These include measuring: the colligative property (osmotic coefficients) relationship, the junction potentials, the freezing point depression, or deviations from ideal solution theory of only one electrolyte. The osmotic coefficient method presented here can be used to determine activity coefficients of a 1:1 electrolyte in water. A vapor pressure osmometer (i.e., dew point osmometer) measures vapor pressure depression.

The osmotic coefficient ψ is defined by:

$$\psi = \frac{\text{mOsm}}{2000\, m} \tag{2.85}$$

where mOsm is the milliosmolality in mmol/kg and m is the molality of the solution in mol/kg. Osmolality is the total number of particles in moles per 1000 g of solvent. If the solute behaves ideally, the ideal osmolality would be $2\, m$. However, ψ is not the activity coefficient for the solute.

The relationship between the osmotic coefficient and activity coefficient is given by:

$$\ln \gamma_{\pm} = \psi - 1 - \int_0^m \frac{1-\psi}{m}\, dm \tag{2.86}$$

The osmotic coefficient is expressed by:

$$\psi = 1 - \frac{0.39\sqrt{m}}{1 + C_1\sqrt{m}} - C_2 m \tag{2.87}$$

where C_1 and C_2 are adjustable constants. Figure 2.8 shows ψ versus the molality of KNO_3. Experiments were carried out from 0.1 to 1 m. However, the equation requires including $\psi = 1$ at 0.0 m, even though that is not an actual experimental point. Numerical integration of $(1 - \psi)/m$ is carried out in steps of 0.002 m. But the integration from 0.0 to 0.002 m cannot be performed because of the infinite number. In this situation, the integral should be changed to:

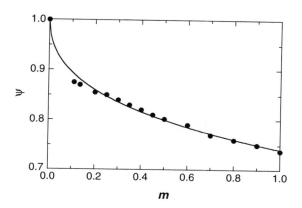

FIGURE 2.8 Osmotic coefficients vs. molality of KNO_3 solutions. [Graph reconstructed from data by Bonicamp et al. *J. Chem. Ed.,* 78, 1541 (2001).]

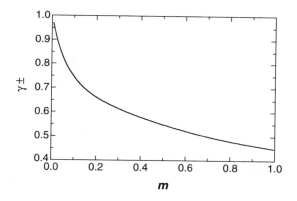

FIGURE 2.9 The mean activity coefficients vs. molality of KNO_3 solutions. [Graph reconstructed from data by Bonicamp et al. *J. Chem. Ed.,* 78, 1541 (2001).]

$$\int_0^{\sqrt{m}} \frac{1-\psi}{\sqrt{m}} \, d\sqrt{m} \qquad (2.88)$$

Figure 2.9 presents the activity coefficient vs. the molality of the KNO_3 solution.

2.2.7 Solubility of Weak Electrolytes and Ampholytes

Acidic or basic drugs are less soluble at low or high pH, respectively, because these drugs are not ionized at either pH. Un-ionized drugs are less hydrated in water than ionized ones. Let us now denote S_o for the solubility of the un-ionized species (HA) and S for the total solubility of the un-ionized and ionized species (A⁻). Then,

$$S = [HA] + [A^-] = S_o + [A^-] \qquad (2.89)$$

The dissolved un-ionized species undergoes ionization as:

$$HA + H_2O \rightleftharpoons H^+ + A^- \qquad (2.8)$$

Substituting Equation (2.89) into Equation (2.9) and taking the logarithm of the resulting equation yields:

$$pH = pK_a + \log\left(\frac{S - S_o}{S_o}\right) \qquad (2.90a)$$

or

$$\frac{K_a}{[H^+]} = \left(\frac{S}{S_o}\right) - 1 \qquad (2.90b)$$

Likewise, the solubility of a weak base can be derived as:

$$pH = pK_a + \log\left(\frac{S_o}{S - S_o}\right) \qquad (2.91a)$$

or

$$[H^+] = K_a\left(\frac{S}{S_o}\right) - K_a \qquad (2.91b)$$

The solubility of a weak acid (un-ionized) or a weak base can be determined graphically. A plot of the reciprocal of the hydrogen ion concentration vs. the total solubility of the weak acid yields the intercept of $-1/K_a$ and the slope of $1/K_aS_o$, as shown in Figure 2.10a. Plotting $[H^+]$ versus the total solubility of the weak base for Equation (2.91b) yields a straight line with a y-intercept of $-K_a$ and a slope of K_a/S_o, as shown in Figure 2.10b.

Some drugs have both anionic and cationic properties (amphoteric); examples include amino acids [e.g., levocarnitine: $CH_3 - N^+(CH_3)_2 CH_2CH(OH)CH_2COO^-$]. The ampholytes act as acids or bases depending on the pH of the solution. At high pH,

$$\begin{array}{ccc} \underset{\underset{NH_2}{|}}{R-Y-COOH} & + \quad H_2O \rightleftharpoons & \underset{\underset{NH_2}{|}}{R-Y-COO^-} & + \quad H^+ \end{array}$$

At low pH,

$$\begin{array}{ccc} \underset{\underset{NH_2}{|}}{R-Y-COOH} & + \quad H_2O \rightleftharpoons & \underset{\underset{NH_3^+}{|}}{R-Y-COOH} & + \quad OH^- \end{array}$$

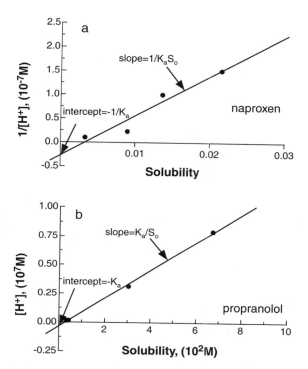

FIGURE 2.10 Plot of $1/[H^+]$ versus S for a weak acid (a) and $[H^+]$ versus S for a weak base (b). [Data taken from Avdeef et al. *Pharm. Res.*, 17, 85 (2000).]

At a specific pH, cationic and anionic groups in a drug coexist as:

$$R-Y-COO^-$$
$$|$$
$$NH_3^+$$

A chemical structure having both anionic and cationic charges on the same molecule is called a zwitterion. At a specific pH, the degree of the ionization of the zwitterion to an anionic electrolyte or to a cationic electrolyte is the same. The pH is called the isoelectric point (IEP). At the IEP, the same amount of anionic and cationic electrolytes exist. The zwitterion has the lowest solubility, denoted as S_o. One can write the ionization of an ampholyte simply as:

$$HAH^+ \underset{H^+}{\overset{K_{a1}}{\rightleftharpoons}} HA^\pm \underset{H^+}{\overset{K_{a2}}{\rightleftharpoons}} A^- \qquad (2.92a)$$

The two ionization constants are given by:

$$K_{a1} = \frac{[HA^\pm][H^+]}{[HAH^+]} \qquad (2.92b)$$

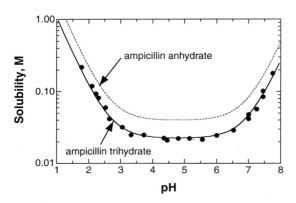

FIGURE 2.11 pH–solubility profile for ampicillin anhydrate and ampicillin trihydrate ($pK_{a1} = 2.67$ and $pK_{a2} = 6.95$) at 37°C and $\mu = 0.5\ M$ and simulated lines. [Graph reconstructed from data by Tsuji et al. *J. Pharm. Sci.*, 78, 1059 (1978).]

$$K_{a2} = \frac{[A^-][H^+]}{[HA^\pm]} \tag{2.92c}$$

Then, the following equations can be derived:

$$S = S_o\left(\frac{[H^+]}{K_{a1}} + 1\right) \quad \text{at pH} < \text{IEP} \tag{2.93a}$$

$$S = S_o\left(\frac{K_{a2}}{[H^+]} + 1\right) \quad \text{at pH} > \text{IEP} \tag{2.93b}$$

The total solubility of the ampholyte over the entire pH range can be given by:

$$S = S_o\left(\frac{[H^+]}{K_{a1}} + 1 + \frac{K_{a2}}{[H^+]}\right) \tag{2.93c}$$

Equation (2.93c) shows a U-shaped pH–solubility curve as shown in Figure 2.11 for ampicillin trihydrate and anhydrate.

Example 2.11

Calculate the lowest solubility of amoxicillin trihydrate. pK_{a1} and pK_{a2} are 2.67 and 7.11, respectively. The saturated concentration of the drug at pH 2 is 0.073 *M*.

Solution

$$0.073 = S_o\left(\frac{10^{-2}}{10^{-2.67}} + 1 + \frac{10^{-7.11}}{10^{-2}}\right) = 5.677 S_o, \quad S_o = 1.3 \times 10^{-2}\ M$$

2.3 POLYPROTIC WEAK ACIDS AND WEAK BASES

2.3.1 pH OF THE SOLUTION OF A DIPROTIC WEAK ACID, WEAK BASE, OR AMPHOLYTE

It has been considered in previous sections that acidic or basic drugs (compounds) accept or give up a single hydrogen ion. Many acids or bases can donate or receive more than one hydrogen ion; these compounds are called polyprotic acids or bases. When an un-ionized diprotic acid donates one hydrogen ion in water, the conjugate base can also act as a weak acid (the conjugate base of a monoprotic weak acid acts only as a weak base). When a diprotic weak acid H_2A is dissolved in water, the following equilibria can be established:

$$H_2A + H_2O \rightleftharpoons H^+ + HA^-$$

$$HA^- + H_2O \rightleftharpoons H^+ + A^{-2}$$

There are five species at equilibrium: H_2A, HA^-, A^{-2}, H^+, and OH^-, and five equations are needed to calculate the concentrations of the five species. These five equations can be derived as shown in Section 2.1:

1. Equilibrium:

$$K_{a1} = \frac{[H^+][HA^-]}{[H_2A]} \tag{2.94a}$$

$$K_{a2} = \frac{[H^+][A^{-2}]}{[HA^-]} \tag{2.94b}$$

$$K_w = [H^+][OH^-] \tag{2.2}$$

where K_{a1} and K_{a2} are the first and second ionization constants, respectively.

2. Material balance: Since H_2A, HA^-, and A^{-2} coexist at equilibrium, the sum of the concentrations of H_2A, HA^-, and A^{-2} should be equal to the amount of the diprotic weak acid initially added to the solution, C_a.

$$C_a = [H_2A] + [HA^-] + [A^{-2}] \tag{2.95}$$

3. Electroneutrality: The sum of the concentration of positively charged species must be equal to the sum of the concentration of negatively charged species in the solution.

$$[H^+] = 2[A^{-2}] + [HA^-] + [OH^-] \qquad (2.96a)$$

$[A^{-2}]$ is multiplied by a factor of two because each mole of A^{-2} requires two moles of H^+. Equation (2.96a) is rearranged as:

$$[HA^-] = [H^+] - 2[A^{-2}] - [OH^-] \qquad (2.96b)$$

Substituting Equation (2.96b) into Equation (2.94a) and Equation (2.94b) for $[HA^-]$ yields:

$$K_{a1} = \frac{[H^+]([H^+] - [OH^-] - 2[A^{-2}])}{[H_2A]} \qquad (2.97a)$$

$$K_{a2} = \frac{[H^+][A^{-2}]}{[H^+] - [OH^-] - 2[A^{-2}]} \qquad (2.97b)$$

Substituting Equation (2.95) into Equation (2.97a) for $[H_2A]$ yields:

$$K_{a1} = \frac{[H^+]([H^+] - [OH^-] - 2[A^{-2}])}{C_a - [HA^-] - [A^{-2}]} \qquad (2.98)$$

Substituting Equation (2.96b) into Equation (2.98) for $[HA^-]$ yields:

$$K_{a1} = \frac{[H^+]([H^+] - [OH^-] - 2[A^{-2}])}{C_a - [H^+] + [OH^-] + [A^{-2}]} \qquad (2.99)$$

Rearranging Equation (2.97b) for $[A^{-2}]$ yields:

$$[A^{-2}] = \frac{K_{a2}[H^+ - OH^-]}{[H^+] + 2K_{a2}} \qquad (2.100)$$

Substituting Equation (2.100) into Equation (2.99) yields:

$$K_{a1} = \frac{[H^+]([H^+] - [OH^-] - 2\dfrac{K_{a2}[H^+ - OH^-]}{[H^+] + 2K_{a2}})}{C_a - [H^+] + [OH^-] + \dfrac{K_{a2}[H^+ - OH^-]}{[H^+] + 2K_{a2}}} \qquad (2.101)$$

Equation (2.101) can be approximated under certain conditions where some terms are negligible compared to others. Here are some assumptions:

1. $[H^+] \gg [OH^-]$: Equation (2.101) becomes:

$$K_{a1} = \frac{[H^+]([H^+] - 2\dfrac{K_{a2}[H^+]}{[H^+] + 2K_{a2}})}{C_a - [H^+] + \dfrac{K_{a2}[H^+]}{[H^+] + 2K_{a2}}} \qquad (2.102)$$

2. Assuming $2K_{a2} \ll [H^+]$, Equation (2.102) can be further approximated to:

$$K_{a1} = \frac{[H^+]^2}{C_a - [H^+]} \qquad (2.103)$$

3. $C_a \gg [H^+]$: Equation (2.103) is simplified to:

$$[H^+] = \sqrt{K_{a1}C_a} \qquad (2.104)$$

Equation (2.103) and Equation (2.104) for diprotic weak acids are identical to Equation (2.13) and Equation (2.17) for monoprotic weak acids, respectively. The pH of a solution of a diprotic acid is governed by a first ionization process. When $C_a > 0.1\ M$ and $K_{a1} < 10^{-5}$, Equation (2.104) is a valid one.

A similar equation for a diprotic weak base can be derived as:

$$K_{b1} = \frac{[OH^-]\left([OH^-] - [H^+] - 2\dfrac{K_{b2}[OH^- - H^+]}{[OH^-] + 2K_{b2}}\right)}{C_b - \left([OH^-] - [H^+] - \dfrac{K_{b2}[OH^- - H^+]}{[OH^-] + 2K_{b2}}\right)} \qquad (2.105)$$

where K_{b1} and K_{b2} are the first and second ionization constants for the diprotic weak base, respectively and C_b is the concentration of the diprotic weak base initially present.

The approximate equations can be given by:

Assumption   *Equation*

$[OH^-] \gg [H^+]$ $K_{b1} = \dfrac{[OH^-]\left([OH^-] - 2\dfrac{K_{b2}[OH^-]}{[OH^-] + 2K_{b2}}\right)}{C_b - \left([OH^-] - \dfrac{K_{b2}[OH^-]}{[OH^-] + 2K_{b2}}\right)}$ $\qquad (2.106a)$

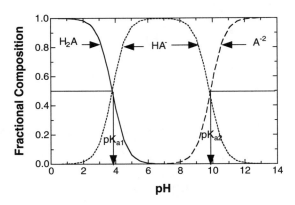

FIGURE 2.12 Equilibrium composition curves of captopril ($pK_{a1} = 3.8$ and $pK_{a2} = 9.8$).

$$2K_{b2} \ll [OH^-] \qquad K_{b1} = \frac{[OH^-]^2}{C_b - [OH^-]} \qquad (2.106b)$$

$$C_b \gg [OH^-] \qquad [OH^-] = \sqrt{K_{b1}C_b} \qquad (2.106c)$$

Since the pH of the solution from Equation (2.102), Equation (2.103), or Equation (2.104) is known, the concentrations of other species in terms of [H⁺] can be determined from Equation (2.94a), Equation (2.94b), and Equation (2.95) as follows:

$$[H_2A] = \alpha_{H_2A}C_a \qquad \alpha_{H_2A} = \frac{[H^+]^2}{[H^+]^2 + K_{a1}[H^+] + K_{a1}K_{a2}} \qquad (2.107a)$$

$$[HA^-] = \alpha_{HA^-}C_a \qquad \alpha_{HA^-} = \frac{K_{a1}[H^+]}{[H^+]^2 + K_{a1}[H^+] + K_{a1}K_{a2}} \qquad (2.107b)$$

$$[A^{-2}] = \alpha_{A^{-2}}C_a \qquad \alpha_{A^{-2}} = \frac{K_{a1}K_{a2}}{[H^+]^2 + K_{a1}[H^+] + K_{a1}K_{a2}} \qquad (2.107c)$$

Fractional mole equilibrium composition curves of captopril ($pK_{a1} = 3.8$ and $pK_{a2} = 9.8$) are shown in Figure 2.12. If $K_{a1} \gg K_{a2}$, the diprotic weak acid can be treated as two monoprotic weak acids, and Equation (2.107a), Equation (2.107b), and Equation (2.107c) can be expanded in series:

$$\alpha_{H_2A} = \frac{[H^+]}{[H^+] + K_{a1}} - \frac{K_{a1}K_{a2}}{([H^+] + K_{a1})^2} + \frac{(K_{a1}K_{a2})^2}{[H^+]([H^+] + K_{a1})^3} + \cdots \qquad (2.108a)$$

$$\alpha_{HA^-} = \frac{K_{a1}}{[H^+]+K_{a1}} - \frac{K_{a1}^2 K_{a2}}{[H]([H^+]+K_{a1})^2} + \cdots \qquad (2.108b)$$

$$\alpha_{A^{-2}} = \frac{K_{a2}}{[H^+]+K_{a2}} - \frac{[H^+]^2 K_{a2}}{K_{a1}([H^+]+K_{a2})^2} + \cdots \qquad (2.108c)$$

Example 2.12

Calculate the pH of a 0.005 M solution of H_2A and the concentration of HA^-. $K_{a1} = 10^{-4.4}$ and $K_{a2} = 10^{-7.2}$.

Solution

First, use Equation (2.104),

$$[H^+] = \sqrt{K_{a1}C_a} = \sqrt{10^{-4.4} \times 0.0005} = 4.46 \times 10^{-4} M$$

The assumption ($C_a \gg [H^+]$) is not a valid one. Use Equation (2.103) instead.

$$10^{-4.4} = \frac{[H^+]^2}{0.005 - [H^+]} \quad \text{or} \quad [H^+] = 4.27 \times 10^{-4} M$$

The assumption $[H^+] \gg 2K_{a2}$ is a valid one. Therefore, pH = 3.37.
Using Equation (2.96b) and Equation (2.100), one can obtain $[HA^-]$ as:

$$[HA^-] = [H^+] - [OH^-] - 2\frac{K_{a2}[H^+ - OH^-]}{[H^+]+2K_{a2}} \approx [H^+] - 2K_{a2} \approx [H^+]$$

$$= 4.27 \times 10^{-4} M$$

Example 2.13

Calculate the pH of a 0.005 M solution of sodium hydrogen captoprilate (NaHA).

Solution

Mass balance and charge balance equations can be given by:

Mass balance: $\qquad C_a = [Na^+] = [H_2A] + [HA^-] + [A^{-2}] \qquad (2.109a)$

Charge balance: $\qquad [Na^+] + [H^+] = [OH^-] + [HA^-] + 2[A^{-2}] \qquad (2.109b)$

Substituting Equation (2.109b) for $[HA^-]$ into Equation (2.94a) and Equation (2.109a) for $[H_2A]$ yields:

$$K_{a1} = \frac{[H^+][C_a + [H^+] - [OH^-] - 2[A^{-2}])}{C_a - [HA^-] - [A^{-2}]} \qquad (2.110a)$$

Once again substituting Equation (2.109b) for [HA⁻] into Equation (2.110a) gives:

$$K_{a1} = \frac{[H^+][C_a + [H^+] - [OH^-] - 2[A^{-2}])}{[OH^-] - [H^+] + [A^{-2}]} \tag{2.110b}$$

Equation (2.94b) can be used to obtain $[A^{-2}]$ after substituting Equation (2.109b) for [HA⁻]:

$$[A^{-2}] = \frac{K_{a2}(C_a + [H^+] - [OH^-])}{[H^+] + 2K_{a2}} \tag{2.111}$$

Substituting Equation (2.111) into Equation (2.110b) yields:

$$K_{a1} = \frac{[H^+]^2\left(\dfrac{(C_a + [H^+] - [OH^-])}{[H^+] + 2K_{a2}}\right)}{[OH^-] - [H^+] + \dfrac{K_{a2}(C_a + [H^+] - [OH^-])}{[H^+] + 2K_{a2}}} \tag{2.112}$$

NaHA is a proton-donating salt, in which the concentration of $[H^+] \gg [OH^-]$ and HA⁻ is the predominant species. Therefore, the fractional composition of HA⁻ is located at the upper portion of the ascending parabolic curve of HA⁻ and the concentration of H⁺ is much greater than K_{a2}. If $C_a \gg [H^+]$, Equation (2.112) becomes:

$$K_{a1} = \frac{[H^+]C_a}{-[H^+] + \dfrac{K_{a2}C_a}{[H^+]}}, \quad [H^+] = \sqrt{\frac{K_{a1}K_{a2}C_a}{K_{a1} + C_a}} \tag{2.113}$$

Thus, substituting $C_a = 0.005\,M$, $K_{a1} = 10^{-3.8}$, and $K_{a2} = 10^{-9.8}$ into Equation (2.113) gives:

$$[H^+] = \sqrt{\frac{10^{-3.8} \times 10^{-9.8} \times 0.005}{10^{-3.8} + 0.005}} = 1.56 \times 10^{-7}\,M$$

$$pH = -\log(1.56 \times 10^{-7}) = 6.81$$

The same approach can be employed in the solution of ampholytes, and one can derive a similar solution to Equation (2.112). In this case, the ampholyte is represented by $NH_3^+RCOO^-$ $(HY^{\pm})$. The dissociation occurs as follows:

$$H_2Y^+ + H_2O \rightleftharpoons H^+ + HY^\pm$$

$$HY^\pm + H_2O \rightleftharpoons H^+ + Y^-$$

1. Equilibrium:

$$K_{a1} = \frac{[H^+][HY^\pm]}{[H_2Y^+]} \qquad (2.114a)$$

$$K_{a2} = \frac{[H^+][Y^-]}{[HY^\pm]} \qquad (2.114b)$$

$$K_w = [H^+][OH^-] \qquad (2.2)$$

2. Mass balance:

$$C_a = [H_2Y^+] + [HY^\pm] + [Y^-] \qquad (2.115)$$

3. Electroneutrality:

$$[H_2Y^+] + [H^+] = [Y^-] + [OH^-] \qquad (2.116)$$

From Equation (2.115) and Equation (2.116), one can obtain:

$$[H_2Y^+] = [Y^-] + [OH^-] - [H^+] \qquad (2.117a)$$

$$[HY^\pm] = C_a - [H_2Y^+] - [Y^-] = C_a - [OH^-] + [H^+] - 2[Y^-] \qquad (2.117b)$$

Substituting Equation (2.117b) into Equation (2.114b) and solving the resulting equation for [Y⁻] yields:

$$[Y^-] = \frac{K_{a2}(C_a + [H^+] - [OH^-])}{[H^+] + 2K_{a2}} \qquad (2.118)$$

Substituting Equation (2.117a) into Equation (2.114a) along with Equation (2.118) yields:

$$K_{a1} = \frac{[H^+]^2 \left(\dfrac{C_a - [OH^-] + [H^+]}{[H^+] + 2K_{a2}} \right)}{[OH^-] - [H^+] + \dfrac{K_{a2}(C_a - [OH^-] + [H^+])}{[H^+] + 2K_{a2}}} \qquad (2.119)$$

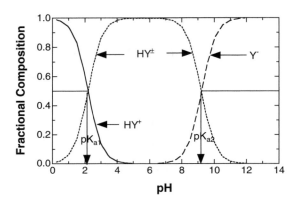

FIGURE 2.13 Fractional equilibrium composition curves of serine ($pK_{a1} = 2.2$ and $pK_{a2} = 9.22$).

Equation (2.119) is identical to Equation (2.112) for NaHA, and can be approximated under given conditions.

If $C_a \gg [H^+] - [OH^-]$ and $[H^+] \gg 2K_{a2}$, Equation (2.119) becomes:

$$[H^+] = \sqrt{\frac{K_{a1}K_{a2}C_a + K_{a1}K_w}{K_{a1} + C_a}} \tag{2.120a}$$

When $K_{a2}C_a \gg K_w$, Equation (2.120a) becomes:

$$[H^+] = \sqrt{\frac{K_{a1}K_{a2}C_a}{K_{a1} + C_a}} \tag{2.120b}$$

If $C_a \gg K_{a1}$, Equation (2.120b) becomes:

$$[H^+] = \sqrt{K_{a1}K_{a2}} \tag{2.120c}$$

Figure 2.13 shows the fractional equilibrium concentration curves for serine ($pK_{a1} = 2.2$ and $pK_{a2} = 9.22$). One can use the same equations, Equation (2.107a), Equation (2.107b), and Equation (2.107c), if H_2A, HA^-, and A^{-2} are substituted by HY^+, $HY^\pm$, and Y^-, respectively. The isoelectric point (IEP) is the pH at which the amino acid does not move in an electrical field or possesses a net charge of zero. It is obtained from $\frac{1}{2}(pK_{a1} + pK_{a2})$.

2.3.2 pH of the Solution of a Triprotic Weak Acid, Weak Base, or Polyprotic Amino Acid

There are a number of compounds that yield more than two protons and a number of amino acids that have an unequal number of amino and carboxylic acid groups.

First, let us consider triprotic weak acids H_3A such as H_3PO_4 or H_3AsO_4. In water, the following three equilibria can be established:

$$H_3A + H_2O \rightleftharpoons H^+ + H_2A^-$$

$$H_2A^- + H_2O \rightleftharpoons H^+ + HA^{-2}$$

$$HA^{-2} + H_2O \rightleftharpoons H^+ + A^{-3}$$

There are six species present in equilibrium. Six equations are needed to solve for pH or for the concentration of H^+. The same approach used for mono- and diprotic weak acids is employed here:

1. Equilibrium:

$$K_{a1} = \frac{[H^+][H_2A^-]}{[H_3A]} \tag{2.121a}$$

$$K_{a2} = \frac{[H^+][HA^{-2}]}{[H_2A^-]} \tag{2.121b}$$

$$K_{a3} = \frac{[H^+][A^{-3}]}{[HA^{-2}]} \tag{2.121c}$$

2. Mass balance:

$$C_a = [H_3A] + [H_2A^-] + [HA^{-2}] + [A^{-3}] \tag{2.122}$$

3. Electroneutrality:

$$[H^+] = [H_2A^-] + 2[HA^{-2}] + 3[A^{-3}] + [OH^-] \tag{2.123}$$

Rearranging Equation (2.123) for H_2A^- and Equation (2.122) for H_3A yields Equation (2.124a) and Equation (2.124b). Substituting these equations with Equation (2.121c) and Equation (2.121b) yields Equation (2.124c) and Equation (2.124d).

$$[H_3A] = C_a - [H_2A^-] - [HA^{-2}] - [A^{-3}] \tag{2.124a}$$

$$[H_2A^-] = [H^+] - 2[HA^{-2}] - 3[A^{-3}] - [OH^-] \tag{2.124b}$$

$$[HA^{-2}] = \frac{[H^+]K_{a2}([H^+]-[OH^-])}{[H^+]^2 + 2K_{a2}[H^+]+3K_{a2}K_{a3}} \tag{2.124c}$$

$$[A^{-3}] = \frac{K_{a2}K_{a3}([H^+]-[OH^-])}{[H^+]^2 + 2K_{a2}[H^+]+3K_{a2}K_{a3}} \tag{2.124d}$$

Substituting Equation (2.124a) through Equation (2.124d) into Equation (2.121a) gives:

$$K_{a1} = \frac{[H^+]\left([H^+]-[OH^-]-2\dfrac{K_{a2}[H^+ - OH^-]}{[H^+]+2K_{a2}} -3\dfrac{K_{a2}K_{a3}[H^+ - OH^-]}{[H^+]^2 + 2K_{a2}[H^+]+3K_{a2}K_{a3}}\right)}{C_a -[H^+]+[OH^-]-\dfrac{[H^+]K_{a2}[H^+ - OH^-]}{[H^+]^2 + 2K_{a2}[H^+]+3K_{a2}K_{a3}} -2\dfrac{K_{a2}K_{a3}[H^+ - OH^-]}{[H^+]^2 + 2K_{a2}[H^+]+3K_{a2}K_{a3}}} \tag{2.125}$$

Equation (2.125) can be further simplified under certain circumstances and some of its terms ignored. The value for $K_{a2}K_{a3}$ is negligible when compared to the other terms. For example, for H_3PO_4, $K_{a2}K_{a3} = 10^{-19.53}$, which is much smaller than the values of $K_{a2}[H^+]$ and $[H^+]^2$, even at pH 8. In this case, Equation (2.125) is equivalent to Equation (2.101) for diprotic weak acids. If other approximations (i.e., $[H^+] >> [OH^-]$ and $[H^+] >> 2K_{a2}$) are made, then the triprotic weak acid behaves as if it were a monoprotic weak acid.

The concentrations of other species in terms of $[H^+]$ can be obtained by algebraic manipulations of Equation (2.121a), Equation (2.121b), Equation (2.121c), and Equation (2.122):

$$\frac{[H_3A]}{C_a} = \alpha_{H_3A} = \frac{[H^+]^3}{[H^+]^3 + K_{a1}[H^+]^2 + K_{a1}K_{a2}[H^+]+K_{a1}K_{a2}K_{a3}} \tag{2.126a}$$

$$\frac{[H_2A^-]}{C_a} = \alpha_{H_2A^-} = \frac{K_{a1}[H^+]^2}{[H^+]^3 + K_{a1}[H^+]^2 + K_{a1}K_{a2}[H^+]+K_{a1}K_{a2}K_{a3}} \tag{2.126b}$$

$$\frac{[HA^-]}{C_a} = \alpha_{HA^{-2}} = \frac{K_{a1}K_{a2}[H^+]}{[H^+]^3 + K_{a1}[H^+]^2 + K_{a1}K_{a2}[H^+]+K_{a1}K_{a2}K_{a3}} \tag{2.126c}$$

$$\frac{[A^{-3}]}{C_a} = \alpha_{A^{-3}} = \frac{K_{a1}K_{a2}K_{a3}}{[H^+]^3 + K_{a1}[H^+]^2 + K_{a1}K_{a2}[H^+]+K_{a1}K_{a2}K_{a3}} \tag{2.126d}$$

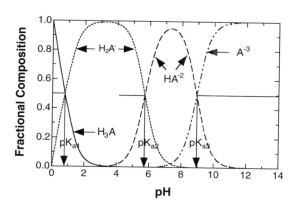

FIGURE 2.14 Fractional mole composition curves of miproxifene phosphate ($pK_{a1} = 0.80$, $pK_{a2} = 5.72$, and $pK_{a3} = 8.90$).

The fractional mole composition curves of miproxifene phosphate ($pK_{a1} = 0.80$, $pK_{a2} = 5.72$, and $pK_{a3} = 8.90$) are shown in Figure 2.14.

Example 2.14

Calculate the hydrogen ion concentrations in 0.01 M NaH_2PO_4, 0.01 M Na_2HPO_4, and 0.01 M Na_3PO_4.

Solution

The same equilibrium and electroneutrality equations shown above are used with the $pK_{a1} = 2.23$, $pK_{a2} = 7.21$, and $pK_{a3} = 12.32$. However, mass balance equations are different for each salt:

1. NaH_2PO_4:
   At the concentration of NaH_2PO_4, C_a, the mass balance equations are:

$$[Na^+] = C_a \tag{2.127a}$$

$$C_a = [H_3PO_4] + [H_2PO_4^-] + [HPO_4^{-2}] + [PO_4^{-3}] \tag{2.127b}$$

and the electroneutrality is:

$$[H^+] + [Na^+] = [H_2PO_4^-] + 2[HPO_4^{-2}] + 3[PO_4^{-3}] + [OH^-] \tag{2.127c}$$

Combining Equation (2.121a), Equation (2.121b), and Equation (2.127a) through Equation (2.127c) yields a full, cumbersome equation similar to Equation (2.125). In addition, the third ionization can be neglected in this pH range (≈ 3). The resulting equation is similar to Equation (2.119) but another approximation is made before the full equation is obtained.

Rearranging Equation (2.127b) for $[H_2PO_4^-]$ and substituting this equation along with Equation (2.127a) into Equation (2.127c) gives:

$$[H^+] + [H_3PO_4] = [HPO_4^{-2}] + 2[PO_4^{-3}] + [OH^-] \qquad (2.128a)$$

The range in the values of the concentrations of the other species is as follows: $[H_2PO_4^-] \gg [HPO_4^{-2}] \gg [OH^-] \gg [PO_4^{-3}]$. The first term in the right-hand side of Equation (2.128a) is most important and can be simplified to:

$$[H^+] + [H_3PO_4] = [HPO_4^{-2}] \qquad (2.128b)$$

Substituting Equation (2.121a) and Equation (2.121b) into Equation (2.128b) yields:

$$[H^+] + \frac{[H^+][H_2PO_4^-]}{K_{a1}} = \frac{K_{a2}[H_2PO_4^-]}{[H^+]} \qquad (2.128c)$$

Note that in this concentration or pH range, $[H_2PO_4^-] \approx C_a$. Then, Equation (2.128c) is solved for $[H^+]$:

$$[H^+]^2 \left(1 + \frac{C_a}{K_{a1}}\right) = K_{a2}C_a \quad \text{or} \quad [H^+] = \sqrt{\frac{K_{a1}K_{a2}C_a}{K_{a1} + C_a}} \qquad (2.129)$$

Equation (2.129) is identical to Equation (2.120b).

$$[H^+] = \sqrt{\frac{10^{-2.23} \times 10^{-7.21} \times 10^{-2.00}}{10^{-2.23} + 10^{-2.00}}} = 10^{-4.82}\, M$$

2. Na_2HPO_4:
    The mass balance equations are:

$$[Na^+] = 2C_a \qquad (2.130)$$

$$C_a = [H_3PO_4] + [H_2PO_4^-] + [HPO_4^{-2}] + [PO_4^{-3}] \qquad (2.127b)$$

The electroneutrality equation is the same as Equation (2.127c). Rearrangement of Equation (2.127b) for $[HPO_4^{-2}]$ and Equation (2.130) for $[Na^+]$ and substitution into Equation (2.127c) gives:

$$[H^+] + 2[H_3PO_4] + [H_2PO_4^-] = [PO_4^{-3}] + [OH^-] \qquad (2.131a)$$

At the pH range (≈ 10), the only dominant term on the left–hand side of Equation (2.131a) is $[H_2PO_4^-]$. Equation (2.131a) then becomes:

$$[H_2PO_4^-] = [PO_4^{-3}] + [OH^-] \tag{2.131b}$$

The dominant species in 0.01 M Na$_2$HPO$_4$ is HPO_4^{-2}. Substituting Equation (2.121b) and Equation (2.121c) into Equation (2.131b) yields:

$$\frac{[H^+][HPO_4^{-2}]}{K_{a2}} = \frac{K_{a3}[HPO_4^{-2}]}{[H^+]} + \frac{K_w}{[H^+]} \tag{2.131c}$$

or

$$[H^+] = \sqrt{K_{a2}K_{a3} + \frac{K_{a2}K_w}{C_a}} \tag{2.131d}$$

$$[H^+] = \sqrt{10^{-7.21} \times 10^{-12.32} + \frac{10^{-7.21} \times 10^{-14.00}}{10^{-2.00}}} = 10^{-9.52} M$$

3. Na$_3$PO$_4$:

The mass balance equations are:

$$[Na^+] = 3C_a \tag{2.132a}$$

and Equation (2.127b).

The same electroneutrality equation, Equation (2.127c), is used. From Equation (2.127b), Equation (2.132a), and Equation (2.127c), the terms $[Na^+]$ and $[PO_4^{-3}]$ are eliminated:

$$[H^+] + 3[H_3PO_4] + 2[H_2PO_4^-] + [HPO_4^{-2}] = [OH^-] \tag{2.132b}$$

At the pH range (≈ 12), $[H^+]$, $[H_3PO_4]$, and $[H_2PO_4^-]$ are negligible in comparison to $[HPO_4^{-2}]$. Then,

$$[HPO_4^{-2}] = [OH^-] \tag{2.132c}$$

Even if $[PO_4^{-3}]$ is dominant, the concentration of HPO_4^{-2} cannot be ignored. Thus, $[PO_4^{-3}] + [HPO_4^{-2}] = C_a$. This leads to:

$$[HPO_4^{-2}] = \frac{C_a[H^+]}{K_{a3} + [H^+]} \tag{2.132d}$$

Equating Equation (2.132d) into Equation (2.132c) gives:

$$\frac{C_a[H^+]}{K_{a3} + [H^+]} = \frac{K_w}{[H^+]}$$

or

$$[H^+] = \frac{K_w / C_a + \sqrt{(K_w / C_a)^2 + 4K_{a3}K_w / C_a}}{2} \qquad (2.132e)$$

$$[H^+] = \frac{10^{-14} / 10^{-2} + \sqrt{(10^{-14} / 10^{-2})^2 + 4 \times 10^{-12.31} \times 10^{-14} / 10^{-2}}}{2} = 10^{-11.88} M$$

The dependence of the equilibrium constants of polyprotic weak acids and weak bases on ionic strength allows them to be treated in exactly the same manner as monoprotic weak acids and weak bases. The first, second, and third ionization constants for triprotic weak acids in terms of activity coefficient are given by:

$$K_{a1}^o = \frac{[H^+]\gamma_+[H_2A^-]\gamma_-}{[H_3A]\gamma_o} = K_{a1}\frac{\gamma_+\gamma_-}{\gamma_o} \qquad (2.133a)$$

$$K_{a2}^o = \frac{[H^+]\gamma_+[HA^{-2}]\gamma_=}{[H_2A^-]\gamma_-} = K_{a2}\frac{\gamma_+\gamma_=}{\gamma_-} \qquad (2.133b)$$

$$K_{a3}^o = \frac{[H^+]\gamma_+[A^{-3}]\gamma_{3-}}{[HA^{-2}]\gamma_=} = K_{a3}\frac{\gamma_+\gamma_{3-}}{\gamma_=} \qquad (2.133c)$$

Taking the logarithm of Equation (2.133a), Equation (2.133b), and Equation (2.133c), applying the Davies equation to each equation in order to evaluate the activity coefficients of the ionic species, and setting the $\log \gamma_o = 0.1\,\mu$ then gives:

$$pK_{a1} = pK_{a1}^o - (2)(0.51)\left(\frac{\sqrt{\mu}}{1 + \sqrt{\mu}} - 0.2\mu\right) - 0.1\mu \qquad (2.134a)$$

$$pK_{a2} = pK_{a2}^o - (4)(0.51)\left(\frac{\sqrt{\mu}}{1 + \sqrt{\mu}} - 0.2\mu\right) \qquad (2.134b)$$

$$pK_{a3} = pK_{a3}^o - (6)(0.51)\left(\frac{\sqrt{\mu}}{1 + \sqrt{\mu}} - 0.2\mu\right) \qquad (2.134c)$$

At higher ionic strengths, the values determined by Equation (2.134b) and Equation (2.134c) are significantly higher than the experimental data. Therefore, the last terms of the equations should be adjusted.

TABLE 2.4
Ionization Constants for
Several Amino Acids at 25°C

Amino acid	pK$_{a1}$	pK$_{a2}$	pK$_{a3}$
Alanine	2.35	9.83	
Arginine	1.82	8.99	12.5
Asparagine	2.02	8.80	
Aspartic acid	2.05	3.87	10.00
Cysteine	1.7?	8.39	10.76
Glutamic acid	2.16	4.27	9.36
Glutamine	2.17	9.13	
Glycine	2.35	9.78	
Histamine	1.82	6.00	9.17
Leucine	2.36	9.60	
Lysine	2.18	8.95	10.53
Phenylalanine	1.83	9.39	
Serine	2.19	9.21	
Tryptophan	2.38	9.39	
Tyrosine	2.20	9.11	10.07

As described in Section 2.3.1, all amino acids are ampholytes. They have at least two dissociating groups (one amino group and one carboxyl group). However, a number of amino acids possess two carboxyl groups and one amino group or two amino groups and one carboxyl group (e.g., aspartic acid, cysteine, glutamic acid, arginine), as shown in Table 2.4. These amino acids are ionized at three different pK$_a$ values. For example, a dicarboxylic amino acid has the following species present at equilibrium:

$$H_3Y^{+2} \underset{K_{a1}}{\rightleftarrows} H_2Y^+ \underset{K_{a2}}{\rightleftarrows} HY^{\pm} \underset{K_{a3}}{\rightleftarrows} Y^- \qquad (2.135)$$

One would expect to apply the same basic approach as with a triprotic weak acid, with the exception of the charge balance.

1. Equilibrium:

$$K_{a1} = \frac{[H^+][H_2Y^+]}{[H_3Y^{+2}]} \qquad (2.136a)$$

$$K_{a2} = \frac{[H^+][HY^{\pm}]}{[H_2Y^+]} \qquad (2.136b)$$

$$K_{a3} = \frac{[H^+][Y^-]}{[HY^\pm]} \tag{2.136c}$$

2. Mass balance:

$$C_a = [H_3Y^{+2}] + [H_2Y^+] + [HY^\pm] + [Y^-] \tag{2.136d}$$

3. Electroneutrality:

$$2[H_3Y^{+2}] + [H_2Y^+] + [H^+] = [Y^-] + [OH^-] \tag{2.136e}$$

Rearranging Equation (2.136a), Equation (2.136b), and Equation (2.136c) for $[H_3Y^{+2}]$, $[Y^-]$, and $[HY^\pm]$, respectively, and substituting them into Equation (2.136e) yields:

$$[H_2Y^+] = \frac{K_{a1}([OH^-] - [H^+])}{K_{a1} + 2[H^+]} \tag{2.137a}$$

$$[HY^\pm] = \frac{K_{a1}K_{a2}([OH^-] - [H^+])}{[H^+](K_{a1} + 2[H^+])} \tag{2.137b}$$

$$[Y^-] = \frac{K_{a1}K_{a2}K_{a3}([OH^-] - [H^+])}{[H^+]^2(K_{a1} + [H^+])} \tag{2.137c}$$

Assume that the term $K_{a1}K_{a2}K_{a3}$ in the above equation is negligible and ignore it. Substituting Equation (2.137a), Equation (2.137b), Equation (2.137c), and Equation (2.136d) into Equation (2.136a) gives:

$$K_{a1} = \frac{[H^+]K_{a1}([OH^-] - [H^+])}{C_a - \dfrac{([OH^-] - [H^+])K_{a1}([H^+] + K_{a2})}{[H^+](2[H^+] + K_{a1})}} \tag{2.138}$$

The fractional equilibrium concentration of glutamic acid ($pK_{a1} = 2.2$, $pK_{a2} = 4.3$, and $pK_{a3} = 9.4$) or any other dicarboxylic amino acid is similar to Figure 2.14.

Example 2.15

Calculate the isoelectric point (IEP) of arginine.

Solution

Arginine is a diaminomonocarboxylic acid with $pK_{a1} = 1.82$, $pK_{a2} = 8.99$, and $pK_{a3} = 12.5$. Arginine dissociates according to Equation (2.135). From four species present in solution, the following electroneutrality among arginine species should be met:

$$2[Arg^{+2}] + [Arg^+] = [Arg^-] \tag{2.139a}$$

Substituting Equation (2.136a), Equation (2.136b), and Equation (2.136c) into Equation (2.139a) yields:

$$2\frac{[H^+][Arg^+]}{K_{a1}} + \frac{[H^+][Arg^\pm]}{K_{a2}} = \frac{K_{a3}[Arg^\pm]}{[H^+]} \tag{2.139b}$$

Substituting Equation (2.136b) into Equation (2.139b) for Arg$^+$ gives:

$$2\frac{[H^+]^2[Arg^\pm]}{K_{a1}K_{a2}} + \frac{[H^+][Arg^\pm]}{K_{a2}} = \frac{K_{a3}[Arg^\pm]}{[H^+]} \tag{2.139c}$$

Equation (2.139c) is simplified to:

$$2\frac{[H^+]^2}{K_{a1}K_{a2}} + \frac{[H^+]}{K_{a2}} = \frac{K_{a3}}{[H^+]} \tag{2.139d}$$

Rearranging Equation (2.139d) yields:

$$2\,pH - \log\left(1 + \frac{2[H^+]}{K_{a1}}\right) = pK_{a2} + pK_{a3} \tag{2.139e}$$

However, $1 \gg 2[H^+]/K_{a1}$, resulting in:

$$pH = \frac{pK_{a2} + pK_{a3}}{2} = \frac{8.99 + 12.5}{2} = 10.75$$

The deprotonation of the polyprotic amino acid mentioned above occurs in a series. However, polyprotic amino acids may either give up or take up protons in a combination of parallel and series ways. For example, an asymmetrical dibasic amino acid may undergo ionization in parallel followed by further ionization in series. The same basic approach for polyprotic amino acids is applied to the asymmetrical ionization process, then:

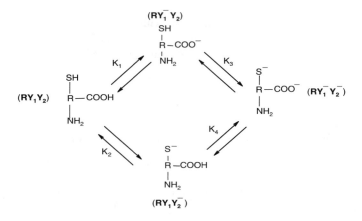

1. Equilibrium:

$$K_1 = \frac{[H^+][RY_1^-Y_2]}{[RY_1Y_2]} \tag{2.140a}$$

$$K_2 = \frac{[H^+][RY_1Y_2^-]}{[RY_1Y_2]} \tag{2.140b}$$

$$K_3 = \frac{[H^+][RY_1^-Y_2^-]}{[RY_1^-Y_2]} \tag{2.140c}$$

$$K_4 = \frac{[H^+][RY_1^-Y_2^-]}{[RY_1Y_2^-]} \tag{2.140d}$$

2. Mass balance:

$$C_a = [RY_1Y_2] + [RY_1^-Y_2] + [RY_1Y_2^-] + [RY_1^-Y_2^-] \tag{2.140e}$$

3. Electroneutrality:

$$[H^+] = [RY_1^-Y_2] + [RY_1Y_2^-] + [RY_1^-Y_2^-] + [OH^-] \tag{2.140f}$$

Rearranging Equation (2.140a) and Equation (2.140b) for $[RY_1^-Y_2]$ and $[RY_1Y_2^-]$, respectively, and multiplying Equation (2.140a) by Equation (2.140e) gives:

$$[RY_1^-Y_2] = \frac{K_1[RY_1Y_2]}{[H^+]}, \quad [RY_1Y_2^-] = \frac{K_2[RY_1Y_2]}{[H^+]}, \quad [RY_1^-Y_2^-] = \frac{K_1K_3[RY_1Y_2]}{[H^+]^2} \tag{2.141}$$

Substituting Equation (2.141) into Equation (2.140e) yields:

$$[RY_1Y_2] = C_a \frac{[H^+]^2}{[H^+]^2 + [H^+](K_1 + K_2) + K_1K_3} \tag{2.142a}$$

$$[RY_1^-Y_2] = C_a \frac{[H^+]K_1}{[H^+]^2 + [H^+](K_1 + K_2) + K_1K_3} \tag{2.142b}$$

$$[RY_1Y_2^-] = C_a \frac{[H^+]K_2}{[H^+]^2 + [H^+](K_1 + K_2) + K_1K_3} \tag{2.142c}$$

$$[RY_1^-Y_2^-] = C_a \frac{K_1K_3}{[H^+]^2 + [H^+](K_1 + K_2) + K_1K_3} \tag{2.142d}$$

Note that there is a relationship $K_1K_3 = K_2K_4$. Substituting Equation (2.142b), Equation (2.142c), and Equation (2.142d) into Equation (2.140f) yields a cumbersome cubic equation with respect to $[H^+]$ and thus solving for $[H^+]$ with a given value of C_a is complicated. However, the reverse calculation is easy:

$$C_a = \frac{([H^+] - [OH^-])([H^+]^2 + [H^+](K_1 + K_2) + K_1K_3)}{[H^+](K_1 + K_2) + 2K_1K_3} \tag{2.143}$$

The pH of the solution can be determined by first assuming $[H^+]$ and then calculating the given value of C_a (a trial-and-error process).

Figure 2.15 shows the concentration of sulfide intermediates of cysteine including the starting intermediate $^+NH_3R(COO^-)SH(= RY_1Y_2)$. The concentrations of the two middle intermediate species will increase to a maximum and then fall, depending on the pK_{a1} and pK_{a2} values, as the system is deprotonated to $NH_3R(COO^-)S^-(= RY_1^-Y_2^-)$ at the end.

Example 2.16

Figure 2.16 shows the fractional composition of a tetraprotonic weak acid (e.g., deferoxamine succinamide), denoted H_4A ($pK_{a1} = 5.13$, $pK_{a2} = 8.60$, $pK_{a3} = 9.24$, $pK_{a4} = 9.98$). Calculate the pH of zpa 0.01 M NaH_3A solution.

Solution

The mass balance equations are given by:

$$[Na^+] = C_a \tag{2.144a}$$

$$C_a = [H_4A] + [H_3A^-] + [H_2A^{-2}] + [HA^{-3}] + [A^{-4}] \tag{2.144b}$$

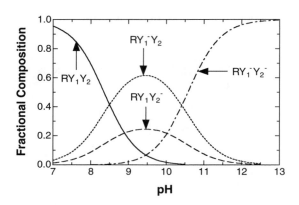

FIGURE 2.15 Fractional concentration of sulfide intermediate species of cysteine ($pK_1 = 8.5$, $pK_2 = 8.9$, $pK_3 = 10.4$, and $pK_4 = 10.0$).

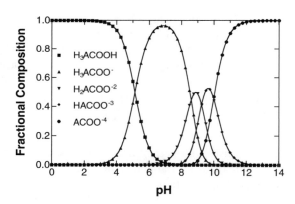

FIGURE 2.16 The concentration distribution of deferoxamine succinamide species ($pK_{a1} = 5.13$, $pK_{a2} = 8.60$, $pK_{a3} = 9.24$, and $pK_{a4} = 9.98$). [Graph reconstructed from data by Inhat et al. *J. Pharm. Sci.*, 91, 1733 (2002).]

The electroneutrality is given by:

$$[H^+] + [Na^+] = [H_3A^-] + 2[H_2A^{-2}] + 3[HA^{-3}] + 4[A^{-4}] + [OH^-] \quad (2.145a)$$

Substituting Equation (2.144b) for $[H_3A^-]$ and Equation (2.144a) into Equation (2.145a) yields:

$$[H^+] + [H_4A] = [H_2A^{-2}] + 2[HA^{-3}] + 3[A^{-4}] + [OH^-] \quad (2.145b)$$

At $pH \approx 7$, the middle two terms of the right-hand side are small, and $[H^+]$ is much smaller than $[H_4A]$, so Equation (2.145b) becomes:

$$[H_4A] = [H_2A^{-2}] + [OH^-] \qquad (2.145c)$$

The concentrations of species in solution can be derived as for other polyprotic acids:

$$\alpha_{H_4A} = \frac{[H^+]^4}{[H^+]^4 + K_{a1}[H^+]^3 + K_{a1}K_{a2}[H^+]^2 + K_{a1}K_{a2}K_{a3}[H^+] + K_{a1}K_{a2}K_{a3}K_{a4}} \qquad (2.146)$$

At pH < 6, the last three terms in the denominator are much smaller than the other terms and then,

$$\alpha_{H_4A} = \frac{[H^+]^4}{[H^+]^4 + K_{a1}[H^+]^3} = \frac{[H^+]}{[H^+]^2 + K_{a1}[H^+]} \qquad (2.147a)$$

$$\alpha_{H_3A^-} = \frac{K_{a1}}{[H^+] + K_{a1}} \qquad (2.147b)$$

$$\alpha_{H_2A^{-2}} = \frac{K_{a1}K_{a2}}{[H^+]^2 + K_{a1}[H^+]} \qquad (2.147c)$$

Substituting Equation (2.147a) and Equation (2.147c) into Equation (2.145c) gives:

$$\frac{C_a[H^+]}{[H^+] + K_{a1}} = \frac{C_a K_{a1} K_{a2}}{[H^+]^2 + K_{a1}[H^+]} + \frac{K_w}{[H^+]} \qquad (2.148)$$

Equation (2.148) can be rearranged:

$$C_a[H^+]^2 - K_w[H^+] - C_a(K_{a1}K_{a2} + K_w K_{a1}) = 0$$

$$[H^+] = \frac{K_w + \sqrt{K_w^2 + 4 \times C_a^2(K_{a1}K_{a2} + K_w K_{a1})}}{2C_a} \cong \sqrt{K_{a1}K_{a2}} = 10^{-6.87}$$

$$pH = 6.87$$

2.3.3 TITRATION CURVES OF A POLYPROTIC WEAK ACID, WEAK BASE, OR POLYAMPHOLYTE

The titration curve of a polyprotic acid can be obtained by using the same approach as for monoprotic weak acids or weak bases. The mass and charge balance equations for the triprotic weak acid (H_3A, C_a, and V_a) and the titrant strong base (NaOH, C_b, and V_b) are:

Mass balance:

$$[H_3A]+[H_2A^-]+[HA^{-2}]+[A^{-3}]=\frac{C_aV_a}{V_a+V_b} \qquad (2.149a)$$

$$[Na^+]=\frac{C_aV_b}{V_a+V_b} \qquad (2.149b)$$

Charge balance:

$$[H^+]+[Na^+]=[H_2A^-]+2[HA^{-2}]+3[A^{-3}]+[OH^-] \qquad (2.149c)$$

Substituting Equation (2.2), Equation (2.149a), and Equation (2.149b) into Equation (2.144c) gives:

$$[H^+]+\left(\frac{C_bV_b}{V_a+V_b}\right)=\left(\alpha_{H_2A^-}+2\alpha_{HA^{-2}}+3\alpha_{A^{-3}}\right)\left(\frac{C_aV_a}{V_a+V_b}\right)+\frac{K_w}{[H^+]} \qquad (2.149d)$$

where αs are given by Equation (2.126a) through Equation (2.126d). Rearranging Equation (2.149d) yields:

$$V_b = V_a\frac{\dfrac{(K_{a1}[H^+]^2+2K_{a1}K_{a2}[H^+]+3K_{a1}K_{a2}K_{a3})C_a}{[H^+]^3+K_{a1}[H^+]^2+K_{a1}K_{a2}[H^+]+K_{a1}K_{a2}K_{a3}}+\dfrac{K_w}{[H^+]}-[H^+]}{C_b-\dfrac{K_w}{[H^+]}+[H^+]} \qquad (2.150)$$

Figure 2.17 shows the titration curve of phosphoric acid in terms of equivalent of alkali.

In the titration curve of H_3PO_4, as shown in Figure 2.17, the pK_a values are far away from each other, causing the equivalence points to look like flat plateaus. For the dicarboxylic amino acids or diamino carboxylic acids, two pK_a values are in close proximity to each other and thus the plateaus are not flat, as shown in Figure 2.18. The isoelectric species is not the one that is abundantly present at a neutral pH. The isoelectric point is one half of ($pK_{a1} + pK_{a2}$) for dicarboxylic amino acids and one half of ($pK_{a2} + pK_{a3}$) for diamino carboxylic acids. The isoelectric species $H_2Y^{\pm}$ is the highest concentration halfway between H_3Y^+ and $H_2Y^{\pm}$. At the isoelectric point of 3.2, the three species (H_3Y^+, $H_2Y^{\pm}$, and HY^-) coexist and the ratio of $H_2Y^{\pm}$ to H_3Y^+ and $H_2Y^{\pm}$ to HY^- is approximately 10:1.

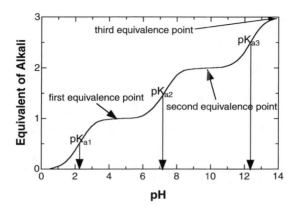

FIGURE 2.17 Titration curve of phosphoric acid ($pK_{a1} = 2.23$, $pK_{a2} = 7.21$, and $pK_{a3} = 12.32$).

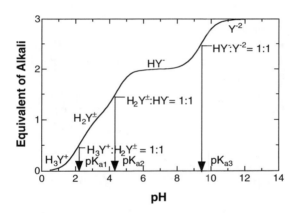

FIGURE 2.18 Titration curve of glutamic acid ($pK_{a1} = 2.2$, $pK_{a2} = 4.3$, and $pK_{a3} = 9.4$).

Thus, in the titration of a diprotic weak acid H_2A, Equation (2.150) reduces to:

$$V_b = V_a \frac{\dfrac{(K_{a1}[H^+] + 2K_{a1}K_{a2})C_a}{[H^+]^2 + K_{a1}[H^+] + K_{a1}K_{a2}} + \dfrac{K_w}{[H^+]} - [H^+]}{C_b - \dfrac{K_w}{[H^+]} + [H^+]} \qquad (2.151)$$

Consider the titration of a concentration C_a and a volume V_a of a weak acid salt KH_2A with a concentration C_b and a volume V_b of the strong base NaOH. The electroneutrality equation and the mass balance equation are given by:

$$[H^+] + [K^+] + [Na^+] = [H_2A^-] + 2[HA^{-2}] + 3[A^{-3}] + [OH^-] \qquad (2.152a)$$

$$[K^+] = [H_2A^-] + [HA^{-2}] + [A^{-3}] = \frac{C_a V_a}{V_a + V_b} \qquad (2.152b)$$

$$[Na^+] = \frac{C_b V_b}{V_a + V_b} \qquad (2.152c)$$

Combining Equation (2.152a), Equation (2.152b), and Equation (2.152c) yields:

$$V_b = V_a \frac{\dfrac{(K_{a1}[H^+]^2 + 2K_{a1}K_{a2}[H^+] + 3K_{a1}K_{a2}K_{a3})C_a}{[H^+]^3 + K_{a1}[H^+]^2 + K_{a1}K_{a2}[H^+] + K_{a1}K_{a2}K_{a3}} - 1 + \dfrac{K_w}{[H^+]} - [H^+]}{C_b - \dfrac{K_w}{[H^+]} + [H^+]} \qquad (2.152d)$$

2.3.4 Buffer Capacity of a Buffer Solution Containing a Polyprotic Weak Acid or Weak Base and Its Conjugate Base or Acid

In the same manner as described in Section 2.2.5, mathematical expressions for the buffer capacity of polyprotic weak acid/base systems can be developed. When one adds a strong base such as NaOH to an aqueous buffer solution containing a polyprotic weak acid (H_nA), the electroneutrality would be:

$$[Na^+] + [H^+] = n[A^{-n}] + (n-1)[HA^{1-n}] + \cdots + 2[H_{n-2}A^{-2}] + [H_{n-1}A^-] + [OH^-] \qquad (2.153a)$$

or

$$C_B = n[A^{-n}] + (n-1)[HA^{1-n}] + \cdots + 2[H_{n-2}A^{-2}] + [H_{n-1}A^-] + [OH^-] - [H^+] \qquad (2.153b)$$

The ionization constant of the polyprotic weak acid is written as:

$$K_j = \frac{[H^+][H_{n-j}A^{-j}]}{[H_{n-j+1}A^{-j+1}]} \qquad (2.154)$$

The concentration of each acid species is given by:

$$[H_{n-j}A^{-j}] / \psi = \left(\prod_{i=0}^{j} K_i \right)[H^+]^{n-j} \qquad (2.155a)$$

where

$$\psi = \frac{[H_nA]}{[H^+]^n} \qquad (2.155b)$$

and $K_0 = 1$ is assigned. The total concentration of the acid (TA) is equal to the sum of each acid species.

$$TA / \psi = \sum_{j=0}^{n}\left[\left(\prod_{i=0}^{j} K_i\right)[H^+]^{n-j}\right] \qquad (2.156)$$

The degree of protolysis for the jth species (α_j) is then given by:

$$\alpha_j = \frac{[H_{n-j}A^{-j}]}{TA} \qquad (2.157)$$

The buffer capacity can be determined by taking the derivative of Equation (2.153b) with respect to pH:

$$\beta = \frac{dC_B}{dpH} = nTA\frac{d\alpha_n}{dpH} + \cdots + 2TA\frac{d\alpha_2}{dpH} + TA\frac{d\alpha_1}{dpH} + \frac{d[OH^-]}{dpH} - \frac{d[H^+]}{dpH} \qquad (2.158)$$

Taking the derivative of Equation (2.157) with respect to pH yields:

$$\frac{d\alpha_j}{dpH} = -2.303\alpha_j\sum_{i=0}^{n}\left[(i-j)\alpha_i\right] \qquad (2.159)$$

Substituting Equation (2.157), Equation (2.158), and Equation (2.159) gives the general equation for the buffer capacity of a polyprotic weak acid.

$$\beta = 2.303\left\{[H^+]+[OH^-]-TA\left[\sum_{j=1}^{n} j\alpha_j\sum_{i=0}^{n}((i-j)\alpha_i)\right]\right\} \qquad (2.160)$$

Equation (2.160) can be simplified to:

$$\beta = 2.303\left[[H^+]+[OH^-]+TA\sum_{j=0}^{n}\sum_{i=0}^{j-1}(j-i)^2\alpha_j\alpha_i\right] \qquad (2.161)$$

The αs are given by Equation (2.157) or Equation (2.126a) through Equation (2.126d) for a diprotic weak acid.

Let us apply the above approach for a diprotic weak acid (carbonic acid). Thus,

$$n = 2 \quad \psi = \frac{[H_2CO_4]}{[H^+]^2} \quad \frac{TA}{\psi} = [H^+]^2 + K_1[H^+] + K_1K_2 \qquad (2.162a)$$

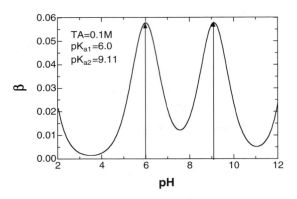

FIGURE 2.19 Buffer capacity as a function of pH for carbonic acid.

$$\beta = 2.303 \left\{ [H^+] + [OH^-] + TA(\alpha_1\alpha_0 + 4\alpha_2\alpha_0 + \alpha_2\alpha_1) \right\} \qquad (2.162b)$$

Figure 2.19 shows a plot of β as a function of pH for carbonic acid. As shown in Figure 2.7 for a monoprotic weak acid, the localized maxima for a diprotic weak acid occur at $pH = pK_{a1}$ and $pH = pK_{a2}$.

2.4   SPARINGLY SOLUBLE SALTS

2.4.1   Solubility Product Constant and Solubility of Sparingly Soluble Salts

The following equilibrium reaction is given for a sparingly soluble ionic salt, M_xY_y, which saturates in water:

$$M_xY_y \rightleftharpoons xM^{+y} + yY^{-x}$$

The mathematical equilibrium expression is given by:

$$K_{sp} = [M^{+y}]^x [Y^{-x}]^y \qquad (2.163)$$

where K_{sp} is the solubility product.

If the product of two ion concentrations (ion product, IP) is equal to the K_{sp}, no precipitation of the salt occurs and the solution is said to be saturated. If $IP > K_{sp}$, the salt precipitates, and if $IP < K_{sp}$, the solution is not saturated. As seen in equilibrium equation, one molar concentration of M_xY_y produces x molar concentration of M^{+y} and y molar concentration of Y^{-x}. When common ions are added to the equilibrium solution, the equilibrium will shift according to Le Chatelier's principle, based on the changes in the concentrations of M^{+y} and Y^{-x}. In this case, the solid does precipitate. Using this principle, quantitative precipitation of the salt will occur. If S_o is the molar solubility of a sparingly soluble salt, S_o can be determined from K_{sp}:

$$K_{sp} = (xS_o)^x (yS_o)^y \qquad (2.164a)$$

$$S_o = \left(\frac{K_{sp}}{x^x y^y}\right)^{1/(x+y)} \qquad (2.164b)$$

Example 2.17

Calculate the solubility of the salt, $PbCl_2$, and the concentration of Pb^{+2} and Cl^- in a saturated solution of $PbCl_2$. When HCl is added to the equilibrium to have 0.4 M of Cl^-, calculate the solubility of the salt. $K_{sp} = 1.6 \times 10^{-5}$.

Solution

Before adding HCl,

$$PbCl_2 \;\rightleftharpoons\; Pb^{+2} + 2Cl^-$$

$$[\, x = 1, \quad y = 2 \,]$$

$$S_o = (1.60 \times 10^{-5}/4)^{1/3} = 1.59 \times 10^{-2} M$$

After adding HCl, the concentration of Cl^- in water is 0.4 M and the solubility of the salt is given by:

$$[Cl^-]^2 [Pb^{+2}] = (0.4)^2 S_o = 1.60 \times 10^{-5}$$

$$S_o = 1.0 \times 10^{-4} M$$

2.4.2 SOLUBILITY OF SPARINGLY SOLUBLE SALTS OF WEAK ACIDS OR WEAK BASES

When the conjugate base of a monoprotic weak acid forms a sparingly soluble salt, the conjugate base will be hydrolyzed as follows:

$$MX(s) \;\rightleftharpoons\; M^+ + X^-$$

$$X^- + H_2O \;\rightleftharpoons\; HX + OH^-$$

There are five species in the solution: M^+, X^-, HX, H^+, and OH^-. The concentration of these species in the solution can be determined as previously described:

1. Equilibrium:

$$K_{sp} = [M^+][X^-] \qquad (2.165a)$$

$$K_b = \frac{K_w}{K_a} = \frac{[OH^-][HX]}{[X^-]} \qquad (2.165b)$$

2. Mass balance:

$$[M^+] = S_o = [HX] + [X^-] \qquad (2.165c)$$

3. Electroneutrality:

$$[M^+] + [H^+] = [X^-] + [OH^-] \qquad (2.165d)$$

Inserting $[X^-]$ from Equation (2.165a) and $[HX]$ from Equation (2.165c) into Equation (2.165b) yields:

$$K_b = \frac{(S_o - K_{sp}/S_o)[OH^-]}{K_{sp}/S_o} \qquad (2.166)$$

or

$$S_o^2 = K_{sp}\left(1 + \frac{K_b}{[OH^-]}\right) = K_{sp}\left(1 + \frac{[H^+]}{K_a}\right) \qquad (2.167)$$

Example 2.18
Calculate the pH of a saturated solution of silver acetate in water. $K_{sp} = 2.3 \times 10^{-3}$ and $K_a = 1.74 \times 10^{-5}$.

Solution

$$AgAc(s) \rightleftharpoons Ag^+ + Ac^-$$

$$Ac^- + H_2O \rightleftharpoons HAc + OH^-$$

$$K_{sp} = [Ag^+][Ac^-] = S^2 = 2.3 \times 10^{-3}$$

$$[Ag^+] = [Ac^-] = 4.8 \times 10^{-2} M$$

Subtracting Equation (2.165) from Equation (2.166) yields:

$$[OH^-]-[H^+]=[HAc]$$

Assuming that $[OH^-]\gg[H^+]$, we obtain $[OH^-]=[HAc]$. Equation (2.165b) becomes:

$$[OH^-]^2 = \left(\frac{K_w}{[H^+]}\right)^2 = K_b[Ac^-] = \frac{K_w}{K_a}[Ac^-] = 2.76\times10^{-11}$$

$$[H^+]=1.90\times10^{-9}M$$

$$pH = 8.72$$

The assumption of $[OH^-]\gg[H^+]$ is a valid one ($5.3\times10^{-6}M \gg 1.90\times10^{-9}M$).

An ampholyte may form a sparingly soluble ionic salt with a metal ion (e.g., silver sulfamethazine and silver sulfamethizole). The salt dissociates as follows:

$$MY(s) \rightleftharpoons M^+ + Y^-$$

$$Y^- + H_2O \rightleftharpoons HY + OH^-$$

$$HY + H^+ \rightleftharpoons H_2^+Y + H_2O$$

The equilibrium and mass balance equations are given by:

$$K_{sp} = [M^+][Y^-] \tag{2.168a}$$

$$K_{a1} = \frac{[H^+][HY]}{[H_2^+Y]} \tag{2.168b}$$

$$K_{a2} = \frac{[H^+][Y^-]}{[HY]} \tag{2.168c}$$

$$[M^+] = S_o = [H_2^+Y]+[HY]+[Y^-] \tag{2.168d}$$

Substituting $[Y^-]$ from Equation (2.168a), $[HY]$ from Equation (2.168c), and $[H_2^+Y]$ from Equation (2.168b) into Equation (2.168d) yields:

$$S_o^2 = K_{sp}\left(\frac{[H^+]^2}{K_{a1}K_{a2}} + \frac{[H^+]}{K_{a2}} + 1\right) \tag{2.169}$$

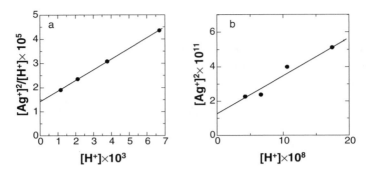

FIGURE 2.20 Equilibrium values of $[Ag^+]^2/[H^+]$ versus $[H^+]$ (a) and $[Ag^+]^2$ versus $[H^+]$ (b) for silver sulfamethazine in 0.1 M nitric acid and 0.05 M 2-(N-morpholino) propanesulfonic acid buffers, respectively, at 0.1 M ionic strength and 25°C. [Graph reconstructed from data by Nesbitt and Sandmann, *J. Pharm. Sci.*, 67, 1012 (1978).]

At low and high pH values, $[Y^-]$ and $[H_2^+Y]$ are negligible when compared to other species and Equation (2.174) becomes:

$$\frac{S_o^2}{[H^+]} = \frac{K_{sp}[H^+]}{K_{a1}K_{a2}} + \frac{K_{sp}}{K_{a2}} \quad \text{for low pH (2–4)} \qquad (2.170a)$$

$$S_o^2 = \frac{K_{sp}[H^+]}{K_{a2}} + K_{sp} \quad \text{for high pH (5–9)} \qquad (2.170b)$$

Figure 2.20a and Figure 2.20b display linear plots of Equation (2.170a) and Equation (2.170b), respectively, for silver sulfamethazine at 0.1 M ionic strength and 25°C.

2.4.3 Effect of Ionic Strength on Solubility of Sparingly Soluble Salts

As shown in Equation (2.164b), the solubility of slightly soluble substances is simply related to the solubility product (K_{sp}). However, the solubility is dependent on the ionic strength of a solution. A slightly soluble salt dissolves in water:

$$AgBr(s) \quad \rightleftharpoons \quad Ag^+ + Br^- \qquad (2.171)$$

The thermodynamic solubility product K_{sp}^o, which is the product of the activities of the ions, is:

$$K_{sp}^o = a_{Ag^+}a_{Br^-} = \left(C_{Ag^+}\gamma_{Ag^+}\right)\left(C_{Br^-}\gamma_{Br^-}\right) = K_{sp}\left(\gamma_{Ag^+}\gamma_{Br^-}\right) \qquad (2.172)$$

where K_{sp} is the apparent solubility product, which is $\left(C_{Ag^+}C_{Br^-}\right)$.

Taking the logarithm of Equation (2.172) yields:

$$-\log\left(\gamma_{Ag^+}\gamma_{Br^-}\right) = \log\left(\frac{K_{sp}}{K_{sp}^o}\right) \tag{2.173}$$

Combining Equation (2.78) and Equation (2.79) into Equation (2.173) gives:

$$-\log\gamma_\pm = \log\left(\frac{K_{sp}}{K_{sp}^o}\right)^{1/2} = 0.51\,z_+z_-\sqrt{\mu} \tag{2.174}$$

For a 1:1 electrolyte such as AgBr, the solubility product is directly related to the solubility of the ions:

$$-\log\gamma_\pm = \log\left(\frac{S}{S^o}\right) = 0.51\,z_+z_-\sqrt{\mu} \tag{2.175}$$

where S and S^o are the apparent and thermodynamic solubilities in mol/L, respectively. S^o is the solubility of the slightly soluble salt for zero ionic strength (i.e., pure solvent) and can be determined by extrapolating log S as $\mu\rightarrow0$. Equation (2.175) shows clearly that an increase in the solubility of the ion results from an increase in the ionic strength of the solution. This is called the "salting-in" effect.

As the ionic strength of the solution increases further, Equation (2.175) may no longer be consistent with the experimental data and thus Equation (2.175) is modified as:

$$\log\left(\frac{S}{S^o}\right) = 0.51\,z_+z_-\sqrt{\mu} - K'\mu \tag{2.176}$$

When the ionic strength of the solution is high, the first term on the right-hand side of Equation (2.176) is negligible and Equation (2.176) then becomes:

$$\log\left(\frac{S}{S^o}\right) = -K'\mu \tag{2.177}$$

where the value of K' is dependent on the size of the solute and the nature of the electrolyte present. Equation (2.177) shows that the solubility decreases with an increase in the ionic strength. This is called the "salting-out" effect.

The effect of ionic strength on the solubility of sparingly soluble salts can be applied to the solubility of proteins. Figure 2.21 shows the effect of the ionic strength of various salts on the solubility of horse hemoglobin. The solubility of the protein increases as the ionic strength increases [Equation (2.175)]. Then, the solubility goes through a plateau and a maximum [Equation (2.176)] before decreasing with increasing

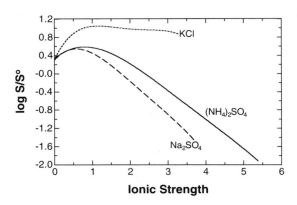

FIGURE 2.21 Effect of ionic strength on the solubility of horse hemoglobin. [Graph reconstructed from E. J. Cohn, *Chem. Rev.,* 19, 241 (1936).]

ionic strength [Equation (2.177)]. However, the shape of the solubility curve is dependent on ionic species [i.e., Na_2SO_4 and $(NH_4)_2SO_4$ show pronounced effects]. The salting-out effect is an invaluable technique in the purification of proteins from solutions. Individual proteins may have different salting-out characteristics. A single protein from a mixture of proteins can be precipitated out by carefully selecting the ionic strength of the protein solution.

SUGGESTED READINGS

1. J. M. Bonicamp, A. Loflin, and R. W. Clark, The Measurement of Activity Coefficients in Concentrated Electrolyte Solutions, *J. Chem. Ed.,* 78, 1541 (2001).
2. J. N. Butler, *Ionic Equilibrium: Solubility and pH Calculations,* Wiley Interscience, New York, 1998.
3. R. Chang, *Physical Chemistry with Applications to Biological Systems,* 2nd Ed., Macmillan, New York, 1981, Chapters 9 and 12.
4. S. Glasstone and D. Lewis, *Elements of Physical Chemistry,* 2nd Ed., Van Nostrand Co., Maruzen Asian Ed., Tokyo, 1960, Chapter 14.
5. D. W. King and D. R. Kester, A General Approach for Calculating Polyprotic Acid Specification and Buffer Capacity, *J. Chem. Ed.,* 67, 932 (1990).
6. H. Kuhn and H.-D. Forsterling, *Principles of Physical Chemistry,* John Wiley & Sons, New York, 2000, Chapters 17, 18, and 20.
7. K. J. Laidler and J. H. Meiser, *Physical Chemistry,* Benjamin/Cummings, Menlo Park, CA, 1982, Chapter 6.
8. R. D. Levie, Explicit Expressions of the General Form of the Titration Curve in Terms of Concentration, *J. Chem. Ed.,* 70, 209 (1993).
9. A. Martin, *Physical Pharmacy,* 4th Ed., Lea and Febiger, Philadelphia, 1993, Chapters 6, 7, and 8.
10. O. Robbins, Jr., *Ionic Reactions and Equilibria,* Macmillan, New York, 1967.
11. W. Stumm and J. J. Morgan, *Aquatic Chemistry,* Wiley Interscience, New York, 1981, Chapter 3.
12. V. R. Williams, W. L. Mattice, and H. B. Williams, *Basic Physical Chemistry for the Life Sciences,* 3rd ed., W. H. Freeman and Co., San Francisco, 1978, Chapter 4.

PROBLEMS

1. Calculate the pH of a mixture containing 0.001 M HCl and 0.01 M benzoic acid ($pK_a = 4.2$).

2. 1.3×10^{-4} M of HCl is added to a mixture containing 10^{-4} M NaOH and 10^{-5} M benzoic acid ($pK_a = 4.2$). Find the pH of the resulting solution.

3. Find the pH of a buffer that is prepared by mixing 100 mL of 0.2 M NaOH and 150 mL of 0.4 M acetic acid.

4. How many mL of 0.45 M NaOH solution should be added to 45 mL of 0.12 M H_3PO_4 to prepare a buffer of pH 6.8? Calculate the buffer capacity of the buffer solution.

5. Derive the buffer capacity equation of a solution containing a weak base and conjugate acid.

6. Calculate the pH of a 0.005 M solution of sodium captoprilate (Na_2A); $pK_{a1} = 3.8$ and $pK_{a2} = 9.8$.

7. Derive the buffer capacity equation of a solution containing two weak acids.

8. Determine the isoelectric point of cystine ($pK_{a1} = 1.65$, $pK_{a2} = 2.26$, $pK_{a3} = 7.85$, $pK_{a4} = 9.85$).

9. When 10 mL of a 0.02 M KH_2PO_4 are added to 10 mL of Na_2HPO_4 solution, the resulting solution has a pH of 6.85. What was the molarity of the Na_2HPO_4 solution?

10. 0.01 M NaOH was added to a buffer containing 0.1 M sodium acetate and 0.1 M acetic acid. What is the buffer capacity of the solution?

11. Calculate the pH of the resulting solution after adding 10 mL, 25 mL, and 50.2 mL of 0.1 M NaOH to 50 mL of 0.1 M acetic acid.

12. Find the pH of a 5×10^{-3} M solution of an ampholytic drug ($pK_{a1} = 4.6$, $pK_{a2} = 9.1$).

13. Calculate the buffer capacity of 0.1 M sodium carbonate and 0.1 sodium bicarbonate.

14. Calculate the pH of 0.1 M $(NH_4)_2HPO_4$.

15. Find the pH of 0.01 M Na_4A (e.g., sodium deferoxamine succinamide: $pK_{a1} = 5.13$, $pK_{a2} = 8.60$, $pK_{a3} = 9.24$, $pK_{a4} = 9.98$).

16. Calculate the isoelectric point of aspartic acid ($pK_{a1} = 2.05$, $pK_{a2} = 3.87$, $pK_{a3} = 10.00$).

17. Calculate the solubility of AgAc ($pK_{sp} = 2.64$, $pK_a = 4.8$) in dilute HCl as a function of $[H^+]$.

18. Derive the buffer capacity equation of a solution containing a weak base B and its conjugate acid BH^+.

19. Calculate the pHs of 0.1 M aspartic acid (acidic amino acid), 0.1 M glycine (neutral amino acid), and 0.1 M arginine (basic amino acid) in pure water.

20. Calculate the hydroxyl ion concentration of a 0.1 g/1000 mL monoprotic weak base in 0.9g /100 mL NaCl solution. The molecular weight of the base is 547 and $pK_a = 8.6$.

3 Solutions and Distribution

Pharmaceutical products can be classified as liquid solutions, disperse systems (e.g., emulsions, suspensions), semisolids (e.g., ointments), and solid dosage forms. Liquid solutions are homogeneous mixtures of one or more substances in pharmaceutical liquids. The understanding of the physicochemical properties of liquid solutions and processes to prepare the liquid solutions is an important step in preparing final liquid solution dosage forms. In this chapter, the solutions of gases in liquids, liquids in liquids, and solids in liquids, as well as colligative properties of solutions and their application to pharmacy, are discussed. Disperse systems will be discussed in Chapter 4.

3.1 SOLUTIONS OF SOLIDS AND NONVOLATILE LIQUIDS IN LIQUIDS

3.1.1 IDEAL SOLUTIONS

Consider a system consisting of a completely miscible solution of solute and solvent in all proportions. One should consider dissolution of solids in liquids as occurring in four steps:

1. The solid is heated to its melting temperature
2. The solid is liquefied
3. The liquefied solid is super-cooled to the experimental temperature
4. The super-cooled liquid is mixed with the solvent.

When it is placed at a temperature below the melting point of the solute (i.e., the solute becomes a solid), the solubility of this solid in a given liquid solvent is therefore limited. Thus, the two phases at equilibrium are the saturated solution containing the solute and the solid solute. At equilibrium, the chemical potentials of the solute in the saturated solution and the solid are equal to:

$$\mu_2^l(T,P,x) = \mu_2^s(T,P) \tag{3.1}$$

where the subscript 2 denotes the solute (i.e., the solvent is denoted by subscript 1), the superscripts l and s represent the saturated solution and solid, respectively, and T, P, and x are the temperature, pressure, and mole fraction, respectively. For an ideal solution, the chemical potential of the solute in the solution can be given by:

$$\mu_2^l(T,P,x) = \mu_2^o(T,P) + RT \ln x_2 \tag{3.2}$$

113

where μ_2° is the chemical potential of the pure liquid solute. Substituting Equation (3.2) into Equation (3.1) yields:

$$\mu_2^s(T,P) = \mu_2^\circ(T,P) + RT \ln x_2 \tag{3.3a}$$

or

$$\ln x_2 = \frac{\mu_2^s(T,P) - \mu_2^\circ(T,P)}{RT} \tag{3.3b}$$

Differentiating Equation (3.3b) with respect to T at constant P yields:

$$\frac{d \ln x_2}{dT} = -\frac{1}{R}\left(\frac{\partial}{\partial T}\left(\mu_2^s(T,P) - \mu_2^\circ(T,P)\right)/T\right)_p \tag{3.4}$$

Substituting the Gibbs–Helmholtz Equation (see Chapter 1) into Equation (3.4) gives:

$$\frac{d \ln x_2}{dT} = \frac{\Delta H_f}{RT^2} \tag{3.5}$$

where ΔH_f is the enthalpy change of fusion of the solute and is independent of T over a moderate change in temperature. Integration of Equation (3.5) from the melting temperature T_m to T yields:

$$-\ln x_2 = \frac{\Delta H_f}{R}\left(\frac{1}{T} - \frac{1}{T_m}\right) = \frac{\Delta H_f}{R}\left(\frac{T_m - T}{T_m T}\right) \tag{3.6}$$

Equation (3.6) illustrates that the solubility of a solid in a liquid depends on the enthalpy change at T_m and the melting temperature of the solid. Equation (3.6) is a valid one when $T > T_m$ because the liquid solute in an ideal solution is completely miscible in all proportions. Table 3.1 shows the ideal solubilities of compounds and their heat of fusion. Equation (3.6) is the equation for ideal solubility. The relationship of $\ln x_2$ (ideal or nonideal solubility) vs. $1/T$ is shown in Figure 3.1.

Example 3.1

Calculate the solubility of phenanthrene at 20°C in an ideal solution. The heat of fusion of the solute at 20°C is 18.6 kJ/mole; the melting temperature of the solute is 96°C.

Solution

Using Equation (3.6),

TABLE 3.1
Heats of Fusion and Ideal Solubilities

Compounds	T_m (K)	ΔH_f (kcal/mol)	Ideal Solubility (mole fraction)	Solvents
Biphenyl	299.2	4.02	0.39	0.39[a]
Naphthalene	353.4	4.56	0.30	0.24[a]
				0.26[b]
				0.22[c]
				0.21[d]
				0.09[e]
Phenanthrene	373	3.94	0.25	0.19[a]
Anthracene	490	6.88	0.011	0.006[a]

[a] In benzene.
[b] In chloroform.
[c] In toluene.
[d] In carbon tetrachloride.
[e] In water.

Source: Taken from data by Letcher and Battino, *J. Chem. Ed.,* 78, 103 (2001).

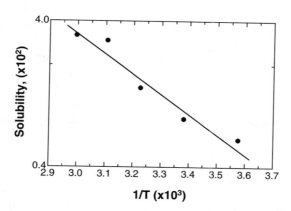

FIGURE 3.1 Solubility of amoxicillin trihydrate in 0.5 M KCl vs. temperature. [Graph reconstructed from data by Tsuji et al., *J. Pharm. Sci.,* 78, 1059 (1978).]

$$-\ln x_2 = \frac{\Delta H_f}{R}\left(\frac{T_m - T}{T_m T}\right) = \frac{18.6\times10^3(96-20)}{8.315\times293\times369} = 1.572$$

ideal solubility by mole fraction = $x_2 = 0.21$

Because there is a difference between the heat capacities of the solid and the liquid solute, the heat of fusion at any temperature can be expressed in terms of the heat of fusion at the melting temperature:

$$\Delta H_f = \Delta H_m - \Delta C_p (T_m - T) \tag{3.7}$$

where ΔH_m and ΔC_p are the heat of fusion at the melting temperature and the heat capacity, respectively. Substituting Equation (3.7) into Equation (3.5) and integrating the resulting equation yields:

$$-\ln x_2 = \frac{\Delta H_m (T_m - T)}{RT_m T} - \frac{\Delta C_p (T_m - T)}{RT} - \Delta C_p \ln \frac{T_m}{T} \tag{3.8}$$

As the temperature gets closer to the melting temperature, the second and third terms on the right-hand side of Equation (3.8) become negligible. Equation (3.8) becomes equivalent to Equation (3.6), and ΔH_m replaces ΔH_f.

3.1.2 Nonideal Solutions and the Solubility Parameter

In solvents that are chemically similar to the solute (i.e., naphthalene/toluene), the experimental solubility of the solute is very close to the ideal value. Either negative or positive deviation from the ideal value occurs when the solute and the solvent are chemically dissimilar. The nonideal behavior results from the differences in the interactions between the solute and the solvent molecules (i.e., solute–solute, solvent–solvent, and solute–solvent). The sum of these interactions usually becomes positive, and having an incomplete mixing of all components results in a finite solubility of the solute in the solvent. These deviations from ideal solution behavior can be expressed by the activity coefficient of the nonideal solution. The activity, a_2, of a solute in a nonideal solution is the product of concentration, x_2^r, and the activity coefficient, γ_2, as:

$$a_2 = x_2^r \gamma_2 \tag{3.9}$$

For an ideal solution, $\gamma_2 = 1$ and $a_2 = x_2^r = x_2$. For a nonideal solution, the solubility of the solute using the mole fraction is:

$$-\ln x_2^r \gamma_2 = \frac{\Delta H_m (T_m - T)}{RT_m T} - \frac{\Delta C_p (T_m - T)}{RT} + \Delta C_p \ln \frac{T_m}{T} \tag{3.10}$$

Intermolecular forces of attraction among the solute and the solvent (cohesion) must be broken while intermolecular forces of attraction between the solute and solvent (adhesion) must be required. Work must be done to randomly distribute the solute in the solution. As the difference between the cohesive and adhesive forces becomes larger, the solubility of the solute will be lower. The activity of a nonideal solution is dependent on the energy of mixing, which is small and provided by the heat of its surroundings.

Theoretical treatments for the energy of mixing have been evaluated based on several models (i.e., unexpanded gas, quasi-crystalline, distribution function). However, similar results can be obtained as:

$$\Delta E_m = -\left(\frac{\Delta E_1^v}{V_1} + \frac{\Delta E_2^v}{V_2} - 2\frac{\Delta E_{12}^v}{V_1 V_2}\right)\varphi_1 \varphi_2 \tag{3.11}$$

where ΔE_m is the total energy of mixing, ΔE_1^v is the energy of vaporization of the compound 1, and φ is the volume fraction defined by $\varphi_1 = n_1 V_1 / (n_1 V_1 + n_2 V_2)$, where n is the number of moles, V is the molar volume at temperature T, and the subscripts 1 and 2 represent the solvent and the solute, respectively.

The partial energy of mixing of the solute, $\Delta \overline{E}_{m,2}$, can be calculated by differentiating the total energy of mixing with respect to the number of moles of the solute, n_2, at a constant n_1:

$$\Delta \overline{E}_{m,2} = \left(\frac{\partial \Delta E_m}{\partial n_2}\right)_{n_1} = -\left(\frac{\Delta E_1^v}{V_1} + \frac{\Delta E_2^v}{V_2} - 2\frac{\Delta E_{12}^v}{V_1 V_2}\right)\varphi_1^2 V_2 \tag{3.12}$$

The cohesive forces between the solvent and the solute are expressed as the geometric mean of the adhesive forces of the solute and the solvent as:

$$\Delta E_{12}^v = \sqrt{\Delta E_1^v \Delta E_2^v} \tag{3.13}$$

Substituting Equation (3.13) into Equation (3.12) gives:

$$\Delta \overline{E}_{m,2} = -\varphi_1^2 V_2 \left[\left(\frac{\Delta E_1^v}{V_1}\right)^{1/2} - \left(\frac{\Delta E_2^v}{V_2}\right)^{1/2}\right]^2 \tag{3.14}$$

The term in the square root in Equation (3.14) is equal to $a^{1/2} / V$ in the van der Waals equation for a nonideal gas and liquid. A new term known as the solubility parameter is defined as:

$$\delta = \left(\frac{\Delta E^v}{V}\right)^{1/2} = \left(\frac{\Delta H^v - RT}{V}\right)^{1/2} = \left(\frac{a}{V^2}\right)^{1/2} \tag{3.15}$$

where ΔH^v is the heat of vaporization. Substituting Equation (3.15) into Equation (3.14) yields:

$$\Delta \overline{E}_{m,2} = -\varphi_1^2 V_2 (\delta_1 - \delta_2)^2 \tag{3.16}$$

The Helmholtz's net free energy of mixing, $\Delta A_{m,2}$, of a solute in a solvent is given by:

$$\Delta A_{m,2} = \Delta \overline{E}_{m,2} - T\Delta S_2 = -RT \ln \gamma_2 \qquad (3.17)$$

where ΔS_2 is the entropy change transferred from a solute in a nonideal solution to an ideal one of the same composition. The entropy of mixing is ideal because the solute and the solvent molecules are randomly dispersed by sufficient thermal energy (i.e., $\Delta S_2 = 0$). Then Equation (3.17) becomes:

$$\Delta \overline{E}_{m,2} = -RT \ln \gamma_2 \qquad (3.18)$$

Substituting Equation (3.18) into Equation (3.16) and Equation (3.10) yields:

$$\ln \gamma_2 = -\frac{\varphi_1^2 V_2 (\delta_1 - \delta_2)^2}{RT} \qquad (3.19)$$

$$-\ln x_2^r = \frac{\Delta H_m (T_m - T)}{RT_m T} - \frac{\Delta C_p (T_m - T)}{RT} + \Delta C_p \ln \frac{T_m}{T} - \frac{\varphi_1^2 V_2 (\delta_1 - \delta_2)^2}{RT} \qquad (3.20)$$

When $\delta_1 = \delta_2$, the heat of mixing becomes zero and Equation (3.20) reduces to Equation (3.10). The solution then becomes ideal. If the difference of the solubility parameters between the solute and the solvent is large, the solubility of the solute will be less. One can intuitively use Equation (3.20) to choose a solvent or solvent systems to dissolve the drug. Water is commonly chosen as the pharmaceutical solvent. Thus, for a given drug, δ_2 and δ_1 are fixed. In order to increase or decrease the solubility of the drug, the solubility parameter of the solvent can be changed by using an additional solvent. When the additional solvent has a solubility parameter smaller than that of water, the solubility parameter of the mixed solvents is less than the one for water and the additive:

$$\delta_{mixture} = \sum_{i=1}^{n} \varphi_i \delta_i \qquad (3.21)$$

where φ_i is the volume fraction of component i and δ_i is the solubility parameter of component i in the solvent mixture. As δ_1 of the solvent mixture gets closer to δ_2 of the solute, the solubility of the solute in the mixed solvent increases. When $\delta_1 = \delta_2$, the maximum solubility is obtained. Figure 3.2 shows the variation in the solubility of a nonelectrolyte solute in a water–cosolvent mixture.

Example 3.2
Calculate the solubility of naphthalene in carbon tetrachloride at 20°C. The melting temperature of naphthalene is 80.2°C, the heat of fusion is 4562 cal/mole, and the

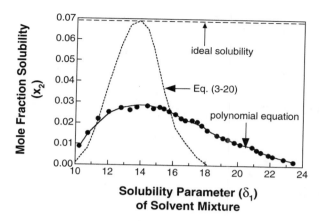

FIGURE 3.2 Variation of the solubility of a nonelectrolyte solute (caffeine) in a water–dioxane mixture. [Graph reconstructed from data by Djei et al., *J. Pharm. Sci.*, 69, 659 (1980).]

molecular weight is 128.6 g/mole. Assume $\Delta C_p = 0$. The molar volumes of naphthalene and carbon tetrachloride are 123 and 97 cm^3, respectively. The heats of vaporization of naphthalene and carbon tetrachloride are 11,500 cal/mole and 7810 cal/mole, respectively.

Solution

Equation (3.15) is used to determine the solubility parameters of the solute and the solvent:

$$\delta_1 = \left(\frac{\Delta H^v - RT}{V_1} \right)^{1/2} = \left(\frac{11,500 - 1.987 \times 293.2}{123} \right)^{1/2} = 9.421$$

$$\delta_2 = \left(\frac{\Delta H^v - RT}{V_2} \right)^{1/2} = \left(\frac{7810 - (1.987 \times 293.2)}{97} \right)^{1/2} = 8.632$$

The solubility of naphthalene in carbon tetrachloride is calculated by Equation (3.20). However, the volume fraction of the solvent, φ_1, is unknown until x_2^r is determined. First, $\varphi_1 = 1$ is approximated. Then,

$$-\ln x_2^r = \frac{\Delta H_m (T_m - T)}{RT_m T} + \frac{\varphi_1^2 V_2 (\delta_1 - \delta_2)^2}{RT}$$

$$= \frac{4562}{1.987} \left(\frac{353.4 - 293.2}{353.4 \times 293.2} \right) + \frac{1 \times 123 \times (8.632 - 9.421)^2}{1.987 \times 293.2}$$

$$-\ln x_2^r = 1.334 + 0.131 = 1.465 \qquad x_2^r = 0.231$$

Substitute x_2^r into Equation (3.21) to estimate φ_1:

$$\varphi_1 = \frac{(1-x_2^r)V_1}{(1-x_2^r)V_1 + x_2^r V_2} = \frac{97 \times (1-0.231)}{97 \times (1-0.231) + 0.231 \times 123} = 0.724$$

Substituting φ_1 into Equation (3.20) gives:

$$-\ln x_2^r = 1.334 + \frac{123 \times (0.724)^2 \times 9.193^2}{582.6} = 1.403 \qquad x_2^r = 0.246$$

After the fifth iteration, the solubility of naphthalene in carbon tetrachloride is:

$$x_2^r = 0.248$$

$$\text{mole concentration} = \frac{m}{1000} = \frac{x_2^r}{x_1^r M_1} = \frac{0.248}{153.8 \times (1-0.248)}$$

$$= 2.144 \text{ mole / kg solvent}$$

The solubilities of the solutes in an aqueous system determined from Equation (3.20) are usually larger than experimental values, as shown in Figure 3.2. This normally occurs for solutes (especially crystalline solids) in polar solvents. There are many interactions between the solute and the polar solvent: self-association of the solute or the solvent, solvation of the solute by the polar solvent, complexation in solution, etc. A modification of Equation (3.20), known as the extended Hildebrand solubility approach, has been developed. In this approach, it is assumed that the activity coefficient is partitioned into two forces: van der Waals forces and residual forces (dipole–dipole and hydrogen-bonding forces).

A solubility parameter based on dispersion forces (δ_D) can be calculated as the summation of the intermolecular attraction forces (F) for all functional groups as:

$$\delta_D = \frac{d \sum F}{M_r} \qquad (3.22)$$

where M_r is the molecular weight of a compound and d is the density of the compound. The molar attraction constants are expressed by ($\Delta e \cdot v_1$) where v_1 and Δe are the contributions of the functional groups to the molar volume in the liquid state and the molar energy of vaporization, respectively. Table 3.2 lists the F values for functional groups of the compounds.

Intermolecular forces in the presence of water include the dispersion forces as well as the dipole–dipole forces and the hydrogen-bonding forces. The hydrogen-bonding component to the solubility parameter (δ_H) can be estimated as:

TABLE 3.2
Molar Attraction Constants *F* for Functional Groups of Chemical Compounds

Group	F $(cal/cm^3)^{1/2}/mol$
$-CH_3$	179
$-CH_2-$	133
$CH-$	67
$-CH-$	0
$-CH=CH-$	231
$-C_6H_4-$ (o-, m-, or p-phenylene)	658
Saturated 5- or 6-membered ring	105
$-OH$ Aliphatic hydroxyl	240
$-C(=O)O-$ Ester	303
$-O-$ Ether	70

Source: Taken from H. Schott, *J. Pharm. Sci.,* 73, 790 (1984).

$$\delta_H = \sqrt{\frac{5000md}{M_r}} \tag{3.23}$$

where m is the number of functional groups in a compound capable of forming hydrogen bonds (e.g., hydroxyl, ether, and amine groups). For example, if there are a ether groups, b hydroxyl groups, and c primary amine groups in a compound, $m = a + b + c$.

The total solubility parameter δ_T is calculated from the sum of the squares of these three components as:

$$\delta_T = \sqrt{\delta_D^2 + \delta_P^2 + \delta_H^2} \tag{3.24}$$

Table 3.3 lists the molar volume and solubility parameters of pharmaceutical liquids and drug compounds.

The interaction energy of the solute with the solvent is not expressed as the geometric mean of φ_1 and φ_2, as shown in Equation (3.13), but as the polynomial power series of the solubility parameter of the solvent. The coefficients of the polynomial equation are determined experimentally by regression analysis. Figure 3.2 shows that the regressed (calculated) solubilities of caffeine in a mixture of water and dioxane are in good agreement with the experimental values.

In all dissolution processes, the undissolved solid is dispersed in the solvent. First, the undissolved solids are separated from one another; the process is always endothermic. Second, the separated solid molecules are associated with the solvent molecules; this process is always exothermic. The overall enthalpy, called the

TABLE 3.3
Molar Volume and Solubility Parameters for Some
Liquid Compounds and Crystalline Drug Compounds

Compounds	Molar Volume (L/mole)	Solubility Parameter $(cal/cm^3)^{1/2}$			
		δ_D	δ_P	δ_H	δ_T
Benzoic acid	101	8.9	3.4	4.8	10.7
Caffeine	144	10.1	3.5	9.1	14.1
Diethyl ether	105	7.1	1.4	2.5	7.7
Ethanol	59	7.7	4.3	9.5	13.0
Ethyl acetate	99	7.7	2.6	3.5	8.9
Ethylene glycol	56	8.3	5.4	12.7	16.1
Glycerin	73	8.5	5.9	14.3	17.7
Methanol	41	7.4	6.0	10.9	14.5
Methyl paraben	145	9.3	4.4	6.0	11.8
Naphthalene	123	9.4	1.0	1.9	9.6
1-Octanol	158	8.3	1.6	5.8	10.3
Phenobarbital	137	10.3	4.8	5.3	12.6
Sulfadiazine	182	9.5	4.8	6.6	12.5
Tolbutamide	229	9.7	2.9	4.1	10.9

Source: Data from A. Martin, *Physical Pharmacy,* 4th Ed., Lea & Febiger, Philadelphia, 1993.

enthalpy of solution ($\Delta H^{\circ}_{solution}$), which may be positive or negative, is the sum of these two processes. The magnitude and sign of $\Delta H^{\circ}_{solution}$ are responsible for the temperature effect on solubility. If $\Delta H^{\circ}_{solution}$ is positive, the overall process is endothermic and an increase in solution temperature will increase the solubility of the solids. The effect of temperature on solubility is reversed for negative $\Delta H^{\circ}_{solution}$ (i.e., exothermic).

In summary, the solubility of a solid in liquids is dependent greatly on the values of ΔH_f and T_m as well as the characteristics of molecular interactions between the solute and solvent.

3.1.3 INTERMOLECULAR AND INTRAMOLECULAR INTERACTIONS BETWEEN MOLECULES

As described in Section 3.1.2, intermolecular interactions between a solute and a solvent or solvents play an important role to dissolve the solute molecule. A number of intermolecular forces have been proposed that invariably contained the masses of the molecules. The molecular properties of materials depend not on the quantity of molecules but on the forces between molecules in close proximity to each other. Intermolecular forces may be divided into three categories:

1. Coulombic forces (e.g., charge-to-charge interactions), including interactions between charges and dipoles

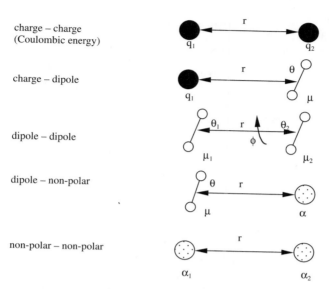

charge – charge
(Coulombic energy)

charge – dipole

dipole – dipole

dipole – non-polar

non-polar – non-polar

FIGURE 3.3 Molecular interactions. [Taken from J. N. Israelachvilli, *Intermolecular and Surface Forces*, Academic Press, London, 1985.]

2. Polarization forces created by the induced dipole moments by the electric fields of charges and dipoles in close proximity to the molecules
3. Quantum mechanical forms in nature, which give rise to covalent bonding and to repulsive forces that are opposite to the attractive forces

When two charged molecules q_1 and q_2 are separated by the distance r (see Figure 3.3), the free energy for the electrostatic or Coulombic forces between the charges, $f(r)$, is given by:

$$f(r) = \frac{q_1 q_2}{4\pi \varepsilon \varepsilon_o r} \qquad (3.25)$$

where ε_o is the permittivity of the vacuum $(= 8.85 \times 10^{-12} C^3 N^{-1} n^{-2})$ and ε is the dielectric constant of the solvent. The Coulombic force, F(r), is given by differentiating Equation (3.25) with respect to r:

$$F(r) = -\frac{df(r)}{dr} = \frac{q_1 q_2}{4\pi \varepsilon \varepsilon_o r^2} \qquad (3.26)$$

For the same charges, the free energy and Coulombic forces are positive, and the charges are repulsive. For opposite charges, the free energy and Coulombic forces are negative, and the charges are attractive. Equation (3.26) shows that the Coulombic

TABLE 3.4
Dielectric Constants of Solvents at 25°C

Solvent	Dielectric constant	Solvent	Dielectric constant
Water	78.5	Glycerin	40.1
Propylene glycol	32.0 (30°)	Methanol	32.6
Ethanol	24.3	N-Propanol	20.1
Acetone	21.2	PEG 400	12.5
Phenol	9.7	Cottonseed oil	6.4
Acetic acid	6.2	Ether	4.3
Ethyl acetate	3.0	Benzene	2.3
Carbon tetrachloride	2.2	Hexane	1.9

forces are inversely dependent on the square of distance. One may consider that NaCl or similar salts do not dissolve readily in water because of the strong Coulombic interactions. However, Equation (3.25) and Equation (3.26) indicate that the Coulombic interaction between ions is much weakened in a solvent by a factor of ε. Furthermore, the logarithm of the solubility of a salt in a solvent is inversely proportional to the negative value of the solvent dielectric constant. The dielectric constant is a function of temperature and ionic radii. Therefore, the large solubilizing power of water for ions such as NaCl comes from its dielectric constant as shown in Table 3.4. The dielectric constant of a solvent links to the ability to store charge in the solvent.

Most molecules are neutral (no net charge) but polar because they possess an electric dipole. For example, there is no net charge in the H_2O molecule, but it is polar because the oxygen atom pulls the hydrogen's electron so that the bonding electrons are localized asymmetrically more on the oxygen than on the hydrogen. Therefore, the oxygen atom shows more characteristics of a negative charge, and the hydrogen atoms are more positively charged. The H_2O molecule has a permanent dipole. The dipoles of molecules vary with the nature of their solvents. The dipole moment of a polar molecule, U, is given by:

$$U = q l \tag{3.27}$$

where l is the distance between the two charges $-q$ and $+q$.

When two polar molecules are approaching each other, a dipole–dipole interaction exists between them as with two magnets. The dipole–dipole interaction energy is given by:

$$f(r,\theta_1,\theta_2,\Phi) = -\frac{u_1 u_2}{4\pi\varepsilon\varepsilon_o r^3}\left[2\cos\theta_1\cos\theta_2 - \sin\theta_1\sin\theta_2\cos\Phi\right] \tag{3.28}$$

where u_1 and u_2 are two dipole moments at a distance r apart, θ is the angle between the dipole and the line intersecting the dipole center, and Φ is the torsion angle rotation.

TABLE 3.5
Heat of Solution at 25°C

Solute	$\Delta H_{solution}$ kcal/mole	Solute	$\Delta H_{solution}$ kcal/mole
HCl (g)	−18.0	KCl	+3.0
NaOH (c)	−10.6	CH_3COOH (l)	−0.4
KI (c)	+4.3	NaCl	+1.0
$Ca(OH)_2$	−2.8	Mannitol (c)	+5.3

Note: c, crystalline.

The dipole–dipole interaction is not as strong as the charge–charge interaction and does not strongly align polar molecules in the liquid state. The solubility of alcohols, the lower organic acids, amines, esters, ketones, etc. in polar solvents such as water are a result of dipole–dipole interaction. If a strong dipole–dipole interaction exists between a solute and a solvent, the solute–solvent interaction may exceed the sum of the solvent–solvent and solute–solute interactions. The excess interaction energy is evolved as heat (e.g., PEG 6000 in water), leading to a negative heat of solution (i.e., negative enthalpy change) (Table 3.5). Commonly, the larger negative heat of solution substances have, the more soluble they are. However, when the sum of the solute–solute and solvent–solvent interaction energies exceeds the solute–solvent interaction energy, heat should be supplied to complete the dissolution process (i.e., positive heat of solution). For example, sorbitol has a positive heat of solution. As sorbitol dissolves in water, thermal energy is absorbed from the surroundings and then the solution becomes cool. However, the magnitude and sign of the heat of solution are solely indicative of the solubility of a molecule. There are other factors affecting the solubility (e.g., spatial arrangement of the molecule).

As an ion and a dipole are separated by the distance r and the intermolecular distance is much larger than the dipole distance, the ion–dipole interaction potential is given by:

$$f(r) = -\frac{qu \cos\theta}{4\pi\varepsilon_o r^2} \qquad (3.29)$$

The ion–dipole interaction energy is usually large so that the ion and the dipole align each other. The dissolution of ionic molecules in polar solvents (e.g., water) is due to the ion–dipole interaction (e.g., ZnCl in polyalcohol). When a dipole attracts toward an oppositely charged ion, the comparable ion–ion bond energy in the solid state is released.

A solvent that has the following properties could be a good solvent for electrolytes:

1. A high dipole moment
2. A small molecular size
3. A high dielectric constant

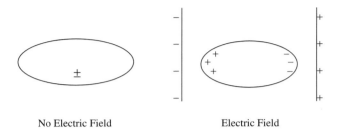

No Electric Field   Electric Field

FIGURE 3.4 Induced polarization.

Water exhibits all these properties for inorganic and organic salts. A highly polar solvent, water tends to orient around small or multivalent ions and the angle θ equals 0 and 180° near cations and anions, respectively. Therefore, water molecules bind to ionic molecules known as solvated or hydrated ions. The bound water molecules tend to interchange slowly with bulk water.

When the ion–dipole interaction energy is larger than the sum of the ion–ion interaction of the solute and the dipole–dipole interaction of the solvent, ionic molecules dissolve in water while giving off heat (i.e., negative heat of solution). A typical example is the dissolution of KOH in water. However, KI dissolves in water by absorbing heat from its surroundings because the sum of the ion–ion and dipole–dipole interaction energies exceeds the ion–dipole interaction energy (i.e., positive heat of solution).

In the absence of an electric field, carbon tetrachloride, CCl_4, possesses the permanent dipole moment of zero because the bonding electrons are symmetrically distributed around the carbon atom. The centers of positive and negative charges coincide. Such molecules are called nonpolar molecules. However, when the molecule is subject to an electric field, the electric charges in CCl_4 are distorted; this is referred to as polarization. The centers of positive and negative charge do not coincide, and a dipole is induced in the molecule by the distortion of the electric charges. CCl_4 is now referred to as having an *induced dipole moment*. When the electric field is removed, the symmetrical distribution of electric charges in CCl_4 is restored (Figure 3.4). The energy of the dipole-induced dipole interaction is given by:

$$f(r) = -\frac{\mu^2\alpha(1+3\cos2\theta)}{2(4\pi\varepsilon\varepsilon_o)^2 r^6} \tag{3.30}$$

The induced dipole moment depends on the electric field strength and the structure of the molecule. Charge-induced dipole interactions occur between a charged ion and polarized molecules. A molecule possessing conjugated double bonds is readily polarized. Examples of solutions due to the dipole-induced dipole interaction are benzene in methanol, chloral hydrate in CCl_4, and phenol in mineral oil.

There are interactions between neutral molecules with zero or small permanent dipole moments, referred to as *induced dipole-induced dipole interactions*. Even though a molecule has no or a small dipole moment, the electric charge distribution in the molecule instantaneously fluctuates. The instantaneous dipole can induce a dipole in a nearby molecule. Interactions between the induced dipole and induced dipoles are called London attractive interactions. As the atoms or molecules are closer, the instantaneous dipole-induced dipole interaction energy is more negative as given by:

$$f(\mathrm{r}) = -\frac{3h\nu\alpha^2}{4(4\pi\varepsilon_o)^2 \mathrm{r}^6} \tag{3.31}$$

Thus, the interaction force between them is always attractive.

If a solvent and solute are nonpolar, the interaction force between them is of the van der Waals type (≈ 1 kJ/mole) where as the distance between them becomes closer, the interaction energy increases rapidly to the twelfth power of the distance. The induced dipole-induced dipole interaction mainly accounts for the dissolution of nonpolar solutes in nonpolar solvents such as paraffin in petroleum benzin or wax in CCl_4. The net heat of solution becomes zero or very small for nonpolar systems when the solute and solvent molecules are of similar size and structure. In this case, the interaction energies of solute–solute, solvent–solvent, and solute–solvent are of the same magnitudes. Materials that can be soluble with zero heat of solution are often called ideal solutions.

An unusual type of bonding by hydrogen is exhibited in certain circumstances where a hydrogen atom covalently bound to one electronegative atom can form a weak bond to the atom (i.e., *hydrogen bond*). The hydrogen atoms tend to be positively polarized and can interact strongly with neighboring electronegative atoms due to their small size. The hydrogen atom in a molecule should be an electron acceptor to be able to form hydrogen bonds. The electron donors are atoms of the most electronegative elements (e.g., O, N, F). Hydrogen atoms bound to small electronegative atoms (e.g., CH_4) do not form hydrogen bonds.

A simple hydrogen compound of oxygen (i.e., H_2O) is anomalous in physical properties from the homologous compounds in the same column of the periodic table. For example, H_2O has a boiling point of 100°C, whereas those of the analogous compounds with sulfur, selenium and tellurium are −62, −42 and 0°C, respectively. The key to this abnormal behavior lies in the hydrogen bond formation of water. Other abnormal properties of hydrogen bond molecules are a high viscosity and a high entropy of vaporization. The high entropy of vaporization results from the breakup energy required for the ordered clustered molecules in liquid water to vaporize. The hydrogen bond energy is around 15–20 kJ/mole, which is stronger than a van der Waals energy but weaker than covalent bonds, which have a bond energy of about 400 kJ/mole. Hydrogen bonds are readily broken by raising the temperature. Hydrogen bonds can be formed intermolecularly (two different molecules) as well as intramolecularly (identical molecules).

The alcohols (i.e., ROH) form hydrogen bonds, but the extent is less notable than that for water because alcohols have only one hydrogen atom in the molecule, whereas water has two. There is no limit to how many molecules can be bound together by hydrogen bonds in alcohol and water. Carboxylic acids (RCOOH) such as formic acid, acetic acid, and benzoic acid, are expected to form double molecules.

In macromolecular and biological systems, such as proteins and nucleic acids, hydrogen bonds occur with O and N possessing unshared-pair electrons. The hydrogen bonds link different segments together within protein molecules and play an important role in the stability of the DNA molecule by holding two helical segments together.

The hydrogen atom of water molecules forms hydrogen bonds with the oxygen atoms of two other water molecules, and the oxygen atom of the water molecule forms hydrogen bonds with two hydrogen atoms of two other water molecules. Therefore the network of water molecules, which is not rigid, is formed. If a nonpolar molecule such as hexane and water are brought together, some hydrogen bonds in the network have to point towards the nonpolar solute molecule and are broken. The hexane does not interact with water and does not form hydrogen bonds. To maintain any of their hydrogen bonds, the water molecules around the hexane must orient themselves and pack around it. Therefore, water molecules around the hexane reorient themselves and become more ordered, resulting in a decrease in entropy, which is thermodynamically unfavorable. So when two nonpolar molecules approach each other in water, they will tend to cluster so that a negative entropy change will be minimized by decreasing the contact area with water.

Such *hydrophobic* interactions are important characteristics of many biological systems. Many biomolecules (e.g., proteins) possess both hydrophilic and hydrophobic features in the same molecule and are therefore called *amphiphilic*. Hydrophobic amino acids of proteins tend to be buried in the interior of the protein. Hydrophilic amino acids are at the surface of the protein, exposed to solvent water.

3.1.4 PREDICTION OF SOLUBILITY

Aqueous solubility has been recognized as an important physicochemical property in the pharmaceutical sciences. During the early stages of a drug discovery, a large number of drug candidates are synthesized in very small quantities. In addition, many homologues of drugs for each category of diseases may be investigated experimentally. Quantitative structure–activity relationships have been employed to develop new drug candidates. It is highly desirable to predict the physicochemical properties (e.g., solubility, partition coefficient, absorption) of the drug candidates without performing experiments when predicted drug structures are dealt with. There are many theoretical approaches; the general solubility equation (GSE), amended solvation energy relationship (ASER), and *in silico* quantitative structure–property relationships (QSPR) are briefly discussed herein.

GSE is used to determine the solubilities of pharmaceutical drugs in water by using their solubility in octanol and the partition coefficient of the drugs in the water–octanol system. Assuming $\Delta C_p = 0$ and/or a negligible difference between the second and third terms in the right-hand side of Equation (3.8) and substituting the enthalpy change at the phase transition with the entropy change at the phase transition (i.e., $\Delta S_m = \Delta H_m / T_m$), Equation (3.8) becomes:

$$-\ln x_2 = \frac{\Delta S_m (T_m - T)}{RT} \tag{3.32}$$

or $$-\ln x_2 = \frac{\Delta S_m (T_m - 298.15)}{RT} \quad \text{at } 25°C \qquad (3.33)$$

Assuming that the entropy change of organic nonelectrolytes at the melting temperature is given by Walden's rule (i.e., $\Delta S_m = 56.6 \text{ J}/\text{mol K}$), Equation (3.33) then becomes:

$$-\ln x_2 = -0.01(T_m - 298.15) = -0.01(t_m - 25) \qquad (3.34)$$

where t_m is the melting temperature in degrees Celsius. If solutes melt below 25°C, the right-hand side term of Equation (3.34) is zero.

In a solute–solvent system of similar polarity (naphthalene in chlorobenzene), Equation (3.34) can estimate the solubility of the liquid solute. If the polarities of the solute and the solvent are very different (naphthalene in n-hexane), Equation (3.34) should be modified. The partition coefficient in the water–octanol system can be used for differences in polarities of the solute and the solvent. The partition coefficient of a liquid solute, K_{wo}, in the water–octanol system is defined as:

$$K_{wo} = \frac{C_o}{C_w} \qquad (3.35a)$$

where C_o and C_w are the equilibrium concentrations of the solute in octanol and water, respectively. When the solute is saturated in two phases, Equation (3.35a) can be approximated by:

$$K_{wo} = \frac{S_o}{S_w} \qquad (3.35b)$$

or $$\log S_w = \log S_o - \log K_{wo} \qquad (3.35c)$$

where S_o and S_w are the solubilities of the solute in octanol and water, respectively.

The solubility of a liquid solute in octanol can be determined in terms of solubility parameters of the solute and octanol, as shown in Equation (3.20). However, the solubility parameters of liquid solutes (i.e., ΔH^v) are generally unknown or are close to that of octanol and thus the liquid solutes are expected to be completely miscible with octanol. The critical solution temperature (T_c) of a nonideal solution of similar size solutes for complete miscibility is given by Hildebrand:

$$T_c = \frac{V(\delta_1 - \delta_2)^2}{2R} \qquad (3.36a)$$

where V is the average molar volume of the solute and octanol. Assuming that V is equal to the molar volume of octanol, Equation (3.36a) becomes:

$$T_c = \frac{138(21.1 - \delta_2)^2}{2R} \tag{3.36b}$$

The complete miscible solution will be obtained when the temperature of the solution is $>T_m$. Equation (3.36b) indicates that any solute having a solubility parameter ranging from 15.1 to 27.1 will be completely miscible with octanol at 25°C. The molar solubility of the liquid solute in octanol is equal to:

$$S_o^{liquid} = \frac{\text{molarity of octanol}}{2} = \frac{827 \text{ g / L}}{2 \times 130 \text{ g / mol}} = 3.18 \tag{3.37a}$$

or
$$\log S_o^{liquid} = 0.50 \tag{3.37b}$$

In Equation (3.37a), it was assumed that complete miscibility relates to a mole fraction of 0.5 for each component.

The ratio of the solubility of a crystalline solute to that of its liquid is equal to the ideal solubility and thus, in octanol:

$$S_o^{solid} = S_o^{liquid} \frac{x_2^{solid}}{x_2^{liquid}} = S_o^{liquid} x_2 \tag{3.38}$$

Substituting Equation (3.34) and Equation (3.37b) into Equation (3.38) and taking the logarithm of the resulting equation yields:

$$\log S_o^{solid} = 0.5 - 0.01(t_m - 25) \tag{3.39}$$

The solubility of a liquid solute in water can be calculated by substituting Equation (3.37b) into Equation (3.35c):

$$\log S_w^{liquid} = 0.5 - \log K_{wo} \tag{3.40}$$

Similar to Equation (3.38), the solubility of a crystalline solute in water is given by:

$$S_w^{solid} = S_w^{liquid} \frac{x_2^{solid}}{x_2^{liquid}} = S_w^{liquid} x_2 \tag{3.41a}$$

or
$$\log S_w^{solid} = 0.5 - 0.01(t_m - 25) - \log K_{wo} \tag{3.41b}$$

It is observed in Figure 3.5 that the experimental solubilities of solutes in water are expressed by a regression equation [Equation (3.41c)] remarkably similar to Equation (3.41b):

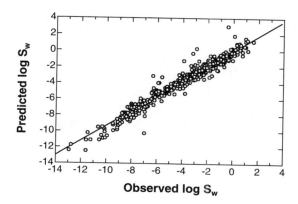

FIGURE 3.5 Experimental aqueous solubility vs. calculated solubility using Equation (3.39). [Graph reconstructed from data by Jain and Yalkowsky, *J. Pharm. Sci.*, 90, 234 (2001).]

$$\log S_w^{solid} = 0.424 - 0.0102 \times (t_m - 25) - 1.031 \times \log K_{wo} \qquad (3.41c)$$

ASER relates a property of a series of drug substances in a given condition, such as solubility in water (S_w) and partition coefficient in water-octanol mixture (K_{wo}), to a sum of solute descriptors as given by:

$$\log S_w = c + rR_2 + s\pi_2^H + a\sum \alpha_2^H + b\sum \beta_2^H + k\sum \alpha_2^H \times \sum \beta_2^H + vV_x \qquad (3.42)$$

where c is a constant, R_2 is an excess molar refraction [(cm³/mol)/10], π_2^H is a combined dipolarity/polarizability, $\sum \alpha_2^H$ is the overall hydrogen bond acidity, $\sum \beta_2^H$ is the overall hydrogen bond basicity, and V_x is the McGowan's characteristic molecular volume [(cm³/mol)/100]. Hydrogen bond interactions between acidic and basic sites in the compound, $\sum \alpha_2^H \times \sum \beta_2^H$, are incorporated in Equation (3.42). R_2 and V_x are determined by a separate formula based on structure, and other descriptors (π_2^H, $\sum \alpha_2^H$, $\sum \beta_2^H$) are obtained from experimental data.

The *in silico* QSPR is similar to the ASER but uses different molecular descriptors. The descriptors are calculated directly from chemical structures and relate to the solubility as:

$$\log S_w = \beta_0 + \sum_{i=1}^{8} \beta_i x_i \qquad (3.43)$$

where β_0 is a constant and β_i is the coefficient for i^{th} descriptor, and x_i is the ith descriptor. Eight descriptors include dipole moment, molecular surface area, molecular volume, molecular weight, number of rotatable bonds/total bonds, number of hydrogen bond acceptors, number of hydrogen bond donors, and density.

These models can predict the solubility of drugs in water with a satisfactory degree of accuracy. These models can serve as a guide in the early stage of drug development of appropriate analogs. However, there are advantages and disadvantages to each model depending on how easily one can obtain the values of descriptors and how complex the drug molecules are.

3.1.5 SOLUBILIZATION OF WEAK ACIDS OR WEAK BASES IN COSOLVENT SYSTEMS

When cosolvents are added to water, they usually increase the solubility of drugs. In some cases the addition of a cosolvent into water will decrease the solubility of a drug. Cosolvent systems have been used in the design of topical, oral, and parenteral dosage forms. Unlike the solubilization of drugs by micelle or inclusion complexation (see Section 3.5.4 and Section 3.5.5), cosolvent systems form homogeneous solutions with water. The increase or decrease in the solubility of the drug will be dependent on the polarity of the drug with respect to water and the cosolvent. Thus, the polarity of the mixture is between that of water and that of the pure cosolvent. The molar solubility of a solute in pure water can be written as:

$$-\ln x_{2,w}^r = \frac{\Delta H_m(T_m - T)}{RT_m T} + \ln \gamma_{2,w} \tag{3.44a}$$

where $x_{2,w}^r$ and $\gamma_{2,w}$ are the solubility of the solute and its activity coefficient in water, and ΔC_p of Equation (3.10) is assumed to be very small. The molar solubility in a pure cosolvent can be written similarly as:

$$-\ln x_{2,c}^r = \frac{\Delta H_m(T_m - T)}{RT_m T} + \ln \gamma_{2,c} \tag{3.44b}$$

When the solubility of a mixed solvent is logarithmically additive, the solubility of the solute in a mixed cosolvent system, $x_{2,m}^r$, is given by:

$$-\ln x_{2,m}^r = \varphi_c \ln x_{2,c}^r + (1-\varphi_c) \ln x_{2,w}^r \tag{3.45}$$

where φ_c is the volume fraction of the cosolvent.

Substituting Equation (3.44a) and Equation (3.44b) into Equation (3.45) yields:

$$-\ln x_{2,m}^r = \frac{\Delta H_m(T_m - T)}{RT_m T} + \ln \gamma_{2,w} + \sigma\varphi_c = -\ln x_{2,w}^r - \sigma\varphi_c \tag{3.46a}$$

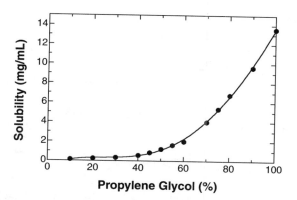

FIGURE 3.6 Solubilization of hydrocortisone butyrate in water/propylene at 25°C. [Graph reconstructed from data by Yip et al., *J. Pharm. Sci.,* 72, 776 (1983).]

where
$$\sigma = \ln \gamma_{2,c} - \ln \gamma_{2,w} \qquad (3.46b)$$

Equation (3.46a) indicates that the solubility of the solute in a mixed solvent system increases as the volume fraction of the cosolvent increases. Figure 3.6 shows the solubilization of hydrocortisone butyrate in a water/propylene glycol system. From the plot of Equation (3.46a), $\ln x_{2,m}^{r}$ vs. φ_c, the slope is defined as the solubilizing power, σ, of the cosolvent for the solute. The solubilizing power is related to the partition coefficient of the solute in a water/octanol system, K_{wo}, as follows:

$$K_{wo} = \frac{S_o}{S_w} = \frac{\gamma_{2,w}}{\gamma_{2,o}} \qquad (3.47)$$

where $\gamma_{2,o}$ is the activity coefficient of the solute in octanol. Taking the logarithm of Equation (3.47) and combining the resulting equation into Equation (3.46b) yields:

$$\sigma = \log K_{wo} + (\log \gamma_{2,o} - \log \gamma_{2,c}) \qquad (3.48a)$$

Equation (3.48a) can also be rewritten as:

$$\sigma = \log K_{wo} - \log K_{co} \qquad (3.48b)$$

where K_{co} is the cosolvent/octanol partition coefficient of the solute. Equation (3.48b) is further simplified to:

$$\sigma = S \log K_{wo} + C \qquad (3.48c)$$

where S and C are the constants for the cosolvent. It was assumed in Equation (3.48c) that for nonpolar drugs the partition coefficient of the drug in the octanol/cosolvent system is much smaller than that in the octanol/water system and log K_{co} is directly proportional to log K_{wo}. For the propylene glycol system, S = 0.89 and C = 0.03 for nonpolar and slightly polar solutes, respectively.

If a drug is a weak acid, the concentrations of the un-ionized species, $[HA]^c$, and the ionized species, $[A^-]^c$, in a water/cosolvent system are in equilibrium and the total solubility, $[HA]^c_{tot}$, in the water/cosolvent system is given by:

$$[HA]^c_{tot} = [HA]^c + [A^-]^c \tag{3.49a}$$

Using Equation (3.46a), the solubility of the un-ionized and the ionized drug in a mixed solvent system is given by:

$$[HA]^c = [HA]_w 10^{\sigma_{HA}\varphi_c} \tag{3.49b}$$

$$[A^-]^c = [A^-]_w 10^{\sigma_{A^-}\varphi_c} \tag{3.49c}$$

where σ_{HA} and σ_{A^-} are the solubility powers of the un-ionized and the ionized drug, respectively, and $[HA]_w$ and $[A^-]_w$ are the concentrations of the un-ionized and the ionized drugs in water, respectively. Incorporating Equation (2.9) into Equation (3.49c) and substituting the resulting equation into Equation (3.49a) yields:

$$[HA]^c_{tot} = [HA]_w 10^{\sigma_{HA}\varphi_c} + [HA]_w 10^{\sigma_{A^-}\varphi_c}\frac{[H^+]}{K_a} \tag{3.49d}$$

The total solubility of weak acid in a water/cosolvent system $[HA]^c_{tot}$ can be determined by the solubility of the un-ionized species in water, the solubilizing powers, the hydrogen ion concentration, and the dissociation constant of the weak acid. Equation (3.49d) illustrates that the total solubility of the weak acid will increase exponentially with respect to the volume fraction of the cosolvent. Even though the solubilizing power of the cosolvent for the un-ionized species is usually larger than that of the ionized species, the solubilization of the ionized species is very important in determining the total solubility when $pH - pK_a > \sigma_{HA} - \sigma_{A^-}$.

For weakly basic drugs (i.e., B), Equation (3.49d) becomes:

$$[B]^c_{tot} = [B]_w 10^{\sigma_B\varphi_c} + [B^+H]_w 10^{\sigma_{B^+H}\varphi_c}\frac{K_a}{[H^+]} \tag{3.49e}$$

Figure 3.7 demonstrates that the total drug solubility of flavopiridol increases exponentially as the volume fraction of the cosolvent (i.e., ethanol) increases. As expected from Equation (3.49e), the solubility lines at the different pHs are parallel to one another.

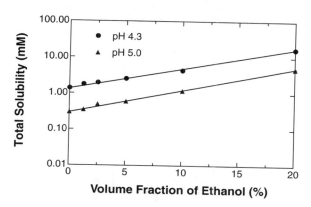

FIGURE 3.7 The total solubility of flavopiridol in a water/ethanol system. [Graph reconstructed from data by Li et al., *J. Pharm. Sci.*, 88, 507 (1999).]

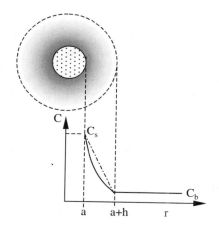

FIGURE 3.8 Pseudo–steady state concentration gradient within a diffusional boundary layer.

3.1.6 Dissolution Kinetics of Solids in Liquids

When a solid dosage form is introduced into the gastrointestinal tract, it disintegrates into fine particles. The effectiveness of the systemic absorption of a drug is strongly dependent on the dissolution rate of the solid drug. The dissolution of the drug in the gastrointestinal fluid is the rate-limiting step in the bio-absorption of low-solubility drugs. The dissolution process of the spherical particles is illustrated in Figure 3.8. In order to establish the mathematical expressions for the dissolution of the solid particle, the following assumptions are made: the particles are spherical and dissolve isotropically; there is a stationary boundary layer of constant thickness around the solid particle; the bulk concentration (C_b) is kept at zero (i.e., sink condition); and there is no accumulation of the dissolved drug within the boundary layer (i.e., pseudo–steady state approximation).

The rate at which the solid drug dissolves may be written as:

$$\frac{dM}{dt} = -DS\frac{\partial C}{\partial r} \tag{3.50}$$

where dM/dt is the dissolution rate, D is the diffusion coefficient, S is the surface area, and r is the radial distance.

Integration of Equation (3.50) yields:

$$\int_a^{a+h} \frac{\partial r}{r^2} = -\frac{4\pi D}{dM/dt} \int_{C_s}^0 \partial C \tag{3.51}$$

where a and h are the particle radius and the boundary layer thickness, respectively. Equation (3.51) results in:

$$\frac{dM}{dt} = -4\,\pi DC_s\left(\frac{1}{a+h} - \frac{1}{a}\right)^{-1} \tag{3.52}$$

where C_s is the solubility.

Given a drug of density ρ, the mass balance expression for the dissolving particle is given by:

$$\frac{dM}{dt} = -4\,\pi a^2 \rho \frac{da}{dt} \tag{3.53}$$

Substituting Equation (3.53) into Equation (3.52) and rearranging the resulting equation gives:

$$\frac{DC_s}{\rho} dt = a^2\left(\frac{1}{a+h} - \frac{1}{a}\right)da \tag{3.54}$$

Integrating Equation (3.54) yields:

$$\frac{DC_s}{\rho h} t = a_o - a - h\,\ln\left(\frac{a_o+h}{a+h}\right) \tag{3.55}$$

where a_o is the original particle radius.

Equation (3.55) is the relationship between the dissolution time and the particle radius. The weight of a particle, w, is given by:

$$w = \frac{4}{3}\pi a^3 \rho \tag{3.56}$$

Substituting Equation (3.56) into Equation (3.55) yields:

$$\frac{DC_s}{\rho h}t = \left(\frac{3w_o}{4\pi\rho}\right)^{1/3} - \left(\frac{3w}{4\pi\rho}\right)^{1/3} - h\ln\frac{\left(\frac{3w_o}{4\pi\rho}\right)^{1/3} + h}{\left(\frac{3w}{4\pi\rho}\right)^{1/3} + h} \tag{3.57}$$

where w_o is the initial weight of a single particle.

If $a_o \gg h$ and $a \gg h$, Equation (3.55) becomes:

$$\frac{DC_s}{\rho h}t = a_o - a = \left(\frac{3w_o}{4\pi\rho}\right)^{1/3} - \left(\frac{3w}{4\pi\rho}\right)^{1/3} \tag{3.58}$$

When $h \gg a_o$, Equation (3.55) is transformed to:

$$\frac{DC_s}{\rho h}t = a_o - a - h\left[\ln\left(1 + \frac{a_o}{h}\right) - \ln\left(1 + \frac{a}{h}\right)\right] \tag{3.59}$$

Applying the Taylor series expansion to Equation (3.59) and using only its first two terms yields:

$$\frac{DC_s}{\rho h}t \approx a_o - a - h\left[\frac{a_o}{h} - \frac{1}{2}\left(\frac{a_o}{h}\right)^2 - \frac{a}{h} + \frac{1}{2}\left(\frac{a}{h}\right)^2\right] = \frac{1}{2}\frac{a_o^2 - a^2}{h} \tag{3.60}$$

Rearranging Equation (3.60) yields:

$$\frac{2DC_s}{\rho}t = a_o^2 - a^2 = \left(\frac{3w_o}{4\pi\rho}\right)^{2/3} - \left(\frac{3w}{4\pi\rho}\right)^{2/3} \tag{3.61}$$

Equation (3.58) and Equation (3.61) are the Hixson and Crowell cube-root and the Higuchi and Hiestand two-thirds–root expressions, respectively. The cube-root and the two-thirds–root expressions are approximate solutions to the diffusional boundary layer model. The cube-root expression is valid for a system where the thickness of the diffusional boundary layer is much less than the particle radius whereas the two-thirds–root expression is useful when the thickness of the boundary layer is much larger than the particle radius. In general, Equation (3.57) is more accurate when the thickness of the boundary layer and the particle size are comparable.

The total time required for the complete dissolution of a particle (i.e., $a = 0$), T, is given by:

$$T = \frac{\rho h}{DC_s}\left(a_o - h\ln\left(a_o + h\right) + h\ln h\right) \tag{3.62}$$

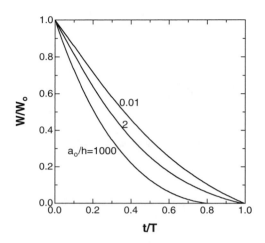

FIGURE 3.9 Simulated particle dissolution profiles with various values of a_o / h.

The dimensionless time, t/T, can be given by:

$$\frac{t}{T} = 1 - \frac{\dfrac{a}{a_o} - \dfrac{h}{a_o} \ln\left(1 + \dfrac{a}{a_o}\dfrac{a_o}{h}\right)}{1 - \dfrac{h}{a_o} \ln\left(1 + \dfrac{a_o}{h}\right)} \qquad (3.63a)$$

Substituting Equation (3.56) into Equation (3.63a) yields:

$$\frac{t}{T} = 1 - \frac{\left(\dfrac{w}{w_o}\right)^{1/3} - \dfrac{h}{a_o} \ln\left[1 + \dfrac{a_o}{h}\left(\dfrac{w}{w_o}\right)^{1/3}\right]}{1 - \dfrac{h}{a_o} \ln\left(1 + \dfrac{a_o}{h}\right)} \qquad (3.63b)$$

Figure 3.9 shows simulated dissolution profiles using Equation (3.63a) and different values of a_o / h. There are deviations from linearity as a_o / h decreases. The linearity usually extends to about 80% dissolution or higher.

For N monodispered particles, Equation (3.57) becomes:

$$\frac{DC_s}{\rho h} t = \left(\frac{3W_o}{4N\pi\rho}\right)^{1/3} - \left(\frac{3W}{4N\pi\rho}\right)^{1/3} - h \ln \frac{\left(\dfrac{3W_o}{4N\pi\rho}\right)^{1/3} + h}{\left(\dfrac{3W}{4N\pi\rho}\right)^{1/3} + h} \qquad (3.64)$$

where W and W_o are the total weight of the particles at time t and t = 0, respectively.

Example 3.3

A drug powder has uniform particle sizes of 500 μm diameter and 75 mg weight. If the solubility of the drug in water = 3 mg/mL, the density of the drug = 1.0 g/mL, and the diffusion coefficient of the drug in water = 5 × 10⁻⁶ cm²/sec, calculate the diffusion layer thickness when it takes 0.3 hours for the complete dissolution.

Solution

Substituting the information given above into Equation (3.62) yields:

$$T = \frac{\rho h}{DC_s}\left(a_o - h\ \ln(a_o + h) + h\ \ln h\right)$$

$$= \frac{1.0 \times h}{5 \times 10^{-6} \times 3 \times 10^{-3}}\left(2.5 \times 10^{-3} - h\ \ln\frac{2.5 \times 10^{-3} + h}{h}\right) = 0.3 \times 3600 = 1080 \quad \text{sec}$$

By trial and error, h = 0.00072 cm.

3.2 SOLUTIONS OF VOLATILE LIQUIDS IN LIQUIDS

3.2.1 RAOULT'S LAW

In a homogeneous solution of volatile liquids in all proportions (e.g., water/alcohol, trichloromonofluoromethane/acetone), the partial vapor pressure of each liquid in the vapor phase in an ideal solution is directly proportional to the mole fraction of the liquid in the solution and the vapor pressure of the pure liquid (Raoult's law):

$$p_1 = x_1 p_1^o \quad \text{and} \quad p_2 = x_2 p_2^o \tag{3.65}$$

Example 3.4

What is the vapor pressure of a 60:40 w/w mixture of propane (MW = 44.1) and isobutane (MW = 58.1)? Assume an ideal solution. The vapor pressures of propane and isobutane are 110 and 30.4 psig at 70°F, respectively. If the vessel is large enough, what is the vapor pressure and composition of the liquid mixture when the last drop of the liquid mixture vaporizes?

Solution

Let us assume that there is a total of 100 g of the mixture (i.e., propane = 60 g and isobutane = 40 g). Then, the mole fractions of propane (denoted as 1) and isobutane (denoted as 2) are given by:

$$x_1 = \frac{60 / 44.1}{60 / 44.1 + 40 / 58.1} = 0.664 \quad x_2 = 1 - x_1 = 0.336$$

The partial vapor pressure of each liquefied gas is given by:

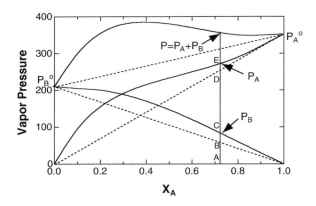

FIGURE 3.10 Vapor pressure–composition curve: ideal (dotted line); positive deviation (solid line) from Raoult's law.

$$\mathrm{p}_1 = x_1\mathrm{p}_1^\circ = 0.664 \times 110 = 73.0 \text{ psig}, \quad \mathrm{p}_2 = x_2\mathrm{p}_2^\circ = 0.336 \times 30.4 = 11.4 \text{ psig}$$

Therefore the total vapor pressure is 73.0 + 11.4 = 84.4 psig. If the two liquids vaporize except for the last drop, the mole fraction of each vapor is 0.664 and 0.336 for y_1 and y_2, respectively.

$$\mathrm{p}_1 = x_1\mathrm{p}_1^\circ = x_1 \times 110 = y_1 P = 0.336 \times P$$

$$\mathrm{p}_2 = x_2\mathrm{p}_2^\circ = x_2 \times 30.4 = y_2 P = 0.664 \times P$$

From the two equations above, P = 60.0 psig, so $x_1 = 0.36$ and $x_2 = 0.64$.

Figure 3.10 shows the vapor pressure/composition curve at a given temperature for an ideal solution. The three dotted straight lines represent the partial pressures of each constituent volatile liquid and the total vapor pressure. This linear relationship is derived from the mixture of two similar liquids (e.g., propane and isobutane). However, a dissimilar binary mixture will deviate from ideal behavior because the vaporization of the molecules A from the mixture is highly dependent on the interaction between the molecules A with the molecules B. If the attraction between the molecules A and B is much less than the attraction among the molecules A with each other, the A molecules will readily escape from the mixture of A and B. This results in a higher partial vapor pressure of A than expected from Raoult's law, and such a system is known to exhibit positive deviation from ideal behavior, as shown in Figure 3.10. When one constituent (i.e., A) of a binary mixture shows positive deviation from the ideal law, the other constituent must exhibit the same behavior and the whole system exhibits positive deviation from Raoult's law. If the two components of a binary mixture are extremely different [i.e., A is a polar compound (ethanol) and B is a nonpolar compound (*n*-hexane)], the positive deviations from ideal behavior are great. On the other hand, if the two liquids are both nonpolar (carbon tetrachloride/*n*-hexane), a smaller positive deviation is expected.

If the attraction between the A and B molecules is stronger than that between like molecules, the tendency of the A molecules to escape from the mixture will decrease since it is influenced by the presence of the B molecules. The partial vapor pressure of the A molecules is expected to be lower than that of Raoult's law. Such nonideal behavior is known as negative deviation from the ideal law. Regardless of the positive or negative deviation from Raoult's law, one component of the binary mixture is known to be very dilute, thus the partial pressure of the other liquid (solvent) can be calculated from Raoult's law. Raoult's law can be applied to the constituent present in excess (solvent) while Henry's law (see Section 3.3) is useful for the component present in less quantity (solute).

The activity coefficient can measure the positive or negative deviation from Raoult's law:

$$p_i = \gamma_i x_i p_i^o \tag{3.66}$$

The activity coefficient can be written as a ratio of real to ideal partial pressures:

$$\gamma_B = \frac{AC}{AB} \quad \text{and} \quad \gamma_A = \frac{AE}{AD} \tag{3.67}$$

When the activity coefficient is greater than 1, a positive deviation from Raoult's law occurs.

3.2.2 TWO-COMPONENT LIQUID SYSTEMS

When a small amount of liquid A is added to a large amount of liquid B at a given temperature, a complete homogeneous solution is obtained. If a two-liquid system has a large positive deviation from Raoult's law, there will be a two-phase separation in the system. When one keeps adding liquid A to a given amount of liquid B, two liquid phases are observed after a certain point, and a homogeneous solution is no longer maintained. Beyond this point, the two liquids are partially miscible with each other: there is limited solubility of liquid A in liquid B and vice versa. The two liquid layers are in equilibrium. In such conjugate solutions, one layer is liquid B–rich (i.e., saturated concentration of A in liquid B) and the other layer is liquid A–rich (i.e., saturated concentration of B in liquid A). For a given temperature and pressure, the composition of A and B in the conjugate solutions is unique. Regardless of the total amount of A and B added to the mixture, the compositions of two liquid layers do not change as long as the experimental temperature does not change. However, the amounts of the A-rich and the B-rich phases are dependent on the total amounts of A and B.

Figure 3.11 shows the partial miscibility of a phenol–water system. At a given temperature (e.g., 45°C), there is initially a homogeneous solution denoted point x, which is an unsaturated solution of phenol in water. When more phenol is added to the solution at the same temperature, the composition line (i.e., tie-line) moves to the right horizontally. When the composition of phenol in water reaches point a, a

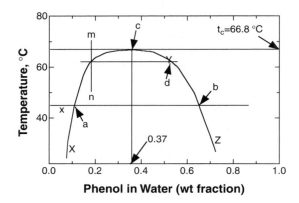

FIGURE 3.11 Partial miscibility curve of phenol–water. [Graph reconstructed from data by Campbell and Campbell, *J. Am. Chem. Soc.,* 59, 2481 (1937).]

second layer, the phenol–rich layer (point b), will start to appear. As more phenol is added to the given volume of water, the relative amount of water-rich phase (i.e., a) decreases while the amount of phenol-rich phase (i.e., b) increases. The composition of each layer (a and b) remains unchanged as long as the same temperature and pressure are maintained at equilibrium. When the composition of phenol in water exceeds b, the two layers disappear and the solution is a one-phase unsaturated solution of water in phenol.

As the temperature increases, the compositions of the two layers come closer together because the solubility of phenol in water or vice versa increases with the increase in temperature. At the temperature of 66.8°C, for example, the compositions of the water-rich phase and the phenol-rich phase are identical. There is one homogeneous solution whose composition is represented by c (e.g., 0.37 weight fraction of phenol). The temperature t_c is known as the critical solution temperature or upper consolute temperature, above which two liquids in all proportions are completely miscible.

The phase diagram shown in Figure 3.11 illustrates that all binary mixtures confined within the composition line XYZ are made up of two layers, and the mixtures outside the XYZ line contain one homogeneous phase solution. By either increasing or decreasing the temperature, a single phase layer may be converted into two phase layers, or vice versa. At a particular temperature, a one-phase homogeneous solution, point m, exists. Without changing the composition of the mixture, the temperature is lowered. When the temperature reaches the XYZ line, the second layer, whose composition is represented by d, will start to appear. Constant, vertical composition lines (e.g., mn) are known as *anisopleths*. As the temperature continues to decrease, the compositions of the conjugate solutions change. For a phenol–water system, as the temperature is lowered, a phenol-rich phase and a water-rich phase are formed. The proportion of the phenol-rich phase will increase as the temperature decreases.

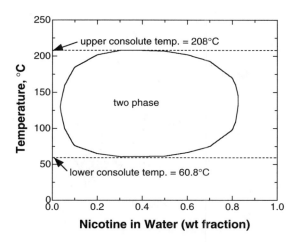

FIGURE 3.12 The partial miscibility of nicotine–water. [Graph reconstructed from data by A. Martin, *Physical Pharmacy,* 4th Ed., Lea & Febiger, Philadelphia, 1995. p. 41.]

Example 3.5

At 50°C, the concentrations of phenol in the water-rich phase and the phenol-rich phase are 11 and 63% w/w (phenol/water), respectively. Then a total of 120 g of a 35:65 w/w (phenol/water) is mixed. Calculate the amount of the phenol-rich and water-rich phases.

Solution

Let the amount of water-rich phase be S. Then the amount of phenol-rich phase is 120 – S. Take a mass balance of phenol:

$$120 \text{ g} \times 0.35 = S \times 0.11 + (120 - S) \times 0.63$$

The weight of the water–rich phase = S = 120 × 0.28 ÷ 0.52 = 64.62 g
The weight of the phenol–rich phase = 120 – 64.62 = 55.38 g

Partially miscible binary systems usually happen at an upper consolute temperature, but one may expect them to occur at a lower consolute temperature. Below the lower consolute temperature, the two liquids become a homogeneous solution in all proportions. In this case, the solubility of the two liquids decreases with an increase in temperature. This large positive deviation from ideality leads to the immiscibility of the two liquids. It may be counterbalanced by a large negative deviation from ideality at the lower temperature, due to the formation of a compound between the two liquids in the liquid state. At a higher temperature, a normal solubility behavior occurs, as shown in Figure 3.11. It is common for binary systems that have a lower consolute temperature to also exhibit an upper consolute temperature. However, the inverse situation is not necessarily true. Outside the temperature contour line, the two liquids are completely miscible but within the line, they are partially miscible. Figure 3.12 illustrates the nicotine–water system, which has both

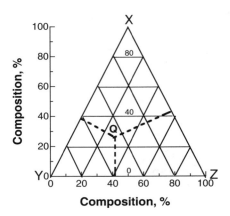

FIGURE 3.13 The triangular diagram for a three-component system.

a lower and an upper consolute temperature. The increase in solubility as the temperature decreases is presumably due to the strong interaction between the two liquids.

3.2.3 THREE-COMPONENT LIQUID SYSTEMS

As a third liquid is added to the partially miscible binary liquid system, the ternary (three-component) system is dependent on the relative solubility of the third liquid in the two liquids. If the third substance is soluble only in one liquid of the original binary mixture or if the solubility of the third in the two liquids is considerably different, the solubility of one liquid in the others will be lowered. The upper consolute temperature should be raised or the lower consolute temperature should be lowered in order to obtain a homogeneous solution. On the other hand, if the third substance is soluble to the same extent in both liquids of the binary system, the complementary solubility of the two liquids is increased. This results in the lowering of an upper consolute temperature or the elevation of a lower consolute temperature.

An equilateral triangle, a symmetrical representation of the three liquids, describes the composition of the third component in the partially miscible binary system in which the third substance is miscible with each of the components of the binary system. The third component is known as the blending agent. Each corner of the X, Y, Z triangle represents the pure component X, Y, or Z, respectively. In the equilateral triangle, the sum of the distances from point Q to the three perpendicular sides is equal to the height of the triangle. Any point within the triangle represents a system of three liquids. One corner of the equilateral triangle represents 100%, parts of each component by weight or mole of one pure component and the other two represent zero, as shown in Figure 3.13. A point located in one of the sides represents two components only. The distance from one corner to the center of the opposite side of the equilateral triangle is divided into 10 or more equal parts and a series of parallel lines are drawn in each side. Figure 3.14 shows a triangular

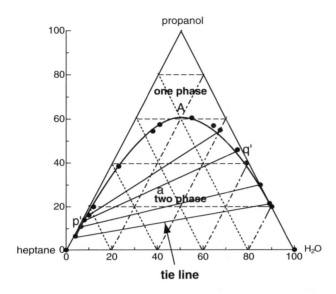

FIGURE 3.14 Phase diagram of a ternary system (water–propranol–heptane) at 25°C. [Graph reconstructed from data by Udale and Wells, *J. Chem. Ed.,* 67, 1106 (1990).]

ternary system of water–propanol–heptane. An added third substance (i.e., heptane) will distribute itself between water and propanol. It results in a two-conjugate ternary system in equilibrium. As shown in a binary system (Figure 3.12), the tie-line can be drawn to connect the compositions of two coexisting liquid phases in equilibrium. The tie-lines need not be parallel to any side of the triangle or each other since the solubilities of heptane in the two liquid phases are different. The tie-lines are constructed experimentally. The phase p′ is in equilibrium with the other phase q′. As the concentrations of the two phases become closer to each other, the tie-lines eventually shorten and meet at one point, A, which is known as the isothermal critical point (or plait point). The plait point is not always at the top of the phase equilibrium curve. The relative amounts of each layer can be determined from the distances, p′a and q′b, based on the gross composition, a, to the points, p′ and q′ (i.e., lever rule).

3.3 SOLUTIONS OF GASES IN LIQUIDS (HENRY'S LAW)

A solution of a gas in a liquid is dependent on the pressure and temperature as well as on the nature of the solvent and the gas. For a given pressure and temperature, the amount of gas dissolved in a given solvent increases with the ease of liquefaction of the gas. If a chemical reaction occurs during the dissolution of the gas in the liquid solvent, the solubility of the gas increases. The solubility of gas is frequently expressed by the Bunsen absorption coefficient, defined as the volume of gas reduced at 0°C and at 1 atm, that is dissolved in a given volume of liquid at a given temperature under a partial pressure of 1 atm for the gas.

Example 3.6

The Bunsen absorption coefficient of carbon dioxide in water at 20°C is 0.88. Calculate the solubility of carbon dioxide in water at 20°C and a partial pressure of carbon dioxide of 0.54 atm.

Solution

The volume of dissolved CO_2 at 0°C under a pressure of 0.54 atm, assuming an ideal gas, is given by:

$$V = 0.88L \times \frac{0.54 \text{ atm}}{1 \text{ atm}} = 0.48L$$

The moles of dissolved CO_2 at 0°C and a pressure of 1 atm are given by:

$$n = \frac{PV}{RT} = \frac{1 \text{ atm} \times 0.48L}{0.082 \times 22.4L \times 273K} = 9.57 \times 10^{-4} \text{ mole} / L$$

The solubility of a gas is denoted in moles per unit volume of the liquid at a constant pressure and considered as the equilibrium constant between the gas molecules in the solution phase and those in the gas phase. When gases dissolve in water, this is accompanied by the generation of heat, resulting in a decrease of gas solubility. If one replaces the equilibrium constant K in the van't Hoff equation, the effect of temperature on the solubility of a gas, α, can be written as:

$$\frac{d \ln \alpha}{dT} = \frac{\Delta H}{RT^2} \tag{3.68a}$$

$$\text{or} \quad \ln\left(\frac{\alpha_2}{\alpha_1}\right) = \frac{\Delta H}{R}\left(\frac{1}{T_1} - \frac{1}{T_2}\right) \tag{3.68b}$$

where α_1 and α_2 are the gas solubilities at temperature T_1 and T_2, respectively, and ΔH is the enthalpy change on evaporation of the pure gas per 1 mole solution of gas.

For the ideal solubilities of gases in liquids, a similar approach to that taken in Section 3.1 for the ideal solubilities of solids in liquids can be used and thus, Equation (3.69), analogous to Equation (3.8), is obtained:

$$-\ln x_2 = \frac{\Delta H_b(T_b - T)}{RT_b T} - \frac{\Delta C_p(T_b - T)}{RT} - \Delta C_p \ln \frac{T_b}{T} \tag{3.69}$$

where ΔH_b is the heat of vaporization at the boiling temperature T_b.

The amount of gas, w, dissolved in a unit volume of solvent at a constant temperature is expressed by Henry's law, which states that the equilibrium solubility of a gas in a liquid is directly proportional to the pressure above the liquid:

$$w = kp \quad \text{or} \quad p_i = x_i H_i \tag{3.70}$$

where p is the equilibrium pressure, k is the constant, x_i is the mole fraction of the gas i, and H_i, is the Henry's constant of the gas i.

Equation (3.70) is applicable to a dilute concentration of the gas. If a mixture of gases is dissolved in a liquid, the amount of each gas in solution is proportional to its partial pressure, independent of the total pressure of the mixture. If the solvent is volatile and the gas (liquefied) is treated as a solute, one can use Raoult's law (Section 3.2) to express the vapor pressure of the gas [Equation (3.65)]. In a dilute solution, the mass of gas dissolved in a given volume (i.e., concentration) is proportional to the mole fraction of the dissolved gas, and Henry's law can be expressed as:

$$x_2 = k' p_2 \tag{3.71}$$

When $k' = 1/p_2^o$, Equation (3.65) and Equation (3.71) are identical and the solution behaves ideally. For example, a liquefied gas has a vapor pressure of 54 atm (p_2^o) at a given temperature. The gas is dissolved in a liquid solvent at a partial pressure of 2 atm for the gas, for which the solubility of the gas is then calculated as:

$$x_2 = \frac{2}{54} = 0.037 \text{ mole fraction} \quad k' = \frac{1}{54} = 0.0185 \text{ atm}^{-1}$$

However, most solutions of gases in liquids do not behave ideally. Again, the activity coefficient can be considered as a measure of the deviation from ideality (Henry's law):

$$p = \gamma_i x_i H_i \tag{3.72}$$

It can be related to vapor pressure as shown in Figure 3.15:

$$\gamma_i (\text{at } x_i = x_A) = \frac{AC}{AB} \tag{3.73}$$

Example 3.7

Estimate the solubility of methane and oxygen in water and *n*-heptane at 25°C, given the following data:

Solute	T_b (K)	ΔH_b (kcal/mol)
CH_4	111.5	8.18
O_2	87.3	6.83

Solution

The ideal solubilities of methane and oxygen in water and *n*-heptane are calculated from Equation (3.66), assuming $\Delta C_p = 0$:

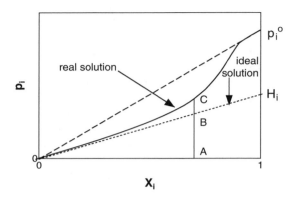

FIGURE 3.15 The partial pessure of gas i in a gas–liquid system.

Solvent	Solute	$x_{2(ideal)}$	$x_{2(real)}$
n-Heptane	CH_4	0.004	0.0051
Water	CH_4	0.004	2.5×10^{-5}
n-Heptane	O_2	0.0013	2.1×10^{-3}
Water	O_2	0.0013	2.3×10^{-5}

The calculated ideal solubilities of the gases in n-heptane are very close to the experimental ones, but the ideal solubilities of the gases in water are too large, giving $\gamma > 1$. For $\gamma > 1$, there is a great difference in intermolecular forces between gas and solvent.

3.4 COLLIGATIVE PROPERTIES

Upon dissolution of a solute in a solvent, the resulting solution will possess different properties than that of the pure solvent. The properties of dilute solutions are dependent only on the concentration of the solute and not on its identity. These are called *colligative* properties (Latin meaning "tied together"). The four colligative properties are freezing point depression, boiling point elevation, osmotic pressure, and vapor pressure lowering.

3.4.1 FREEZING POINT DEPRESSION AND BOILING POINT ELEVATION

On cooling dilute solutions, the solvent usually separates as the solid phase. There are two phases at equilibrium: solid solvent and liquid solution with a solute. Assume that the solute does not dissolve in the solid solvent. The thermodynamic approach to this equilibrium is identical to the one for saturated solutions as described in Section 3.1.1. Following the same reasoning as in Section 3.1.1, Equation (3.1) to Equation (3.6) can be applied to the solvent (component 1), and the freezing point of an ideal solution becomes:

$$\ln x_1 = \frac{\Delta H_{m,l}}{R} \left(\frac{1}{T_{m,l}} - \frac{1}{T} \right) \tag{3.74}$$

where x_1 is the mole fraction of solvent in the solution, $\Delta H_{m,l}$ is the latent heat of melting of the solvent, and $T_{m,l}$ is the melting point of the solvent. Equation (3.74) can be expressed in terms of the mole fraction of the solute:

$$\ln (1 - x_2) = \frac{\Delta H_{m,l}}{R} \left(\frac{T - T_{m,l}}{T_{m,l}T} \right) \tag{3.75}$$

The Taylor expansion is applied to $\ln (1 - x_2) = -x_2 - 1/2x_2^2 - 1/3x_2^3 \cdots$. Since x_2 is much smaller than 1, only the first term of the expansion is kept. Equation (3.75) is then simplified to:

$$\ln (1 - x_2) = -x_2 = \frac{\Delta H_{m,l}}{R} \left(\frac{T - T_{m,l}}{T_{m,l}T} \right) \tag{3.76}$$

Since $\Delta T_f = T_{m,l} - T$, the freezing point depression is small in comparison to $T_{m,l}$ and $T_{m,l}T \approx T_{m,l}^2$. Equation (3.76) becomes:

$$x_2 = \frac{\Delta H_{m,l}}{R} \frac{\Delta T_f}{T_{m,l}^2} \tag{3.77}$$

The mole fraction of the solute in the dilute solution can be approximated by:

$$x_2 \equiv \frac{n_2}{n_1 + n_2} \cong \frac{n_2}{n_1} = \frac{n_2 / W_1}{n_1 / W_1} = \frac{m_2}{W_1 / W_1 / M_1} = m_2 M_1 \tag{3.78}$$

where n is the number of moles, W_1 is the mass of solvent, m is the molality, and M is the molecular weight. Equation (3.78) can be rearranged to:

$$\Delta T_f = \frac{M_1 R T_{m,l}^2}{\Delta H_{m,l}} m_2 \tag{3.79a}$$

Equation (3.79a) can be further simplified as:

$$\Delta T_f = K_f m_2 \tag{3.79b}$$

where K_f is the freezing point depression constant:

$$K_f = \frac{M_1 RT_{m,1}^2}{\Delta H_{m,1}} \qquad (3.80)$$

Each solvent has a different value of K_f, which is independent of the solute identity. Equation (3.79b) can be applied to a mixture of solutes; in this case, the sum of the molalities of all the solutes replaces m_2. If the solute is an ionic species, the total molality of all the species present in the solution must be accounted for.

When a nonvolatile solute is dissolved in a volatile solvent, the solution is at equilibrium with the vapor phase. The thermodynamic condition for this equilibrium is:

$$\mu_1^l(T, P, x) = \mu_1^v(T, P) \qquad (3.81)$$

Equation (3.81) is used in the same manner as Equation (3.1) in Section 3.1.1. The freezing point depression method described above can be analogously applied to the boiling point elevation. Equation (3.79a) then becomes:

$$\Delta T_b = \frac{M_1 RT_{b,1}^2}{\Delta H_{v,1}} m_2 \qquad (3.82a)$$

where ΔT_b is the boiling point elevation, $\Delta H_{v,1}$ is the heat of vaporization of the solvent, and $T_{b,1}$ is the normal boiling point of the solvent. Equation (3.82a) is further simplified:

$$\Delta T_b = K_b m_2 \qquad (3.82b)$$

where K_b is the boiling point elevation constant:

$$K_b = \frac{M_1 RT_{b,1}^2}{\Delta H_{v,1}} \qquad (3.83)$$

Table 3.6 lists K_f and K_b for several solvents. In general, the higher the molar mass of the solvent, the larger the values of K_f and K_b. If the freezing point depression and boiling point elevation constants are known, the molecular weight of the dissolved solute, M_2, can be determined:

$$M_2 = \frac{K_f(\text{or } K_b)W_2}{\Delta T_f(\text{or } \Delta T_b)W_1} \qquad (3.84)$$

where W_2 is the mass of the solute.

Figure 3.16 is a phase diagram of the vapor pressure vs. the temperature in a water–nonvolatile solute system and illustrates the freezing point depression and the

TABLE 3.6

Freezing Point Depression and Boiling Point Elevation Constants for Various Solvents

Solvent	T_m (°C)	K_f (°C/kg mole)	T_b (°C)	K_b (°C/kg mole)
Acetic acid	16.7	3.9	118.0	2.93
Acetone	−94.8	2.4	56.0	1.71
Camphor	178.4	37.7	208.3	5.95
Chloroform	−63.5	4.96	61.2	3.54
Ethanol	−114.5	3	78.4	1.22
Water	0.0	1.86	100.0	0.51

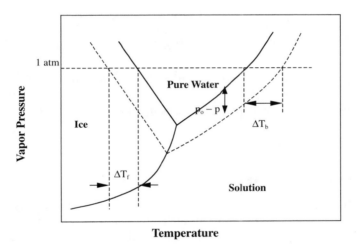

FIGURE 3.16 Phase diagram of pure water (solid lines) and of an aqueous solution containing a nonvolatile solute (dotted lines).

boiling point elevation. The dissolution of the solute in a solvent results in reduction of the vapor pressure (see Section 3.2.1) according to Raoult's law. The boiling point of the solution must be higher than that of the pure solvent in order for the vapor pressure to be equal to 1 atm. Points A and C represent the vapor pressures of the solvent, p_o, (= 1 atm), and the solution, p at temperature T_b, respectively. The lowering of vapor pressure is $p_o - p$. To increase the vapor pressure of the solution to p_o, the temperature of the solution must be raised by ΔT_b. This same analogy can be applied to the freezing point depression.

Example 3.8

Ethylene glycol is a common antifreezing agent. How much weight must be added to water to prevent the formation of ice at −20°C? What is the concentration of ethylene glycol in the solution?

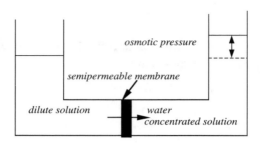

FIGURE 3.17 Osmosis process.

Solution

The freezing point depression constant for water is 1.86. Using equation (3.79b),

$$\Delta T_f = 20 = K_f m_2 = 1.86 m_2$$

$$m_2 = 20 / 1.86 = 10.75$$

$$m_2 = w_2 / M_2 = w_2 / 62 = 10.75 \qquad w_2 = 666.5$$

The concentration of ethylene glycol in the solution is:

$$c_2 = 666.5 / (1000 + 666.5) \times 100 = 40.0\% w / w$$

3.4.2 OSMOTIC PRESSURE

Solvent from a lower concentration solution will move spontaneously to a higher concentration solution across an ideal semipermeable membrane, permeable only to the solvent but impermeable to the solute. Although the solvent flows in both directions, the rate of flow from the dilute concentration (or pure solvent) is much faster than from the concentrated solution. This phenomenon is called osmosis. The flow of the solvent can be reduced by directly applying pressure to the higher concentration side of the membrane as shown in Figure 3.17. At a certain pressure, equilibrium is reached, causing the movement of water to cease. This pressure is called the osmotic pressure and is the sole property of the solution.

When equilibrium is reached, the chemical potentials of the pure solvent (or dilute solution) and the concentrated solution are equal:

$$\mu(T, P + \pi, x_1) = \mu^*(T, P) \tag{3.85}$$

where π is the osmotic pressure. The left-hand side of Equation (3.85) can be rewritten in terms of the pure solvent as:

$$\mu^*(T, P + \pi) + RT \ln x_1 = \mu^*(T, P) \tag{3.86}$$

TABLE 3.7
Typical Osmotic Pressure

Compound	Concentration mg/L	moles/L	Osmotic Pressure (atm at 25°C)
NaCl	35,000	0.5989	27.1
NaCl	1,000	0.0171	0.78
Na_2SO_4	1,000	0.0070	0.41
$MgCl_2$	1,000	0.0105	0.66
Sucrose	1,000	0.0029	0.095
Dextrose	1,000	0.0056	0.14

Source: Data from J. E. Cruver, in *Physicochemical Processes for Water Quality Control* (W. J. Weber, Jr., Ed.), Wiley-Interscience, New York, 1972.

We can express the chemical potential of the concentrated solution in terms of the solvent as:

$$\mu^*(T, P + \pi) = \mu^*(T, P) + \int_p^{\pi + p} V_1 dp \tag{3.87}$$

where V_1 is the volume of solvent. Substitution of Equation (3.86) and Equation (3.87) into Equation (3.85) yields:

$$-RT \ln(1 - x_2) = \int_p^{\pi + p} V_1 dp \tag{3.88}$$

For very dilute solutions, $\ln x_1 = \ln(1 - x_2) = -x_2$. Assuming a constant molar volume of the solvent, the van't Hoff equation can be derived from Equation (3.88):

$$\pi V_1 = n_2 RT \quad \text{or} \quad \pi = cRT \tag{3.89a}$$

where $c = n_2/V_1$ is the molar concentration of the solute.

As shown in Table 3.7, the osmotic pressure is high for various solutes. Ionic salts have a much higher pressure than nonionic solutes. Theoretically the osmotic pressure of an ionic salt is given by:

$$\pi V_1 = i\, n_2 RT \tag{3.89b}$$

where i is the number of ions that compose the salt, known as the van't Hoff factor.

Problem 3.9

Calculate the osmotic pressure of the saturated solution of phenobarbital sodium ($i = 2.0$). $C_s = 100$ g/L, M = 254.2 g/mole, temp.=37°C.

Solution

$$\pi = 2.0 \ \frac{n_2 RT}{V_1} = 2.0 \ \frac{(100)(0.08205)(310)}{254.2} = 20.0 \text{ atm}$$

If the salt completely dissociates, the number of ions present in solution is equal to the number of ionic species in the salt. However, if the salt is incompletely dissociated, the van't Hoff factor is determined as follows:

$$i = \frac{\text{actual number of particles in solution}}{\text{number of particles in solution before dissociation}}$$

If a solution contains N units of a salt (e.g., $M_x X_y$), the salt dissociates as:

$$M_x X_y \rightleftarrows xM^{+y} + yX^{-x} \tag{3.90}$$

If α is the degree of dissociation, $N(1 - \alpha)$ is the undissociated species present at equilibrium with $N(x + y)\alpha$ ions in solution. Then the van't Hoff factor is given by:

$$i = \frac{N(1-\alpha)+N(x+y)\alpha}{N} = 1-\alpha+(x+y)\alpha \tag{3.91}$$

and

$$\alpha = \frac{i-1}{x+y-1} \tag{3.92}$$

Experimentally, the van't Hoff factor is determined as:

$$i = \frac{\text{osmotic pressure of the same concentration of salt}}{\text{osmotic pressure of the nonelectrolyte solution}}$$

3.4.3 VAPOR PRESSURE LOWERING

For a solution containing a nonvolatile solute, the total pressure of the solution is the partial vapor pressure of the solvent and is directly proportional to the mole fraction of the solvent in the solution:

$$P_{\text{vap(total)}} = x_1 p_1^o = (1 - x_2)p_1^o \tag{3.93}$$

$$\frac{p_1^o - P_{vap(total)}}{p_1^o} = x_2 = \frac{n_2}{n_1 + n_2} \cong \frac{n_2}{n_1} = \frac{w_2 / M_2}{w_1 / M_1 + w_2 / M_2} \qquad (3.94)$$

Equation (3.94) says that the relative lowering of the vapor pressure of the solvent is equal to the mole fraction of the solute.

Example 3.10

The vapor pressure of an aqueous solution (118 g) containing a nonvolatile solute (18 g), whose molecular weight is unknown, was determined to be 17.23 mmHg at 20°C. The vapor pressure of water at 20°C is 17.54 mmHg. Calculate the molar mass of the solute.

Solution

Equation (3.81) is used as follows:

$$\frac{p_1^o - P_{vap(total)}}{p_1^o} = \frac{17.54 - 17.23}{17.54} = \frac{w_2 / M_2}{w_1 / M_1 + w_2 / M_2} = \frac{18 / M_2}{100 / 18 + 18 / M_2}$$

$$M_2 = 180$$

3.4.4 ISOTONIC SOLUTIONS

The colligative properties, described in Section 3.4.1 to Section 3.4.3, have been used to determine the molar mass of unknown chemical compounds. Pharmaceutical scientists and pharmacists may apply this concept in the preparation of isotonic (meaning of equal tone) solution dosage forms. These solution dosage forms can be applied to sensitive and delicate organs such as the eye, nose, or ear or directly injected into the body (i.e., blood vessels, muscles, lesions, etc.). They should have, when administered, the same osmotic pressure as body fluids. Otherwise, transport of body fluids inside and outside the cell tissues will occur, causing discomfort and damage to the tissue. Osmolarity of body fluids is approximately 0.307 osmol/L or 307 mosmol/L.

3.4.4.1 Freezing Point Method

The values of K_f and K_b for water are 1.86 and 0.51°C/kg mole, respectively, as shown in Table 3.6. A one molal concentration of a nonelectrolyte lowers the freezing point of water (0°C) by 1.86°C and elevates the boiling point of water (100°C) by 0.51°C.

It has been determined experimentally that the freezing point depression for two body fluids (tears and blood) is −0.52°C. Solution dosage forms should be made to provide this freezing point in water. Many drug compounds and solutes have been tested for freezing point depression in water; their ΔT_f values are shown in Table 3.8. $\Delta T_f^{1\%}$ in Table 3.8 is the freezing point depression of a 1% solution of solute in water. Colligative properties are additive and dependent only on the number of

TABLE 3.8
Isotonicity Values

Drug	M.W.	$\Delta T_f^{1\%}$	$E_{NaCl}^{1\%}$
Aminophylline	456.5	0.10	0.17
Amphetamine chloride	368.5	0.13	0.22
Antopyrine	188.2	0.10	0.17
Ascorbic acid	176.1	0.11	0.18
Atropine sulfate	694.8	0.07	0.13
Barbital sodium	206.2	0.29	0.29
Boric acid	61.8	0.29	0.50
Caffeine	194.2	0.05	0.08
Calcium chloride 2H$_2$O	147.0	0.30	0.51
Calcium gluconate	448.4	0.09	0.16
Camphor	152.2	0.12	0.20
Chlorobutanol	177.5	0.14	0.24
Cocaine HCl	339.8	0.09	0.16
Dextrose H$_2$O	198.2	0.09	0.16
Dibucaine HCl	379.9	0.08	0.13
Diphenhydramine HCl	291.8	0.34	0.20
Ephedrine HCl	201.7	0.18	0.30
Ephedrine sulfate	428.5	0.14	0.23
Epinephrine bitartrate	333.3	0.11	0.18
Epinephrine HCl	219.7	0.17	0.29
Glycerin	92.1	0.20	0.34
Lactose anhydrous	342.3	0.04	0.07
Morphine HCl	375.8	0.09	0.15
Nicotinamide	122.1	0.15	0.26
Penicillin G potassium	372.5	0.11	0.18
Phenobarbital sodium	254.2	0.14	0.24
Pilocarpine HCl	244.7	0.13	0.24
Potassium chloride	74.6	0.45	0.76
Potassium phosphate dibasic	174.2	0.26	0.46
Potassium phosphate monobasic	136.1	0.25	0.45
Procaine HCl	272.8	0.12	0.21
Sodium bicarbonate	84.0	0.38	0.65
Sodium chloride	58.5	0.58	1.00
Sodium phosphate dibasic	142.0	0.30	0.53
Sodium phosphate, monobasic monohydrate	138.0	0.24	0.43
Sucrose	342.3	0.05	0.08
Tetracycline HCl	480.9	0.08	0.14
Urea	60.1	0.35	0.59
Zinc sulfate 7H$_2$O	287.6	0.09	0.15

Source: Taken from J. E. Thompson, *A Practical Guide to Contemporary Pharmacy Practice,* Williams & Wilkins, Baltimore, 1998.

the solute. Therefore, one can calculate the amount of solute in addition to drug needed to make an isotonic solution.

Example 3.11

Make an isotonic solution formulation containing 2% atropine sulfate and boric acid in 15 mL water. How many mg of boric acid should be added to the solution?

Solution

First, calculate the freezing point depression of a 2% atropine sulfate solution:

$$2\% \text{ atropine sulfate} \rightarrow \Delta T_f = 2 \times 0.07°C = 0.14°C \text{ from Table 3.8.}$$

The freezing point depression of body fluids = 0.52°C
The freezing point depression needed from boric acid is $(0.52 - 0.14)°C = 0.38°C$.

$$1\% \text{ boric acid} \rightarrow \Delta T_f = 0.29°C \text{ from Table 3.8}$$

Therefore, one should make a solution of 1.3% boric acid ($=1\% \times 0.38/0.29$). The amount of boric acid needed is:

$$1.3\% \times 15 \text{ mL} = 0.195 \text{ g} = 195 \text{ mg}$$

When using NaCl instead of boric acid, follow the same procedure as outlined above. The freezing point depression of 0.38°C should be made up with NaCl. A 1% NaCl solution gives a freezing point depression of 0.58°C (see Table 3.8). One should make a solution of 0.655% NaCl ($=1\% \times 0.38/0.58$). The amount of NaCl needed is:

$$0.655\% \times 15 \text{ mL} = 0.098 \text{ g} = 98 \text{ mg}$$

3.4.4.2 NaCl Equivalent Method

Instead of using the $\Delta T_f^{1\%}$ method, one can use the NaCl equivalent method. $E_{NaCl}^{1\%}$ in Table 3.8 is the weight of NaCl that lowers the same freezing point to the same extent as 1 g of the drug. Let us use the same example (Example 3.11) for demonstration.

The amount of atropine in the solution = $2\% \times 15$ mL = 0.3 g
One gram of atropine sulfate is equivalent to 0.13 g NaCl (from Table 3.6)
Three tenths of one gram of atropine sulfate is equivalent to 0.13 g × 0.3/1 = 0.039 g NaCl
An isotonic saline solution contains 0.9% NaCl in water
The amount of NaCl needed to make 15 mL of a plain isotonic saline solution is:

$$0.9\% \times 15 \text{ mL} = 0.135 \text{ g NaCl}$$

The amount of NaCl needed to make an isotonic solution of 2% atropine sulfate is:

$$0.135 \text{ g} - 0.039 \text{ g} = 0.096 \text{ g NaCl}$$

This number is very close to the calculated 0.098 g NaCl used in the freezing point depression method.

If one wants to prepare this solution using a normal saline solution (NSS) (0.9% NaCl), the volume of 10.7 mL NSS can be calculated as follows:

If 100 mL NSS contains 0.9 g NaCl, then 0.096 g of NaCl is equivalent to 10.7 mL of NSS (= 100 mL × 0.096/0.9).

This solution dosage form can be formulated by dissolving 0.3 g atropine sulfate in 10.7 mL NSS and then adding sterile water up to a total volume of 15 mL (q.s. 15 mL).

3.5 DISTRIBUTION LAW (PARTITION COEFFICIENT)

3.5.1 NONDISSOCIATED AND NONASSOCIATED SYSTEMS

If a third substance, either liquid or solid, is added to a system of two immiscible liquids, it will distribute itself between the two phases in a definite concentration ratio. The ratio of the concentrations in the two phases is independent of the total amount of the third substance and has a definite value at equilibrium for a given temperature. If C_1 and C_2 are the equilibrium concentrations of the third substance in the two phases, then

$$\frac{C_1}{C_2} = K \qquad (3.95)$$

where K is the equilibrium constant and is known as the distribution ratio or partition coefficient. The distribution law expressed by Equation (3.95) can be applied to dilute solutions. When an excess of solute is added to the immiscible binary mixture, it attains equilibrium, and the two phases are saturated with the dissolved solute. If the solubilities of the solute in the two liquids are C_{s1} and C_{s2}, the distribution law then gives:

$$\frac{C_1}{C_2} = \frac{C_{s1}}{C_{s2}} = K \qquad (3.96)$$

Equation (3.96) is valid when the solute is slightly soluble in the two phases and dilute saturated solutions are obtained.

When two phases are in equilibrium at a constant pressure and temperature, the chemical potentials of the dissolved solute in both phases are the same. The chemical potential of the dissolved solute in both phases is given by Equation (3.97):

$$\mu_1 = \mu_1^\circ + RT \ln a_1 \quad \text{and} \quad \mu_2 = \mu_2^\circ + RT \ln a_2 \qquad (3.97)$$

TABLE 3.9
Distribution of Succinic Acid
between Water and Ether at 15°C

C_1 (mole/L)	0.191	0.370	0.547	0.749
C_2		0.0248	0.0488	0.0736	0.101
C_1/C_2		7.69	7.58	7.43	7.41

Source: Data taken from S. Glasstone and D. Lewis, *Elements of Physical Chemistry,* 2nd Ed., Macmillan, New York, 1960, p. 380.

When the two phases are at equilibrium, $\mu_1 = \mu_2$ and then

$$RT \ln \frac{a_1}{a_2} = \mu_2^\circ - \mu_1^\circ \qquad (3.98)$$

At constant temperature and pressure, the standard chemical potentials are constant, and Equation (3.98) becomes:

$$\frac{a_1}{a_2} = \text{constant} \qquad (3.99)$$

For systems that are ideal or very dilute, Equation (3.99) then reverts back to Equation (3.96). Table 3.9 shows the distribution of succinic acid between water (C_1) and ether (C_2). The ratio (partition coefficient) is relatively constant (≈ 7.53, between 7.41 and 7.67).

The partition coefficient of organic compounds in a number of solvents has been used to predict or correlate their biological activity in a complex biological system. The water–octanol system is commonly accepted as a reference to relate the absorption and distribution of drugs and the quantitative structure–biological activity. As shown in Section 3.1.1, water solubilities of organic compounds can be predicted simply by the partition coefficient (K_{wo}) in the water–octanol system. The K_{wo} can be determined experimentally or predicted by a simple function of molecular properties such as dipole, charge distribution, molecular surface, molecular volume, molecular weight, and molecular shape. It is very important to estimate the partition coefficient, along with the solubility in water, in the new drug design process of a homologous series or series of closely related drugs, in which the biological activities of drugs and K_{wo} have been established.

Equation (3.42), the general solvation equation, can also be used to predict the partition coefficient:

$$\log K_{wo} = c + rR_2 + s\pi_2^H + a\sum \alpha_2^H + b\sum b_2^H + k\sum \alpha_2^H \times \sum \beta_2^H + vV_x \qquad (3.100)$$

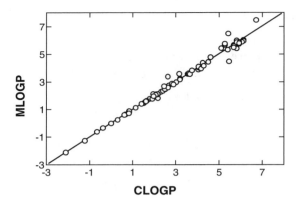

FIGURE 3.18 Water–octanol partition coefficients measured and calculated by CLOGP. [Graph reconstructed from data by Yang et al., *J. Pharm. Sci.,* 91, 517 (2001).]

There are many theoretical expressions to estimate the partition coefficient besides Equation (3.100). The most commonly used one is the CLOGP® program. CLOGP is a fragment method that can be expressed as:

$$\log P = \sum \alpha_n f_n + \sum \beta_m F_m \qquad (3.101)$$

where α is the number of occurrences of fragment f of type n and β is the number of occurrences of fragment interaction correction factor F of type m. A complete description of the CLOGP method is beyond the scope of this book. The CLOGP software program can be referenced for more details (Ref. 2). As shown in Figure 3.18, the K_{wo} values calculated by CLOGP are in good agreement with the experimental ones.

3.5.2 Association of a Solute in One Phase

Suppose a third substance forms dimers in phase 1 and exists as simple molecules in phase 2, (i.e., benzoic acid in a binary mixture of acidified water and benzene). An equilibrium will exist between the dimers and the simple molecules in phase 1:

$$A_2 \rightleftharpoons 2A$$

where A and A_2 are the simple and dimer molecules, respectively. The equilibrium constant in phase 1 is given by:

$$K_d = \frac{C_A^2}{C_{A_2}} \qquad (3.102)$$

where C_A and C_{A_2} are the concentrations of the simple (monomer) molecules and dimer molecules, respectively. If the solute in the phase 1 is mainly dimers, Equation (3.102) becomes:

TABLE 3.10
Distribution of Benzoic Acid in Benzene and
Acidified Water at 25°C

C_1 ($\times 10^{-2}$ mole/L)	C_2 ($\times 10^{-1}$ mole/L)	C_1/C_2	$C_1/\sqrt{C_2}$
4.88	3.64	0.134	0.0256
8.00	8.59	0.093	0.0273
16.0	33.8	0.047	0.0275
23.7	75.3	0.030	0.0273

Source: Data taken from S. Glasstone and D. Lewis, *Elements of Physical Chemistry*, 2nd Ed., Macmillan, New York, 1964, p. 382.

$$C_A = \sqrt{K_d} \times \sqrt{C_{A_2}} \approx \text{constant} \ \times \sqrt{C_1} \tag{3.103}$$

where C_1 is the total concentration of the solute in phase 1. If the simple molecules in phase 1 are at equilibrium with those in phase 2, the distribution law is as follows:

$$\frac{C_2}{C_A} = \text{constant} \tag{3.104}$$

where C_2 is the concentration of the simple molecules in phase 2. Substituting Equation (3.103) into Equation (3.104) yields:

$$\frac{C_2}{\sqrt{C_1}} = \text{constant} \tag{3.105}$$

The modified distribution law of benzoic acid in benzene and acidified water is shown in Table 3.10. It demonstrates that the original distribution ratio (i.e., C_2/C_1) is dependent on the concentration of benzoic acid in water and vice versa, but the modified distribution ratio of 0.0256 to 0.0275 (≈ 0.269) does not change over a concentration range.

3.5.3 DISSOCIATION IN AQUEOUS PHASE AND ASSOCIATION IN OIL PHASE

Most drugs are either weak acids (denoted HA) or weak bases (denoted B). When these drugs are incorporated into two immiscible liquids (i.e., peanut oil and water), the drugs are evenly distributed into both the oil and the water phases. When there are no dimers present in the oil phase, the distribution is:

$$(HA)_w \rightleftarrows (HA)_o \quad \text{oil phase} \tag{3.106a}$$

$$(HA)_w \; \rightleftharpoons \; H^+ + (A^-)_w \quad \text{aqueous phase} \tag{3.106b}$$

where the subscripts w and o refer to the water and oil phases, respectively. The true distribution constant of a weak acid in the oil and water phases (K_d) and the dissociation constant of the weak acid (K_a) are given by:

$$K_d = \frac{[HA]_o}{[HA]_w} \tag{3.107a}$$

$$K_a = \frac{[H^+][A^-]_w}{[HA]_w} \tag{3.107b}$$

The total concentrations of a weak acid in the oil and aqueous phases (C_o and C_w) are given by:

$$C_o = [HA]_o \tag{3.108a}$$

$$C_w = [HA]_w + [A^-]_w \tag{3.108b}$$

The distribution ratio or apparent partition coefficient is experimentally determined as follows:

$$K'_d = \frac{[HA]_o}{[HA]_w + [A^-]_w} = \frac{C_o}{C_w} \tag{3.109}$$

Substituting Equation (3.107a) and Equation (3.107b) into Equation (3.109) yields:

$$\frac{1}{K'_d} = \frac{1}{K_d} + \frac{K_a}{[H^+]K_d} \tag{3.110}$$

A plot of $1/K'_d$ vs. $1/[H^+]$ yields a slope of K_a/K_d and an intercept of $1/K_d$. Assume the volume ratio, $q = V_o/V_w$, for the oil and aqueous phases. The total concentration of the weak acid in the two phases is given by:

$$C_T = qC_o + C_w \tag{3.111}$$

where the total concentration of the substance in the two liquids is based on the volume of the aqueous phase. Substituting for $[A^-]_w$ from Equation (3.107b) into Equation (3.109) yields:

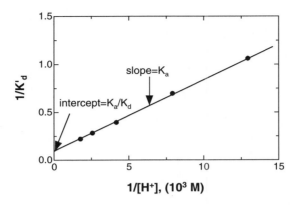

FIGURE 3.19 Apparent partition coefficient of salicylic acid vs. hydrogen ion concentration. [Graph reconstructed from data by Weiner et al., *Am. J. Pharm. Ed.,* 30, 192, (1966).]

$$K'_d = \frac{[HA]_o[H^+]}{([H^+] + K_a)[HA]_w} \tag{3.112}$$

Substituting for $[HA]_o$ from Equation (3.107a) into Equation (3.112) gives:

$$K'_d = \frac{K_d[HA]_w[H^+]}{([H^+] + K_a)[HA]_w} = \frac{C_o}{C_w}, \quad \text{or} \quad C_o = \frac{K_d[H^+]}{K_a + [H^+]}C_w \tag{3.113}$$

Substituting Equation (3.113) into Equation (3.111) results in:

$$C_T = \frac{K_d q[H^+]}{K_a + [H^+]}C_w + C_w = \frac{K_d q[H^+] + K_a + [H^+]}{K_a + [H^+]}C_w \tag{3.114}$$

Rearranging Equation (3.114) yields:

$$\frac{K_a + [H^+]}{C_w} = \frac{K_a}{C_T} + \frac{K_d q + 1}{C_T}[H^+] \tag{3.115}$$

A plot of $(K_a + [H^+])/C_T$ vs. $[H^+]$ should yield a straight line with a slope of $(K_d q + 1)/C_T$ and an intercept of K_a/C_T.

Equation (3.110) is more direct than Equation (3.115). An advantage of Equation (3.115) is that it is not necessary to analyze the concentration of the weak acid in the oil phase. Figure 3.19 shows the effect of the pH on the partition coefficient of a slightly soluble weak acid (i.e., salicylic acid). The apparent partition coefficient becomes the true partition coefficient when the weak acid is essentially in the unionized form (low pH).

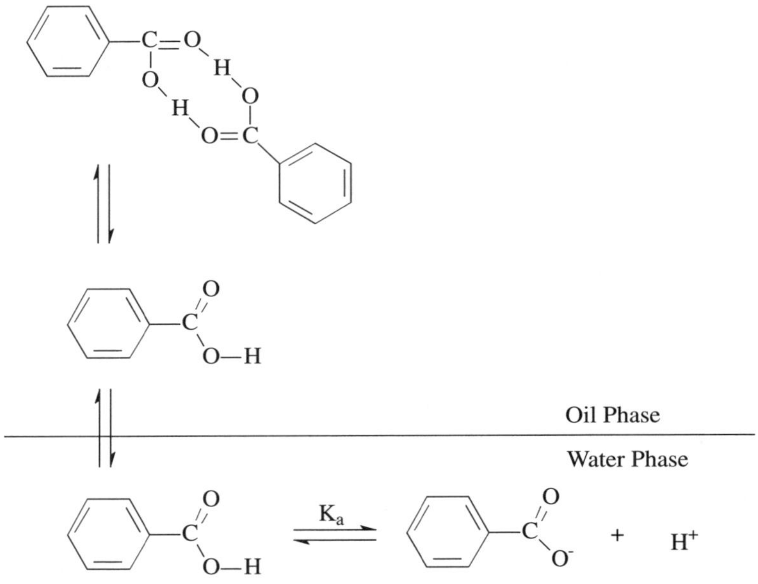

FIGURE 3.20 Distribution of benzoic acid between water and an oil phase.

If a weak acid forms dimers in an oil phase as shown in Figure 3.20, the modified distribution ratio given by Equation (3.105) is used as:

$$K'' = \frac{\sqrt{[HA]_o}}{[HA]_w} \tag{3.116}$$

Substituting Equation (3.115) and Equation (3.107b) into Equation (3.109) yields:

$$\frac{[HA]_w}{K'_d} = \frac{1}{K''^2} + \frac{K_a}{K''^2[H^+]} \tag{3.117}$$

Similar to Equation (3.115), the equation for an immiscible binary system, in which the weak acid in the oil phase exists as a dimer, is in terms of volume ratio:

$$\frac{K_a + [H^+]}{C_w} = \frac{K_a}{C_T} + \frac{K''^2 q[HA]_w + 1}{C_T}[H^+] \tag{3.118}$$

The total concentration of a weak acid in both the water and oil phases provides a final specified concentration of the undissociated acid, $[HA]_w$, in the aqueous phase at specific pH. Therefore, it can be calculated from Equation (3.117) and Equation (3.118). The undissociated acid molecules are soluble in lipid materials and easily penetrate the biological membranes. This concept is applicable to the preservative action of oil–water mixtures. For example, benzoic acid is more effective than its conjugate base, benzoate, because the undissociated acid easily penetrates the living membrane while the ionized conjugate base does not.

Example 3.12

A total of 0.50 g of benzoic acid was added to 200 mL of water at pH 5.2. 100 mL of benzene was then added to the aqueous phase and thoroughly mixed. How much benzoic acid remains in the oil phase of the emulsion as dimers? The pK_a of benzoic acid is 4.2. The apparent distribution ratio is 38.5.

Solution

Equation (3.110) may be rewritten as:

$$C_T = qC_o + C_w = q[HA]_o + [HA]_w + [A^-]_w \tag{3.119}$$

Combining Equation (3.107b) and Equation (3.118) into Equation (3.119) yields:

$$C_T = K''^2 q[HA]_w^2 + [HA]_w + \frac{K_a[HA]_w}{[H^+]} = [HA]_w\left(K''^2 q[HA]_w + 1 + \frac{K_a}{[H^+]}\right)$$

$$C_T = \frac{0.5}{122 \times 0.2} = [HA]_w\left(38.5^2 \frac{100}{200}[HA]_w + 1 + \frac{10^{-4.2}}{10^{-5.2}}\right)$$

$$= 741[HA]_w^2 + 1.1[HA]_w = 0.0205$$

$$[HA]_w = \frac{-2.2 + \sqrt{1.1^2 + 4 \times 741 \times 0.0205}}{2 \times 741} = 3.827 \times 10^{-3} \text{ mole / L}$$

Therefore, the concentration of benzoic acid dimers is given by:

$$[HA]_o = K''^2[HA]_w^2 = 38.5^2 \times 0.003827^2 = 0.02171 \text{ mole / L} = 0.265 \text{ g}$$

$$\text{in } 100 \text{ mL benzene}$$

As shown in Equation (3.49d) and Equation (3.110), the solubility and partition coefficients are dependent on the pH of solution. For weak acid drugs, the solubility increases with the increase in pH, whereas the partition coefficient decreases with the increase in pH. One may postulate that the product of solubility and partition coefficient is independent of pH because the pH effect of the solubility counterbalances out that of the partition coefficient as:

$$S_T \cdot K_D = S_i \cdot K_i = \text{ constant} \tag{3.120}$$

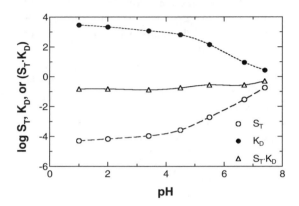

FIGURE 3.21 Plot of $\log S_T$, $\log K_D$, and $\log (S_T \cdot K_D)$ vs. pH for naproxen. [Graph reconstructed from data by Ni et al., *Pharm. Res.*, 19, 1862 (2002).]

where S_T and K_D are the solubility and partition coefficient at any pH, respectively, and S_i and K_i are the intrinsic solubility and intrinsic octanol–water partition coefficient of unionized species, respectively. Figure 3.21 shows the dependence of $\log S_T$, $\log K_D$, and $\log (S_T \cdot K_D)$ upon pH for naproxen. As shown in Figure 3.21, pH has no significant effect on the product of solubility and partition coefficient. The product has been used for predicting the absorption potential of a passively transported drug.

3.5.4 DISTRIBUTION AND SOLUBILIZATION OF WEAK ACIDS OR WEAK BASES IN MICELLES AND THE AQUEOUS PHASE

A surface-active agent is added to an aqueous phase to enhance the concentration of drug compounds when the solubility of the drugs is very low. Due to the presence of dual functional groups (i.e., lipophilic and hydrophilic), the surface-active agent molecules orient themselves to form micelles above the critical micelle concentration. Drugs can be dissolved in both the micelles (see Chapter 4), which are clusters of surface-active agents, and the aqueous phase. Nonpolar drug molecules are effectively dissolved in the core of the micelles. As a result, the total solubility of the drug is increased. If a drug is a weak acid, both the undissociated and dissociated species will be present in the solution. The total solubility of the drug, $[HA]_T$, is expressed as the sum of the concentrations of the drug in the entire solution:

$$[HA]_T = [HA]_w + [A^-]_w + [HA]_m + [A^-]_m$$

where the subscripts w and m represent the aqueous phase and the micelles, respectively. The distribution ratios of the undissociated and the dissociated species in both the aqueous phase and the micelles, K_d^{ud} and K_d^{d}, are defined as:

$$K_d^{ud} = \frac{[HA]_{m,p}}{[HA]_{w,p}} \tag{3.121a}$$

$$K_d^{d} = \frac{[A^-]_{m,p}}{[A^-]_{w,p}} \tag{3.121b}$$

where the subscript p denotes the concentration terms in Equation (3.121a) and Equation (3.121b) based on the individual phase volumes. Equation (3.121a) and Equation (3.121b), in terms of total volume, can be expressed as:

$$K_d^{ud} = \frac{[HA]_m(1-F)}{[HA]_w F} \tag{3.122a}$$

$$K_d^{d} = \frac{[A^-]_m(1-F)}{[A^-]_w F} \tag{3.122b}$$

where F is the volume fraction of the micelles. However, the amount of the surface-active agent added to the entire solution is very small and can be neglected. Equation (3.122a) and Equation (3.122b) reduce to:

$$[HA]_m = K_d^{ud}[HA]_w F \quad \text{and} \quad [A^-]_m = K_d^{d}[A^-]_w F \tag{3.123}$$

The total solubility of a weak acid drug without a surface active agent, $[HA]_T^*$, is defined as:

$$[HA]_T^* = [HA]_w + [A^-]_w \tag{3.124}$$

The fraction of the undissociated species in the aqueous phase, $[HA]_w / [HA]_T^*$, is given by:

$$\frac{[HA]_w}{[HA]_T^*} = \frac{[HA]_w}{[HA]_w + [A^-]_w} = \frac{[HA]_w}{[HA]_w + K_a[HA]_w / [H^+]} = \frac{[H^+]}{K_a + [H^+]} \tag{3.125}$$

The ratio of the drug solubility in the presence of micelles to the drug solubility in the absence of micelles is given by:

$$\frac{[HA]_T}{[HA]_T^*} = \frac{[HA]_m + [A^-]_m}{[HA]_w + [A^-]_w} + 1 \tag{3.126}$$

Substituting Equation (3.123) into Equation (3.126) yields:

$$\frac{[HA]_T}{[HA]_T^*} = 1 + \frac{F}{[HA]_w + [A^-]_w}\left(K_d^{ud}[HA]_w + K_d^d[A^-]_w\right)$$

$$= 1 + F\left[K_d^{ud}\left(1 - \frac{[H^+]}{[H^+]+K_a}\right) + K_d^d\frac{[H^+]}{[H^+]+K_a}\right] \qquad (3.127)$$

$$= 1 + F\left(\frac{K_d^{ud}K_a + K_d^d[H^+]}{K_a + [H^+]}\right)$$

For given values of the distribution ratios of the undissociated and the dissociated species in both the aqueous phase and the micelles, the total drug solubility in the entire solution can be calculated from Equation (3.127). If a drug is a weak base, Equation (3.127) can be transformed to:

$$\frac{[B]_T}{[B]_T^*} = 1 + F\left(\frac{K_d^{ud}K_b + K_d^d[OH^-]}{K_b + [OH^-]}\right) = 1 + F\left(\frac{K_d^{ud}K_w/K_a + K_d^dK_w/[H^+]}{K_w/K_a + K_w/[H^+]}\right)$$

$$= 1 + F\left(\frac{K_d^{ud}[H^+] + K_d^dK_a}{K_a + [H^+]}\right) \qquad (3.128)$$

where $[B]_T$ and $[B]_T^*$ are the total solubility of the weak base in the presence of and absence of micelles, respectively.

Example 3.13

Calculate the amount of surfactant added to an aqueous medium containing sulfisoxazole to increase the concentration to 2.0 g/L at 25°C and pH 5.5. The pK_a is 5.12 and the solubility of undissociated sulfisoxazole is 0.15 g/L at 25°C. The distribution ratios of the undissociated and the dissociated sufisoxazoles in Tween 80 micelles and water are 70 and 15, respectively.

Solution

The total solubility of sulfisoxazole in water at pH 5.5 in the absence of Tween 80 is given by:

$$[HA]_T^* = [HA]_w\frac{K_a + [H^+]}{[H^+]} = 0.15 \text{ g}/L\left(\frac{10^{-5.12} + 10^{-5.5}}{10^{-5.5}}\right) = 0.51 \text{ g}/L$$

From Equation (3.127), the ratio of the solubility of the drug in the presence and the absence of Tween 80 is:

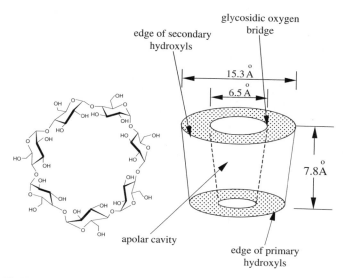

FIGURE 3.22 The shape of β-cyclodextrin.

$$\frac{[HA]_T}{[HA]_T^*} = \frac{2.0}{0.51} = 3.92 = 1 + F\left(\frac{K_d^{ud}K_a + K_d^d[H^+]}{K_a + [H^+]}\right) = 1 + F\left(\frac{70 \times 10^{-5.12} + 15 \times 10^{-5.5}}{10^{-5.12} + 10^{-5.5}}\right)$$

$$F = \frac{3.92 - 1}{53.78} = 0.054$$

Therefore, the volume portion of Tween 80 in the solution containing micelles is 5.4%.

3.5.5 DISTRIBUTION AND SOLUBILIZATION OF DRUG CHEMICALS BY INCLUSION COMPLEX FORMATION

The solubility of a drug in an aqueous solution can be increased by adding cyclodextrin (CD) in the solution. CD is a cyclic oligosaccharide consisting of six, seven, or eight β-D-glucopyranose residues in (β-1,4) linkages, called α-, β-, or γ-, respectively. Figure 3.22 shows the structure of β-CD, and the derivatives of CD are illustrated in Table 3.11. CD is obtained by the enzymatic degradation of starch. It forms a rigid, truncated cone (torus)–shaped molecule with a hollow interior of the torus. The hydroxyl groups of the molecule face to the exterior of the torus, and the skeletal carbons and ether linkages of the glucopyranose are oriented to the interior of the central cavity. Therefore, this configuration yields a polar, hydrophilic exterior and a nonpolar, relatively lipophilic interior. The lipophilic interior of the molecule harbors a good microenvironment to accommodate appropriately sized nonpolar,

TABLE 3.11
Derivatives of Cyclodextrin

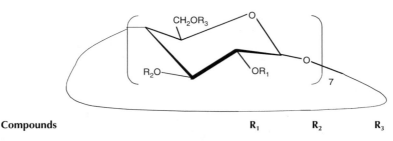

Compounds	R_1	R_2	R_3
Hydrophilic Derivatives			
Methylated Cyclodextrins			
3-Mono-*O*-methylcyclodextrins	H	CH_3	H
2,6-Di-*O*-methylcyclodextrins	CH_3	H	CH_3
Hydroxyalkylated Cyclodextrins			
2-Hydroxyethylcyclodextrins	R_1, R_2, R_3 = H or CH_2CH_2OH		
2-Hydroxypropylcyclodextrins	R_1, R_2, R_3 = H or $CH_2CH(OH)CH_3$		
Hydrophobic Derivatives			
Alkylated Cyclodextrins			
2,6-Di-*O*-ethylcyclodextrins	C_2H_5	H	C_2H_5
2,3,6-Tri-*O*-ethylcyclodextrins	C_2H_5	C_2H_5	C_2H_5
Acylated Cyclodextrins			
2,3-Di-*O*-hexanoylcyclodextrins	COC_5H_{11}	COC_5H_{11}	H
2,3,6-*O*-Hexanoylcyclodextrins	COC_5H_{11}	COC_5H_{11}	COC_5H_{11}
Ionic Derivatives			
6-*O*-(Carboxymethyl)-*O*-ethylcyclodextrins	H	H	H or CH_2COONa
Cyclodextrin sulfate	R_1, R_2, R_3 = H or SO_3Na		
Sulfobutylcyclodextrins	R_1, R_2, R_3 = H or $(CH_2)_4SO_3Na$		

Source: Taken from data by Uekama et al., *Chem. Rev.*, 98, 2045 (1998).

lipophilic moieties or drug molecules that form inclusion complexes such as a benzene ring. When a drug molecule is of the appropriate size and the CD is in an aqueous solution, the nonpolar segment of the drug enters the nonpolar interior portion of the CD. This inclusion complexation separates the nonpolar portion of the drug from the aqueous, polar environment so that the solubility of the drug is further increased. The main driving force for this inclusion complexation is probably the escape of the water molecules from the interior cavity. The water molecules located in the interior of the cavity have a higher enthalpy than the water molecules in solution since the hydrogen bonding potential is not met inside the cavity. As nonpolar drug molecules are bound with nonpolar segments of the CD, the enthalpy-rich water molecules are released and the energy of the system is lowered.

In aqueous solutions, the free drug molecules (denoted as S) that dissolve in water are in equilibrium with those bound to CD, and the successive equilibria are described as:

$$S + CD \rightleftharpoons SCD \qquad K_{1:1} = \frac{[SCD]}{[S][CD]} \qquad (3.129)$$

$$SCD + CD \rightleftharpoons SCD_2 \qquad K_{1:2} = \frac{[SCD_2]}{[SCD][CD]} \qquad (3.130)$$

$$SCD_{n-1} + CD \rightleftharpoons SCD_n \qquad K_{1:n} = \frac{[SCD_n]}{[SCD_{n-1}][CD]} \qquad (3.131)$$

where $K_{1:n}$ is the stability constant.

The total concentrations of the drug and CD, ($[S]_T$ and $[CD]_T$, respectively), are given by the mass balance equations:

$$[S]_T = [S]_o + [SCD] + \cdots + [SCD_n] \qquad (3.132a)$$

$$[CD]_T = [CD] + [SCD] + 2[SCD_2] + \cdots + n[SCD_n] \qquad (3.132b)$$

where $[S]_o$ is the solubility of the drug without the presence of CD.

Substituting Equation (3.129) through Equation (3.131) into Equation (3.132a) and Equation (3.132b) gives:

$$[S]_T = [S]_o \left(1 + K_{1:1}[CD] + \cdots + [CD]^n \prod_{i=1}^{n} K_{1:i} \right) \qquad (3.133)$$

$$[CD]_T = [CD] + K_{1:1}[S]_o[CD] + 2K_{1:1}K_{1:2}[S]_o[CD]^2 + \cdots n[S]_o[CD]^n \prod_{i=1}^{n} K_{1:i} \quad (3.134)$$

In a 1:1 complex, plotting $[S]_T$ vs. $[CD]$ yields an intercept of $[S]_o$ and a slope of $K_{1:1}$. Figure 3.23 shows the increase in solubility of flavopiridol with hydroxypropyl β-CD (HPβCD) at a given pH.

If two or more complexes are formed, the material balance equations, Equation (3.133) and Equation (3.134), become nonlinear, and the determination of the stability constants requires the concentration of free CD, which is not known. However, if the extent of complexation is small or the concentration of the total CD is large,

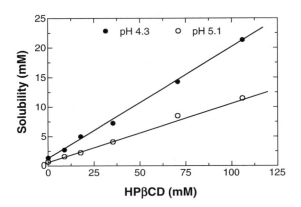

FIGURE 3.23 Solubility of flavopiridol vs. concentration of HPβCD. [Graph reconstructed from data by Li et al., *J. Pharm. Sci.*, 87, 1536 (1998).]

it is reasonable to approximate $[CD] = [CD]_T$. Then, for the formation of the two complexes, Equation (3.133) becomes parabolic and can be rearranged as:

$$\frac{[S]_T - [S]_o}{[CD]_T} = K_{1:1}[S]_o + K_{1:1}K_{1:2}[S]_o[CD]_T \tag{3.135}$$

Plotting $([S]_T - [S]_o)/[CD]_T$ vs. $[CD]_T$ gives the first estimated values for $K_{1:1}$ and $K_{1:2}$ from the intercept and the slope, respectively. The estimated values are substituted to Equation (3.134) to determine $[CD]$. The stability constants are estimated after substituting the estimated $[CD]$ values. Three or four iterations, after the first estimated values of $K_{1:1}$, $K_{1:2}$, and $[CD]$ are calculated from Equation (3.135) and Equation (3.133), yield constant values for the stability constants. However, the determination of the stability constants for higher order complexes is not possible with this approach.

For instance, for the third-order complex system, Equation (3.133) and Equation (3.134) give:

$$[S]_T = [S]_o\left(1 + K_{1:1}[CD] + K_{1:1}K_{1:2}[CD]^2 + K_{1:1}K_{1:2}K_{1:3}[CD]^3\right) \tag{3.136}$$

$$[CD]_T = [CD] + K_{1:1}[S]_o[CD] + 2K_{1:1}K_{1:2}[S]_o[CD]^2 \\ + 3K_{1:1}K_{1:2}K_{1:3}[S]_o[CD]^3 \tag{3.137}$$

Equation (3.136) cannot be linearized as Equation (3.135). Thus a third-order polynomial is employed to estimate the stability constants using $[CD]_T$ as the independent variable for Equation (3.136). The estimated stability constants are then used to calculate the free CD and the solubility of the drug at each solubility data point using Equation (3.136) and Equation (3.137), respectively. Until the residuals

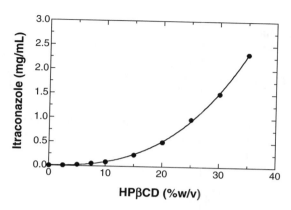

FIGURE 3.24 Solubility of crystalline itraconazole as a function of HPβCD at pH 4. [Graph reconstructed from data by Brewster, et al., 15th AAPS Meeting, Paper No. 2253, Indianapolis, IN, Oct. 29–Nov. 2, 2000.)]

between the experimental and the calculated solubility data are minimized, an iterative nonlinear least-square regression is carried out. Figure 3.24 shows the solubility of crystalline itraconazole as a function of CD at pH 4. When the second-order complexation is assumed, negative stability constants are obtained.

If a drug is a monoprotic weak acid or weak base, the inclusion complexation will occur through un-ionized and ionized species. For a 1:1 complex system, the complexation process can be expressed as:

$$HA + CD \; \rightleftharpoons \; HACD \tag{3.138}$$

$$A^- + CD \; \rightleftharpoons \; A^-CD \tag{3.139}$$

If the drug molecule and CD form a 1:1 complex, the complexation constants are defined as:

$$K_{1:1}^{ud} = \frac{[HACD]}{[HA]_w[CD]} \tag{3.140}$$

$$K_{1:1}^{d} = \frac{[A^-CD]}{[A^-]_w[CD]} \tag{3.141}$$

The distribution of a weak acid (or weak base) in water containing cyclodextrin is given by an equation similar to Equation (3.120):

$$[HA]_T = [HA]_w + [A^-]_w + [HACD] + [A^-CD] \tag{3.142}$$

Substituting Equation (3.106a), Equation (3.140), and Equation (3.141) into Equation (3.142) gives:

$$[HA]_T = [HA]_w + \frac{K_a[HA]_w}{[H^+]} + [HACD] + \frac{K^d_{1:1}[HACD]K_a}{K^{ud}_{1:1}[H^+]} \qquad (3.143)$$

The total concentration of CD, $[CD]_{tot}$, in the solution is the sum of the concentrations of the free CD, $[CD]$, and the concentrations of cyclodextrins bound to $[HA]$ and $[A^-]$, which are $[HACD]$ and $[A^-CD]$, respectively:

$$[CD]_{tot} = [CD] + [HACD] + [A^-CD] \qquad (3.144)$$

Substituting Equation (3.140) and Equation (3.141) into Equation (3.144) yields:

$$[HACD] = [CD]_{tot}\left(\frac{1}{K^{ud}_{1:1}[HA]_w} + 1 + \frac{K^d_{1:1}K_a}{K^{ud}_{1:1}[H^+]}\right)^{-1} \qquad (3.145)$$

Substituting Equation (3.145) into Equation (3.143) gives:

$$[HA]_T = [HA]_w + \frac{K_a[HA]_w}{[H^+]}$$

$$+ [CD]_{tot}\left(\frac{1}{K^{ud}_{1:1}[HA]_w} + 1 + \frac{K^d_{1:1}K_a}{K^{ud}_{1:1}[H^+]}\right)^{-1}\left(1 + \frac{K^d_{1:1}K_a}{K^{ud}_{1:1}[H^+]}\right) \qquad (3.146)$$

If the portion of CD bound to the ionized drug is very small in comparison to the one bound to the un-ionized drug, Equation (3.144) then becomes:

$$[CD]_{tot} = [CD] + [HACD] \qquad (3.147)$$

Equation (3.146) can be simplified to:

$$[HA]_T = [HA]_w + \frac{K_a[HA]_w}{[H^+]} + [CD]_{tot}\left(\frac{1}{K^{ud}_{1:1}[HA]_w} + 1\right)^{-1}\left(1 + \frac{K^d_{1:1}K_a}{K^{ud}_{1:1}[H^+]}\right) \qquad (3.148)$$

If both $K^{ud}_{1:1}[HA]_w$ and $K^d_{1:1}[A^-]_w$ are $<<1$, Equation (3.148) is further simplified to:

$$[HA]_T = [HA]_w + \frac{K_a[HA]_w}{[H^+]} + K^{ud}_{1:1}[CD]_{tot}[HA]_w + K^{ud}_{1:1}K^d_{1:1}K_a\frac{[CD]_{tot}[HA]_w}{[H^+]} \qquad (3.149)$$

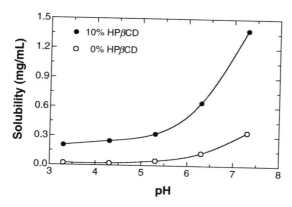

FIGURE 3.25 Solubility of droxicam as a function of pH in the presence and absence of HPβCD. [Graphs reconstructed from data by Park and Choi, *Proceed. Int. Symp. Control. Rel. Bioact. Mater.*, 26, 990 (1999).]

The solubility of the drug in the solution containing CD increases as the pH, K_a, and the complex constants (i.e., $K_{1:1}^{ud}$ and $K_{1:1}^{d}$) increase. It is common for $K_{1:1}^{ud} \gg K_{1:1}^{d}$. The increase in solubility as a result of adding CD is primarily responsible for the inclusion complex formation of the un-ionized drug at low pH. However, as the pH of the solution increases, the ionized species significantly contributes to the total solubility of the drug. Figure 3.25 presents the solubility of droxicam in the presence of 10% HPβCD at the different pH values.

Example 3.14

Flavopiridol, a weakly basic drug (i.e., B), was solubilized by HPβCD with concentrations of free un-ionized, complexed un-ionized, free ionized, and complexed ionized species at pH 4.3 of 0.06, 1.8, 1.5, and 11.3 mmol/L, respectively. The total concentration of HPβCD in the solution was 10% w/v. The pK_a of the drug is 5.68. Calculate the complexation constants and the amount of HPβCD needed to make the total solubility of the drug 10.5 mmole/L at pH 5.1.

Solution

According to Equation (3.144),

$$[CD]_{tot} = 10 \% \text{ w / v} = \frac{100 \text{ g}}{L} = \frac{100 \text{ g}}{1390 \text{ (g / mole) L}} = 71.94 \text{ mmole / L}$$

Then,

$$[CD] = [CD]_{tot} - [BCD] - [B^+HCD] = 71.94 - 1.8 - 11.3 = 58.84 \text{ mmole / L}$$

The complexation constants for the un-ionized and the ionized weakly basic drug at pH 4.3 are given by:

$$K_{1:1}^{ud} = \frac{[BCD]}{[B]_w[CD]} = \frac{1.8}{0.06 \times 58.84} = 508 \text{ L / mole}$$

$$K_{1:1}^{d} = \frac{[B^+HCD]}{[B^+H]_w[CD]} = \frac{11.3}{1.5 \times 58.84} = 128 \text{ L / mole}$$

The total solubility of the weakly basic drug is given by:

$$[B]_T = [B]_w + \frac{K_b[B]_w}{[OH^-]} + [CD]_{tot}\left(\frac{1}{K_{1:1}^{ud}[B]_w} + 1 + \frac{K_{1:1}^d K_b}{K_{1:1}^{ud}[OH^-]}\right)^{-1}\left(1 + \frac{K_{1:1}^d K_b}{K_{1:1}^{ud}[OH^-]}\right)$$

$$= [B]_w + \frac{[H^+][B]_w}{K_a} + [CD]_{tot}\left(\frac{1}{K_{1:1}^{ud}[B]_w} + 1 + \frac{K_{1:1}^d[H^+]}{K_{1:1}^{ud}K_a}\right)^{-1}\left(1 + \frac{K_{1:1}^d[H^+]}{K_{1:1}^{ud}K_a}\right) \quad (3.150)$$

$$10.5 = 0.06 + \frac{0.06 \times 10^{-5.1}}{10^{-5.68}}$$

$$+ [CD]_{tot}\left(\frac{1}{508 \times 0.06} + 1 + \frac{128 \times 10^{-5.1}}{508 \times 10^{-5.68}}\right)^{-1}\left(1 + \frac{128 \times 10^{-5.1}}{508 \times 10^{-5.68}}\right)$$

$$[CD]_{tot} = \frac{10.5 - 0.288}{0.984} = 10.38 \text{ mmole / L} = \frac{10.38 \times 1390}{1000} = 14.4 \text{ \% w / v}$$

If the drug is a polyprotic weak acid or weak base, the inclusion complexation process can be described as (e.g., a diprotic weak base):

The total solubility of the weak base can be represented by the summation of all the species containing B. However, the second or higher order complexes for the

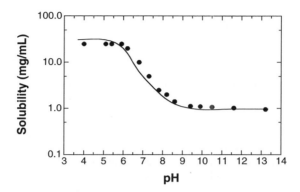

FIGURE 3.26 Solubility of levemopal HCl vs. pH. [Graph reconstructed from data by McCandless and Yalkowsky, *J. Pharm. Sci.*, 87, 1639 (1998).]

ionized species are not likely formed. Thus, the material balance equation can be given by:

$$[S]_T = [B] + [BH^+] + [BH_2^{+2}] + [BCD] + [BCD_2] + [BH^+CD] + [BH_2^{+2}CD] \quad (3.151)$$

where

$$[BCD] = K_{1:1}[B][CD], \quad [BCD_2] = K_{1:1}K_{1:2}[B][CD]^2 \quad (3.152)$$

$$[BH^+] = \frac{[B][H^+]}{K_{a1}}, \quad [BH_2^{+2}] = \frac{[BH^+][H^+]}{K_{a2}} = \frac{[B][H^+]^2}{K_{a1}K_{a2}} \quad (3.153)$$

$$[BH^+CD] = \frac{K_{1:1}^+[B][H^+][CD]}{K_{a1}}, \quad [BH_2^{+2}CD] = \frac{K_{1:1}^{+2}[B][H^+]^2[CD]}{K_{a1}K_{a2}} \quad (3.154)$$

Combining Equation (3.151) through Equation (3.154) yields:

$$[S]_T = [B] + K_{1:1}[B][CD] + K_{1:1}K_{1:2}[B][CD]^2 + \frac{[B][H^+]}{K_{a1}} + \frac{[B][H^+]^2}{K_{a1}K_{a2}}$$

$$+ \frac{K_{1:1}^+[B][H^+][CD]}{K_{a1}} + \frac{K_{1:1}^{+2}[B][H^+]^2[CD]}{K_{a1}K_{a2}} \quad (3.155)$$

It is interesting to point out that Equation (3.155) does not need the pK_a of the complexed drug. Figure 3.26 illustrates the solubility of levemopal HCl, which is a monoprotic weak base that forms a 1:2 complex in the neutral state, in the presence of 20% HPβCD. In this case, the terms containing the second ionization constant are deleted.

3.5.6 DISTRIBUTION OF DRUGS IN PROTEINS (PROTEIN BINDING)

The binding of drugs to proteins in the body influences the biological properties of the drugs because the free drug available for therapeutic action is reduced. Protein binding can alter the distribution of drugs throughout the body, slowing the excretion of a drug and reducing its efficacy. For example, if a drug is highly bound to proteins, the remaining free drug available for therapeutic action is very small. If other agents competitively displace the site in the protein occupied by the drug, the concentration of the free drug increases drastically. Albumin is one of many important proteins involved in the binding of drugs. It exists in high concentration and has the ability to bind both acidic and basic drugs. However, only a limited number of binding sites are available on the albumin molecule. The bound drugs in the protein are in equilibrium with free drugs in the circulation. As the concentration of free drug in the blood decreases, the bound drug is released into the circulation.

The mathematical treatment for protein binding is very similar to the one described in Section 3.5.5. The equilibrium between free drugs and bound drugs can be written as:

$$D + P \quad \rightleftharpoons \quad DP \tag{3.156}$$

where D, P, and DP represent the free drug, the free protein, and the bound drug, respectively.

The equilibrium binding constant is given by:

$$K_{bind} = \frac{[DP]}{[D][P]} \tag{3.157}$$

The total concentration of proteins is given by:

$$[P]_{tot} = [P] + [DP] \tag{3.158}$$

Substituting Equation (3.158) into Equation (3.157) yields:

$$[DP] = K_{bind}[D]([P]_{tot} - [DP]) \tag{3.159}$$

Rearranging Equation (3.159) then gives:

$$\frac{[DP]}{[P]_{tot}} = Y = \frac{K_{bind}[D]}{1 + K_{bind}[D]} \tag{3.160}$$

where Y is the number of moles of the bound drug per mole of the total protein, known as the "fractional saturation of sites." The values of Y vary from 0 to 1. When $Y = 0.5$, half of the drug is bound to the protein and $[D] = 1/K_{bind}$. Taking the reciprocal of Equation (3.160) yields:

$$\frac{1}{Y} = 1 + \frac{1}{K_{bind}[D]} \tag{3.161}$$

Plotting $1/Y$ against $1/[D]$ gives a straight line with a slope of $1/K_{bind}$.

Suppose a protein has n independent equivalent binding sites and each site has the same binding constant, K_{bind}. First, when n = 2:

$$D + P \;\rightleftharpoons\; DP \qquad K_{b,1} = \frac{[DP]}{[D][P]} \tag{3.162a}$$

$$DP + D \;\rightleftharpoons\; D_2P \qquad K_{b,2} = \frac{[D_2P]}{[DP][D]} \tag{3.162b}$$

where $K_{b,1}$ and $K_{b,2}$ are the binding constants. The total protein concentration is given by:

$$[P]_T = [P] + [DP] + [D_2P] \tag{3.163}$$

Then, the fractional saturation of binding sites Y is defined as:

$$Y = \frac{[DP] + 2[D_2P]}{[P] + [DP] + [D_2P]} \tag{3.164}$$

Substituting Equation (3.162a) and Equation (3.162b) into Equation (3.164) yields:

$$Y = \frac{K_{b,1}[D][P] + 2K_{b,1}K_{b,2}[D]^2[P]}{[P] + K_{b,1}[D][P] + K_{b,1}K_{b,2}[D]^2[P]} = \frac{K_{b,1}[D] + 2K_{b,1}K_{b,2}[D]^2}{1 + K_{b,1}[D] + K_{b,1}K_{b,2}[D]^2} \tag{3.165}$$

The general relationship for the successive binding constants ($K_{b,1}$ and $K_{b,2}$) is given by:

$$\frac{1}{K_{b,i}} = \left(\frac{i}{n-i+1}\right)\frac{1}{K} \tag{3.166}$$

where K is an intrinsic binding constant. For i = 1, 2 and n = 2,

$$K_{b,1} = 2K, \quad K_{b,2} = K/2, \quad K = \sqrt{K_{b,1}K_{b,2}} \qquad (3.167)$$

Substituting Equation (3.167) into Equation (3.165) gives:

$$Y = \frac{2K[D] + 2K^2[D]^2}{1 + 2K[D] + K^2[D]^2} = \frac{2K[D]}{1 + K[D]} \qquad (3.168)$$

Equation (3.168) for n = 2 can be generalized for n equivalent sites as:

$$Y = \frac{nK[D]}{1 + K[D]} \qquad (3.169)$$

Taking the reciprocal of Equation (3.169) yields:

$$\frac{1}{Y} = \frac{1}{n} + \frac{1}{nK[D]} \qquad (3.170)$$

Equation (3.170) is called the double reciprocal plot or the *Kloz* plot. The plot of 1/Y against 1/[D] provides a straight line with a slope of 1/nK and an intercept of 1/n.

Rearranging Equation (3.169) gives:

$$Y + KY[D] = nK[D]$$

$$\frac{Y}{[D]} = nK - KY \qquad (3.171a)$$

or

$$\frac{[D]}{Y} = \frac{1}{nK} + \frac{[D]}{n} \qquad (3.171b)$$

Equation (3.171a) is known as the *Scatchard* plot. Plotting Y/[D] against Y gives a straight line with a slope of −K and an intercept of nK. Equation (3.171b) is known as the *Hames* plot. A plot of [D]/Y vs. [D] yields a straight line of slope 1/n and intercept 1/nK.

Figure 3.27 illustrates a rectangular hyperbolic plot [Equation (3.169)], double-reciprocal plot [Equation (3.170)], Scatchard plot [Equation (3.171a)], and Hames plot [Equation (3.171b)] for the binding of NADH to rabbit muscle lactate dehydrogenase.

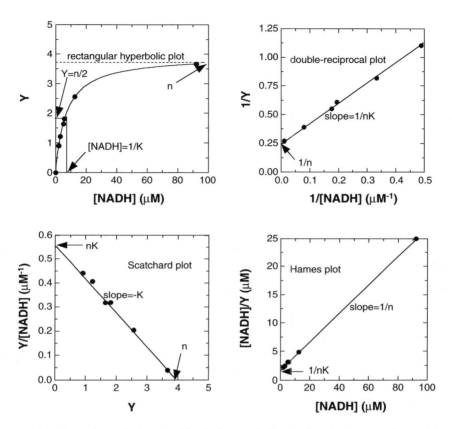

FIGURE 3.27 Binding of NADH with rabbit muscle lactate dehydrogenase using various methods of presenting experimental data. [Graphs reconstructed from data by Ward and Winzor, *Biochem. J.*, 215, 685 (1983).]

Example 3.15

The following binding data have been obtained between cefotaxime and rabbit serum albumin:

Y	0.42	0.75	0.96	1.11	1.25	1.42	1.78	2.62
[D](mM)	260	540	740	920	1150	1430	2070	7280

Calculate the binding constant and number of binding sites.

Solution

The above data are modified as:

Y	0.42	0.75	0.96	1.11	1.25	1.42	1.78	2.62
Y/[D] $(10^{-4}$ mM)	16.1	13.9	13.0	12.1	10.9	9.93	8.60	3.60

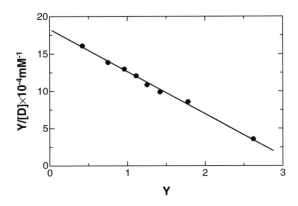

FIGURE 3.28 Scatchard plot of Y/[D] vs. 1/Y for the interaction between cefotaxime and rabbit serum albumin ($5 \times 10^{-5}\,M$) at the ionic strength of $0.17\,M$ at 20°C. [Graph reconstructed from data by Fernandez et al., *J. Pharm. Sci.,* 82, 948 (1993).]

A Scatchard plot is constructed in Figure 3.28. From the y- and x-intercepts, $n = 3.3$ and $K = 5.6 \times 10^{-4}\,mM^{-1}$.

Equation (3.170), Equation (3.171a), and Equation (3.171b) cannot be used if the nature and amount of protein present in the experiment are not known. Even though the concentration of proteins is not known, the drug–protein binding constant can be determined. The extent of drug–protein complex in the plasma may be assumed to be proportional to the concentration of bound drug. Then, Equation (3.171a) can be modified to:

$$Y = \frac{[D_b]}{[P]_{tot}} = \frac{nK[D]}{1+K[D]} \qquad (3.172)$$

where $[D_b]$ is the concentration of the bound drug. Equation (3.172) is rearranged to:

$$\frac{[D_b]}{[D]} = nK[P]_{tot} - K[D_b] \qquad (3.173)$$

The plot of $[D_b]/[D]$ vs. $[D_b]$ gives a straight line with the slope of $-K$ and the intercept of $nK[P]_{tot}$. Concentrations of bound drug and free drug can be easily determined experimentally.

If the binding of a drug on one site of a protein strongly activates the other sites, the sites fill up immediately (i.e., highly cooperative binding). Then, concentrations of all species are negligible except [P] and [D$_n$P]. Equation (3.165) becomes:

$$Y = \frac{nK[D]^n}{1+K[D]^n} \qquad (3.174)$$

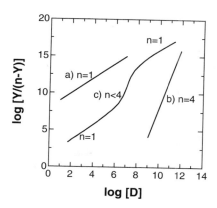

FIGURE 3.29 Hill plot for cooperative binding.

$$\text{or} \quad \frac{Y}{n-Y} = \frac{[\text{sites occupied}]}{[\text{sites vacant}]} = K[D]^n \qquad (3.175)$$

Plotting $\log[Y/(n-Y)]$ vs. $\log[D]$ (called a Hill plot) can easily determine whether highly cooperative binding exists. The independent binding gives a slope of 1 (a in Figure 3.29), whereas a slope of n is obtained for the highly cooperative binding (b in Figure 3.29). However, highly cooperative binding seldom occurs over a wide range of drug concentrations. At higher and lower concentrations, a slope of 1 will be obtained, and a slope of <n will be prevalent at the intermediate range of [D] (c in Figure 3.29). This can be explained by the fact that cooperative binding is not important if there are very few drug molecules available or a very few sites available for binding.

Application of a least–squares method to the linearized plots (e.g., Scatchard and Hames) is not reasonable for analysis of drug–protein binding or other similar cases (e.g., adsorption) to obtain the parameters because the experimental errors are not parallel to the y-axis. In other words, because the original data have been transformed into the linear form, the experimental errors appear on both axes (i.e., independent and dependent variables). The errors are parallel to the y-axis at low levels of saturation and to the x-axis at high levels of saturation. The use of a double reciprocal plot to determine the binding parameters is recommended because the experimental errors are parallel to the y-axis. The best approach to this type of experimental data is to carry out nonlinear regression analysis on the original equation and untransformed data.

If there are two different, independent binding sites, the Scatchard plot becomes nonlinear (curvilinear). The collective curvilinear line results from combining two linear lines (high- and low-binding capacity of sites). This is attributed to the fact that each binding site has its own independent binding sites (n_1 and n_2) and constants (K_1 and K_2). Examples of this type of drug–protein binding are the binding of salicylic acid and bis-hydroxy-coumarin to crystalline bovine and human serum albumins, respectively. This type of drug–protein binding can be expressed by:

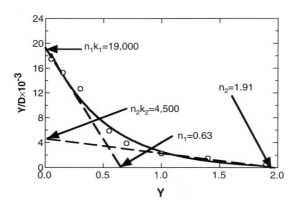

FIGURE 3.30 Hypothetical binding curve of drug to protein. The Ks and ns represent the binding constants and the number of binding sites per protein molecule.

$$Y = \frac{n_1 K_1 [D]}{1 + K_1 [D]} + \frac{n_2 K_2 [D]}{1 + K_2 [D]} + \cdots \tag{3.176}$$

In this case, the binding sites and binding constants can be determined from each linear portion of the curvilinear line as shown in Figure 3.30.

However, it is not easy to obtain two straight lines, especially for those independent binding sites, which have very close binding capacity within a factor of 10. In such cases, the two limiting slopes do not correspond to their drug–protein binding constants. As mentioned before, the untransformed data are used for the analysis of drug–protein binding. When there are two different, independent binding sites in a protein molecule, the concentration of bound drug is given by:

$$[D_b] = \frac{R_1 [D]}{1 + K_1 [D]} + \frac{R_2 [D]}{1 + K_2 [D]} \tag{3.177}$$

where R_1 and R_2 are $n_1 [P]_{tot} K_1$ and $n_2 [P]_{tot} K_2$, respectively. Substituting $[D_b] = [D]_{tot} - [D]$, where $[D]_{tot}$ is the total drug concentration, into Equation (3.177) and rearranging yields:

$$[D]^3 + u[D]^2 + v[D] + w = 0 \tag{3.178}$$

where

$$u = 1 + \frac{1}{K_2} + \frac{R_1}{K_1} + \frac{R_2}{K_2} - [D]_{tot} \tag{3.179a}$$

$$v = \frac{1}{K_1 K_2} + \frac{R_1}{K_1 K_2} + \frac{R_2}{K_1 K_2} - \frac{[D]_{tot}}{K_1} - \frac{[D]_{tot}}{K_2} \tag{3.179b}$$

$$w = -\frac{[D]_{tot}}{K_1 K_2} \tag{3.179c}$$

Let us transform Equation (3.178) by setting $[D] = \beta - u/3$,

$$\beta^3 - \left(\frac{u^2}{3} - v\right)\beta + \left(\frac{2}{27}u^3 - \frac{1}{3}uv + w\right) = 0 \tag{3.180}$$

There are three real roots of Equation (3.180), among which Equation (3.181a) is the unique one because of the definition of β and the physical conditions imposed on the system:

$$[D] = \frac{2}{3}\sqrt{(u^2 - 3v)}\cos\left(\frac{\theta}{3}\right) - \frac{u}{3} \tag{3.181a}$$

or

$$[D_b] = [D]_{tot} - [D] = [D]_{tot} - \frac{2}{3}\sqrt{(u^2 - 3v)}\cos\left(\frac{\theta}{3}\right) + \frac{u}{3} \tag{3.181b}$$

where

$$\theta = \arccos\left(\frac{-2u^3 + 9uv - 27w}{2\sqrt{(u^2 - 3v)^3}}\right) \quad (0 < \theta < \pi) \tag{3.181c}$$

Substitution of Equation (3.181a) into Equation (3.158) and Equation (3.160) allows the determination of the concentrations of protein and bound drug in sites 1 and 2.

A number of experimental methods are used to determine the amount of bound drug and/or free drug in a mixture, including equilibrium dialysis, steady–state dialysis, ultrafiltration, and size exclusion chromatography. Each of the methods is described briefly here.

In the equilibrium dialysis technique, a permeable (dialysis) membrane with a specific molecular weight cutoff point is placed in two solution compartments, as shown in Figure 3.31. A solution of drug in one compartment (A) and a solution of protein in the other compartment (B) are allowed to equilibrate at constant temperature. Compounds with a smaller size than the molecular cutoff point pass through the membrane into the other compartment while proteins with a larger size than the molecular weight cutoff are retained. It may take several hours or several days to obtain thermodynamic equilibrium depending on the experimental setup. At equilibrium, the concentration of the unbound drug in compartment A is equal to that of the unbound drug in compartment B. Based on the concentration of the unbound drug in compartment A and the concentration of the drug–protein complex in compartment B, the drug–protein binding parameters (i.e., binding constant and binding sites) are determined as described above.

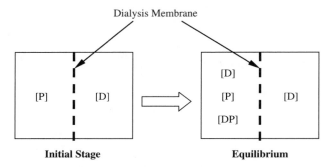

FIGURE 3.31 Equilibrium dialysis method for analysis of drug–protein binding.

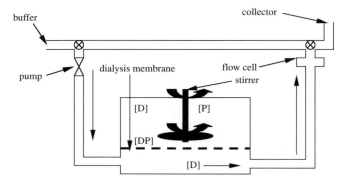

FIGURE 3.32 Steady-state dialysis method for analysis of drug–protein binding.

One problem with the equilibrium dialysis method is the lengthy time required to reach equilibrium across the dialysis membrane. To overcome the problem, a steady-state dialysis method has been developed, as shown in Figure 3.32. The solution of protein and drug in the upper compartment is separated by a dialysis membrane from the buffer solution in the lower compartment, which is circulated continuously at a constant flow rate. Both solutions are stirred to minimize the concentration gradients in each solution. It has been found that it takes several minutes to achieve a steady-state rate of permeation of the drug through the dialysis membrane. The concentration of the drug in the lower compartment can be obtained by periodic withdrawal with an equivalent amount of buffer solution replenished or by the recycling of effluent entailing a constant rate of concentration change.

The data analysis of the steady-state dialysis method is given by:

$$-\frac{d[D]_{tot}}{dt} = k[D] \qquad (3.182)$$

where k is the first-order rate constant depicting the permeability rate constant of the drug through the dialysis membrane. The rate constant can be determined by

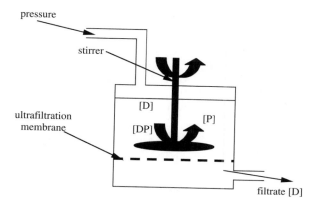

FIGURE 3.33 Ultrafiltration apparatus for drug–protein binding studies.

running a separate experiment without protein in the upper compartment. The total concentration of the drug in the drug–protein solution shows normal curvature even in the semilog plot. Thus, the time-course $[D]_{tot}$ can be expressed by:

$$[D]_{tot} = A_1 e^{-A_2 t} + B_1 e^{-B_2 t} + C_1 e^{-C_2 t} \tag{3.183}$$

Taking the first derivative of Equation (3.183) yields:

$$-\frac{d[D]_{tot}}{dt} = A_1 A_2 e^{-A_2 t} + B_1 B_2 e^{-B_2 t} + C_1 C_2 e^{-C_2 t} \tag{3.184}$$

The concentration of unbound drug in the upper compartment is determined by substituting Equation (3.184) into Equation (3.183) with knowledge of k.

The ultrafiltration method (Figure 3.33) is similar to equilibrium dialysis. The solution of drug–protein mixture is placed in a ultrafiltration membrane chamber. When pressure is applied to the chamber, the unbound drug passes through the membrane. The ultrafiltrate is analyzed for the equilibrium concentration of the unbound drug. Instead of applying pressure to the system, centrifugal force is employed to obtain the ultrafiltrate. These techniques (ultrafiltration or ultracentrifuge) give a much shorter experimental time of 10 to 20 minutes than equilibrium dialysis. One problem common to these methods is the decrease in volume of drug–protein solution in the chamber as liquid is forced to give the ultrafiltrate. As a result, extremely accurate measurements of the volume and drug concentration of the ultrafiltrate are needed. This problem may be overcome by supplementing the drug–protein solution with an equivalent volume of buffer or drug solution. However, because the constant volume of the mixture solution is still approximated, there are errors calculating the amount of buffer/drug solution introduced from the chamber. This problem is further complicated if highly hydrophobic drugs are adsorbed to the ultrafiltration membrane.

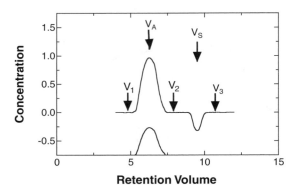

FIGURE 3.34 Elusion profiles of drug–protein complex from gel filtration chromatography. [Graph reconstructed from data by Cann et al., *Arch. Biochem. Biophys.*, 270, 173 (1989).]

In the gel filtration method, gel filtration packing materials such as Sephadex or Bio-Gel P-2 are pre-equilibrated in a drug solution and then placed into a chromatography column. A small volume of drug–protein solution prepared with the same drug solution used for pre-equilibration is applied to the top of the chromatography column. The drug–protein complex is eluted from the column because of size exclusion, as illustrated in Figure 3.34. The area under the peak corresponds to the amount of drug–protein complex, provided that total drug concentration in the presence of protein can be determined. Alternatively, the area under the peak at a trough gives the amount of bound drug because the drug–protein complex has been formed in the pre-equilibrated drug solution.

SUGGESTED READINGS

1. M. H. Abraham and J. Le, The Correlation and Prediction of the Solubility of Compounds in Water Using an Amended Solvation Energy Relationship, *J. Pharm. Sci.,* 8, 868 (1999).
2. Biobyte Corporation, CLOGP for Windows, Claremont, CA.
3. R. Chang, *Physical Chemistry with Applications to Biological Systems,* 2nd Ed., Macmillan, New York, 1981, Chapter 10.
4. X.-Q. Chen et al., Prediction of Aqueous Solubility of Organic Compounds Using a Quantitative Structure–Property Relationship, *J. Pharm. Sci.,* 91, 1838 (2002).
5. K. A. Connors, *Binding Constants: The Measurement of Molecular Complex Stability,* Wiley Interscience, New York, 1987.
6. A. T. Florence and D. Attwood, *Physicochemical Principles of Pharmacy,* 2nd Ed., Chapman and Hall, New York, 1988, Chapters 5 and 10.
7. S. Glasstone and D. Lewis, *Elements of Physical Chemistry,* 2nd Ed., Van Nostrand Co., Maruzen Asian Ed., Tokyo, 1960, Chapters 8 and 11.
8. J. H. Hildebrand and R. L. Scott, *The Solubility of Nonelectrolytes,* 3rd Ed., Dover Publications, New York, 1964.
9. J. N. Israelachvili, *Intermolecular and Surface Forces*, Academic Press, London, 1985.

10. N. Jain and S. H. Yalkowsky, Estimation of the Aqueous Solubility I: Application to Organic Nonelectrolytes, *J. Pharm. Sci.,* 90, 234 (2001).

11. K. C. James, *Solubility and Related Properties,* Marcel Dekker, New York, 1986.

12. K. J. Laidler and J. H. Meiser, *Physical Chemistry,* Benjamin/Cummings, Menlo Park, CA, 1982, Chapter 6.

13. A. Leo, Calculating log P(oct) from Structures, *Chem. Rev.,* 30, 1283 (1993).

14. A. Martin, *Physical Pharmacy,* 4th Ed., Lea and Febiger, Philadelphia, 1993, Chapters 5, 10, and 11.

15. R. G. Mortimer, *Physical Chemistry,* Benjamin/Cummings, Menlo Park, CA, 1993, Chapter 6.

16. K. Shinoda, *Principles of Solution and Solubility,* Marcel Dekker, New York, 1974.

17. K. Uekama, F. Hirayama, and T. Irie, Cyclodextrin Drug Carrier Systems, *Chem. Rev.,* 98, 2045 (1998).

18. J. Wang and D. R. Flanagan, General Solution for Diffusion-Controlled Dissolution of Spherical Particles. 1. Theory, *J. Pharm. Sci.,* 88, 731 (1999).

19. Z.-X. Wang and R.-F. Jiang, A Novel Two-Site Binding Equation Presented in Terms of the Total Ligand Concentration, *FEBS Lett.,* 392, 245 (1996).

20. V. R. Williams, W. L. Mattice, and H. B. Wlliams, *Basic Physical Chemistry for the Life Sciences,* 3rd ed., W. H. Freeman and Co., San Francisco, 1978, Chapter 3.

21. A. G. Williamson, *An Introduction to Non-Electrolyte Solutions,* Oliver and Boyd, London, 1967.

22. D. J. Winzor and W. H. Sawyer, *Quantitative Characterization of Ligand Binding,* Wiley-Liss, Brisbane, Australia, 1995.

23. S. H. Yalkowsky (Ed.), *Techniques of Solubilization of Drugs,* Marcel Dekker, New York, 1981.

PROBLEMS

1. The vapor pressure of pure CCl_4 and $SiCl_4$ at 25°C are 114.9 and 238.3 mmHg, respectively. Assuming ideal behavior, calculate the total vapor pressure of a mixture of 3:2 weight ratio (CCl_4/$SiCl_4$) of the two liquids.

2. Calculate the solubility of a drug at 25°C in (1) a pH 4.23 buffer and (2) the same buffer containing 3.0% (v/v) sodium lauryl sulfate (SLS), and calculate (3) the fraction of the drug solubilized in the SLS micelles in the solution. The aqueous solubility of the nonionized drug at 25°C is 0.21 g/L and its pK_a is 5.09. The apparent partition coefficients (1) between the aqueous solution of un-ionized and the surfactant micelles and (2) between the aqueous solution of the ionized drug and the micelles are 63 and 24, respectively.

3. The following data were obtained for the binding of coumarin to human albumin at 20°C. Determine the binding sites per protein molecule and their binding constants.

Y	0.83	1.09	1.35	1.50	1.92	2.33	3.22	4.00	5.08	6.00
[D] ($\times 10^6$ M)	1.04	1.55	2.25	2.87	4.59	7.19	14.7	33.3	66.7	167.0

4. Derive an expression for the concentration of the free drug for one-site drug–protein binding similar to Equation (3.181a).

5. The following drug–protein binding data were obtained. Calculate the number of binding sites and the binding constant. Prove that the binding occurs independently and is identical.

$$[D] \quad 0.5 \quad 1.0 \quad 2.0 \quad 5.0 \quad 10.0 \quad 20.0 \times 10^3 \, M$$
$$Y \quad \ \ \ 1.6 \quad 2.5 \quad 3.2 \quad 4.0 \quad \ 4.1 \quad \ 4.8$$

6. Calculate the ideal solubility of phenanthracene in benzene.

7. A solution of 1.80 g serum albumin in 100 g water gives 56 mmHg at 25°C. What are the molecular weight of serum albumin and the freezing point of the solution?

8. Methanol is a common antifreezing agent. How much methanol must be added to water to prevent it from being frozen at −10°C? What is the concentration of the solution in w/w%?

9. The following distribution data of quinine $(C_{20}H_{24}O_2N_2)$ were obtained.

| Ether layer | (g/100 mL) | 1.1142 | 1.2901 | 1.4281 |
| Water layer | (g/100 mL) | 0.0547 | 0.0590 | 0.0622 |

What is the molecular structure of quinine in ether, if quinine exists as monomer in water?

10. Oxygen binds to myoglobin to form oxymyoglobin. The standard free energy is $\Delta G° = -30.0 \, kJ / mole$ at 25°C and pH 7. Assume the oxygen behaves as an ideal gas. Calculate the ratio of oxymyoglobin to myoglobin in an aqueous solution at equilibrium at the partial pressure of oxygen = 30 mmHg.

11. An enzyme has four identical and independent binding sites for its substrate. The osmotic pressure of a solution of the enzyme was measured and found to be 2.4×10^{-3} atm at 20°C. The binding equilibrium between the enzyme and its substrate was carried out in a dialysis bag at 20°C. The concentration of unbound substrate outside the dialysis bag and the total substrate concentration inside the bag were found to be 1.0×10^{-4} and $3.0 \times 10^{-4} \, M$, respectively. Calculate the equilibrium constant for the binding of the substrate to the enzyme at 20°C.

12. The binding data of p-*tert*-amylphenol to human serum albumin were obtained by the dynamic dialysis technique as follows:

[D] 1.08   1.19   1.25   1.33   1.41   1.51   1.68   1.82   1.99
Y   0.147 0.154 0.159 0.164 0.168 0.175 0.187 0.196 0.207
[D] 2.12   2.25   2.59   2.71   2.35   2.52 ($\times 10^5$ moles)
Y   0.216 0.224 0.230 0.240 0.246 0.255

Calculate the binding constants and the number of binding sites of human serum albumin.

13. Calculate the total solubility parameter (δ_T) of polyoxyethylated octylphenol:

$$CH_3 - C(CH_3)_2CH_2C(CH_3)_2 - \langle\!\!\!\bigcirc\!\!\!\rangle - (OCH_2CH_2)_3OH$$

4 Surface Chemistry and Colloids

The physicochemical principles involved in homogeneous solutions were discussed in Chapter 3. In some instances, drug solubility is so low that a homogeneous mixture of the drug in a pharmaceutical solvent cannot be achieved or the liquid form of the drug is not miscible in pharmaceutical solvents. In addition, pharmaceutical scientists design uniformly distributed multiphase systems to enhance drug stability and absorption. At least two phases are present. The plane that keeps apart the two phases is described as an *interface* or *interfacial surface*. Interfacial surfaces show different properties from those of bulk phases. Activities of the molecules in the interfacial surface play an important role in pharmaceutical dosage forms. Interfaces of pharmaceutical interest include liquid/solid, liquid/liquid, and liquid/vapor. The liquid/vapor system was discussed in Chapter 3; the liquid/liquid (emulsion) and liquid/solid (suspension) systems will be discussed in this chapter.

4.1 ADSORPTION FROM SOLUTIONS

4.1.1 ADSORPTION PROCESSES

The most pharmaceutical value of adsorption is that of unwanted active materials in solution onto solids such as activated carbon, kaolin, and tannic acid. In addition, adsorption may cause formulation problems when active drugs or inert excipients (i.e., preservatives) adsorb onto containers or medical devices.

Adsorption is the process in which materials of one phase accumulate or concentrate at the interfacial surface of the other phase. It occurs at the interfaces of two phases such as liquid/liquid, gas/solid, gas/liquid, or liquid/solid. We will focus on adsorption in the liquid/solid interface. The materials being adsorbed and the adsorbing materials are called adsorbates and adsorbents, respectively.

Three different types of adsorption processes exist: lyophobicity of the solute against the solvent, physical adsorption (physisorption), and chemical adsorption (chemisorption). The more hydrophobic a material is in an aqueous solution, the more the material will be adsorbed on a solid surface from the solution. The majority of active drugs consist of both hydrophobic and hydrophilic groups, so that the hydrophobic segment of the drug adsorbs on the surface of the solid and the hydrophilic segment extends toward water. In physical adsorption, materials adsorb on the surface of a solid by van der Waals forces, which are relatively weak nonspecific forces. The adsorbed material is not fixed to the surface of the solid but is able to move freely within the interfacial surface. Physisorption is fast and reversible, resulting in multilayer adsorption. In chemisorption, discovered by Langmuir in

1916, substances are held on the surface of a solid by specific covalent forces between the adsorbate and the adsorbent. The chemically adsorbed materials are not free to move on the surface. Chemisorption is slow and not readily reversible, resulting in monolayer adsorption since the chemical forces between adsorbates and adsorbents are very weak once the surfaces of the solid have become saturated with a single layer of adsorbed substances. Most adsorption processes involve organic compounds such as active drugs and incorporate chemical donor–acceptor complex formation between aromatic hydroxyl and nitro-substituted compounds with the active carbon and the carbonyl oxygen groups of the adsorbent surface. Physisorption prevails at low temperature whereas chemisorption is favored at high temperature because chemical reactions between the adsorbate and adsorbent increase with higher temperature. However, most adsorption processes are dominated not by a single process but rather by a combination of the three types of adsorption.

4.1.2 Adsorption Isotherms

When a substance moves away from a solution and accumulates at the surface of a solid, the concentration of the solute remaining in solution is in dynamic equilibrium with the accumulated concentration at the surface. This distribution ratio of the solute in solution and at the surface is a measure of the adsorption equilibrium. A mathematical expression that relates the quantity of the solute adsorbed in a solid surface per unit weight of solid adsorbent to a function of the solute concentration remaining in solution at a fixed temperature is known as the adsorption isotherm.

There have been numerous attempts to assign mathematical isothermal adsorption relations to various experimental data. Among the most frequently used isotherm equations are Langmuir, Freundlich, and BET.

4.1.2.1 Langmuir Isotherm

This is the simplest isotherm equation, proposed in 1916 by I. Langmuir. The Langmuir equation is based on the fact that every active site in the surface acts the same way, and the maximum adsorption occurs at a saturated monolayer of the solutes on the surface. When an adsorbent is added to a solution containing a substance to be removed, the substance adsorbs on the surface of the adsorbent, and equilibrium is established. A fraction α of the adsorbing surface is occupied with adsorbed substance and a fraction $(1 - \alpha)$ of the adsorbing surface will remain unoccupied. The rate of adsorption is proportional to the availability of the adsorbing surface and the concentration [A] of the substance in solution:

$$\text{Rate of adsorption of solute} = k_a[A](1-\alpha) \tag{4.1}$$

where k_a is the adsorption rate constant. The adsorbed substances tend to escape from the surface. The rate of desorption is proportional to the extent of occupied surface:

$$\text{Rate of desorption of solute} = k_d \, \alpha \tag{4.2}$$

where k_d is the desorption rate constant. At equilibrium, the rates of adsorption and desorption are equal and thus:

$$k_a[A](1-\alpha) = k_d \alpha$$

or

$$\alpha = \frac{k_a[A]}{k_a[A]+k_d} \quad (4.3)$$

If a monolayer of the solute covers the surface of the adsorbent, the amount of solute, q_e, adsorbed per unit weight of adsorbent is directly proportional to the fraction α of the surface occupied with the solute:

$$q_e = k'\alpha \quad (4.4)$$

where k' is a constant. Substituting Equation (4.3) into Equation (4.4) and dividing the resulting equation by k_d yields:

$$q_e = \frac{(k_a k' / k_d)[A]}{1+(k_a / k_d)[A]} = \frac{K_1[A]}{1+K_2[A]} \quad (4.5)$$

where $K_1 = k_a k' / k_d$ and $K_2 = k_a / k_d$.

Equation (4.5) can be rearranged in a double-reciprocal form to:

$$\frac{1}{q_e} = \frac{K_1}{K_2} + \frac{1}{K_1}\left(\frac{1}{[A]}\right) \quad (4.6)$$

Hence the plot of $1/q_e$ vs. $1/[A]$ gives a slope of $1/K_1$ and an intercept of K_1/K_2. The Langmuir isotherm is represented by Figure 4.1a.

Figure 4.2 shows the Langmuir isotherms of (a) phenobarbital and (b) mephobarbital adsorption on activated carbon. The maximum adsorption capacity (K_1/K_2) of activated carbon for mephobarbital is lower than that for phenobarbital. The affinity constant $(1/K_2)$ for mephobarbital is higher than that for phenobarbital. This is expected because higher solubility gives a lower adsorption affinity. Table 4.1 illustrates the Langmuir constants of various drugs on carbon black.

4.1.2.2 Freundlich Isotherm

There are two special cases of the Langmuir isotherm. For very low concentrations (i.e., $K_2[A] \ll 1$), the specific adsorption is directly proportional to the remaining concentration of the solute in solution:

$$q_e = K_1[A] \quad (4.7)$$

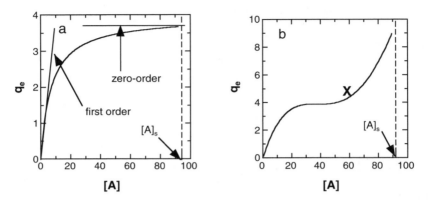

FIGURE 4.1 Langmuir and BET adsorption isotherms.

TABLE 4.1
Langmuir Constants of Various Drugs on Activated Carbon

Drugs	K_1 ($\times 10^{-1}$ L/g)	K_2 ($\times 10^{-4}$ L/mol)
Amitriptyline	4.24	2.07
Carpipramine	3.63	2.36
Chlorhexidine	31.33	0.097
Chlorpromazine	7.43	4.37
Dipiperon	0.20	0.17
Isothipendyl	2.90	2.23
Opipramol	2.67	1.77
Promazine	5.71	3.36

Source: Taken from Nambu et al., *Chem. Pharm. Bull.*, 23, 1404 (1975) and E. Akaho and Y. Fukjumori, *J. Pharm. Sci.*, 90, 1288 (2001).

On the other hand, for high concentrations (i.e., $K_2[A] \gg 1$), the specific adsorption is independent of the concentration of the adsorbate in solution:

$$q_e = \frac{K_1}{K_2} \tag{4.8}$$

The independence of the solute concentrations for adsorption arises when the surface is fully occupied by a monolayer of adsorbate. Equation (4.7) and Equation (4.8) along with the Langmuir isotherm are illustrated in Figure 4.1a.

For the intermediate concentrations, another empirical equation, the Freundlich equation, for adsorption at given temperature can be given as:

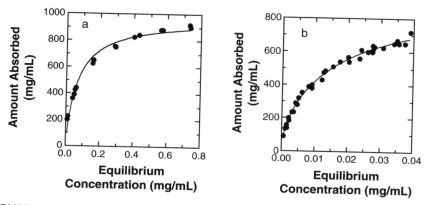

FIGURE 4.2 Langmuir isotherms of (a) phenobarbital and (b) mephobarbital by activated carbon. [Graph reconstructed from data by Wurster et al., *Pharmscitech*, 1(3), 25 (2000).]

$$q_e = k[A]^n \qquad (4.9)$$

where k and n are constants. The value of n ranges from zero to one. In general, the Freundlich equation agrees well with the Langmuir equation [Equation (4.5)]. The constant k is approximated for the adsorption capacity and the nth exponent is an indicator of the adsorption intensity. It is worthwhile to note that when n = 1, the Freundlich equation is identical to the very low concentration case of the Langmuir isotherm [Equation (4.7)] and that when n = 0, the very high concentration case of Equation (4.8) applies. Taking the logarithms of Equation (4.9) yields:

$$\log q_e = \log k + n \log [A] \qquad (4.10)$$

Plotting $\log q_e$ against $\log [A]$ gives a straight line with a slope of n and an intercept of log k.

Example 4.1

The following adsorption data for chlorhexidine on carbon black have been collected. Calculate the Langmuir constants for the adsorption of chlorhexidine on carbon black.

q_e	0.75	0.95	1.10	1.25	1.40	1.55	1.65×10^3 mole/g
[A]	0.25	0.40	0.60	0.70	1.10	1.35	1.95×10^4 mole/L

Solution

From Figure 4.3,

$$\text{slope} = \frac{1}{K_1} = 0.01204 \qquad K_1 = 83.06$$

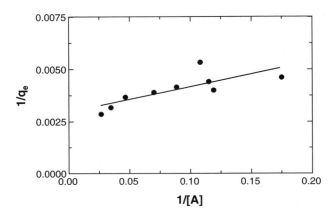

FIGURE 4.3 Linear plots of adsorption isotherms.

$$\text{intercept} = \frac{K_1}{K_2} = 0.002963 \qquad K_2 = \frac{K_1}{0.002963} = \frac{83.06}{0.002963} = 28032$$

4.1.2.3 BET Isotherm

The Langmuir isotherm is based on the formation of a saturated unimolecular layer of adsorbate molecules on the surface of the adsorbent at equilibrium. The BET isotherm (Bruauser, Emmett, and Teller) assumed that a multimolecular layer of adsorbate molecules covers the surface of the adsorbent and that each layer behaves as the Langmuir isotherm. It is not necessary to cover the entire bare surface with the adsorbate to form the multilayers. When using the Langmuir treatment, take into account the multilayer adsorption in which the sequential layers have equal adsorption energies. The BET isotherm is then written in the form of:

$$q_e = \frac{b[A]q^\circ}{([A]_s - [A])[1 + (b-1)([A]/[A]_s)]} \tag{4.11}$$

where $[A]_s$ is the saturated concentration of the adsorbate, q° is the number of moles of the adsorbate adsorbed per unit weight of adsorbent in a monolayer, and b is a constant related to the energy of interaction with the surface:

$$b \propto \exp\left[-\frac{\Delta H_a}{RT}\right] \tag{4.12}$$

where ΔH_a is the net enthalpy change of the adsorption. The BET adsorption isotherm has the form shown in Figure 4.1b. The point X represents the completion of the adsorbed monolayer on the surface of the adsorbent. However, the pattern of the BET isotherm can vary with the value of b. The larger the value of b, the more the sigmoidal shape prevails. The inflection point of the isotherm becomes greater when the value of b is greater than two. Even though the inflection point does not exist for values of b less than or equal to two, a gradual increase in the adsorption is observed. Equation (4.11) can be rearranged to:

$$\frac{[A]}{([A]_s - [A])q_e} = \frac{1}{bq^o} + \left(\frac{b-1}{bq^o}\right)\left(\frac{[A]}{[A]_s}\right) \tag{4.13}$$

Plotting the left-hand side term of Equation (4.13) vs. $[A]/[A]_s$ gives a slope of $(b-1)/bq^o$ and an intercept of $1/bq^o$. From the slope and intercept, one can obtain values of:

$$q^o = \frac{1}{slope + intercept} \tag{4.14}$$

$$b = \frac{slope}{intercept} + 1 \tag{4.15}$$

Equation (4.11) is reduced to the Langmuir equation [Equation (4.6)] if $[A]$ is much smaller than $[A]_s$ and b is much greater than unity. A linear plot for each of three types of adsorption isotherms is illustrated in Figure 4.4. Furthermore, a generalized isotherm equation can be written as:

$$q_e = \frac{q^o b}{(1-x)} \frac{1 - (n+1)x^n + nx^{n+1}}{1 + (b-1)x - bx^{n+1}} \tag{4.16}$$

where $x = [A]/[A]_s$ and n is the number of adsorption layers. Equation (4.16) reduces to the Langmuir equation when n is equal to unity and the BET equation when n is equal to infinity.

Example 4.2
Water vapor absorption into polyvinylpyrrolidone solids was found to obey the BET equation. The following absorption data were obtained. Calculate the values of q^o and b.

Water absorbed (%)	0.06	0.08	0.10	0.10	0.15	0.26	0.39	0.58
Relative pressure	0.11	0.23	0.33	0.44	0.58	0.76	0.85	0.90

Solution
Applying Equation (4.13) to the above data yields the slope of 8.82 and intercept of 2.14 from Figure 4.5.

$$q^o = \frac{1}{slope + intercept} = \frac{1}{8.82 + 2.14} = 0.0912$$

$$b = \frac{slope}{intercept} + 1 = \frac{8.82}{2.14} + 1 = 5.12$$

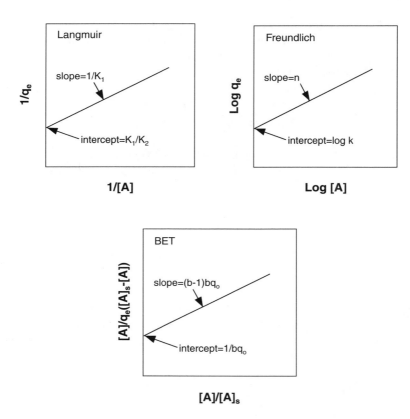

FIGURE 4.4 Reciprocal plot of adsorption of chlorhexidine by carbon black.

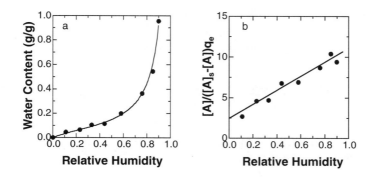

FIGURE 4.5 The BET isotherm of water vapor on highly hydroscopic herbal extracts: (a) regular form; (b) linear form. [Graph reconstructed from data by Chu and Chow, *Pharm. Res.,* 17, 1133 (2000).]

4.1.2.4 Competitive Adsorption

If two substances adsorb onto given active sites of the surface of the adsorbent, the removal of substance A from the solution is highly dependent on the adsorption characteristics of substance B on the adsorbent surface. For example, the efficacy of activated carbon against an overdose of an active drug is subject to the presence of adsorbable substances in the gastrointestinal tract. Let us consider that substance A and substance B adsorbed the fractions of the adsorbent surface α_A and α_B, respectively. The remaining fractions, which can be used for adsorption, are $1 - \alpha_A - \alpha_B$. Then, the rates of adsorption of A and B (i.e., r_A^a and r_B^a, respectively) are given by:

$$r_A^a = k_a^A [A](1 - \alpha_A - \alpha_B) \tag{4.17a}$$

$$r_B^a = k_a^B [B](1 - \alpha_A - \alpha_B) \tag{4.17b}$$

where k_a^A and k_a^B are the adsorption rate constants for substances A and B, respectively. The rates of desorption of substances A and B (i.e., r_A^d and r_B^d, respectively) are given by:

$$r_A^d = k_d^A \alpha_A \tag{4.18a}$$

$$r_B^d = k_d^B \alpha_B \tag{4.18b}$$

where k_d^A and k_d^B are the desorption rate constants for substances A and B, respectively.

At equilibrium, Equation (4.17a) and Equation (4.17b) are equal to Equation (4.18a) and Equation (4.18b), respectively, and then:

$$\frac{\alpha_A}{1 - \alpha_A - \alpha_B} = K_A [A] \tag{4.19a}$$

$$\frac{\alpha_B}{1 - \alpha_A - \alpha_B} = K_B [B] \tag{4.19b}$$

where $K_A = k_a^A / k_d^A$ and $K_B = k_a^B / k_d^B$. Simplifying Equation (4.19a) and Equation (4.19b) yields:

$$\alpha_A = \frac{K_A [A]}{1 + K_A [A] + K_B [B]} \qquad \alpha_B = \frac{K_B [B]}{1 + K_A [A] + K_B [B]} \tag{4.20}$$

The amount of A adsorbed per unit weight of adsorbent, q_e^A, under the assumption of the formation of a monolayer is given by:

$$q_e^A = k_A' \alpha_A = \frac{k_A' K_A [A]}{1 + K_A [A] + K_B [B]} \tag{4.21}$$

where k_A' is a constant.

Equation (4.21) is equal to Equation (4.5) when there is no adsorption of B, even if substance B is present in the solution (i.e., $K_B = 0$). Equation (4.21) shows that the amount of A adsorbed decreases as the amount of B in the solution increases, since both substances, A and B, compete for the same number of active sites. For a multicomponent adsorption, Equation (4.21) can be generalized as:

$$q_e^i = \frac{k_A' K_1 [A_1]}{1 + \sum_i K_i [A_i]} \tag{4.22}$$

In a binary mixture of substances A and B, when the amounts of A and B are high enough, the value of unity can be ignored and Equation (4.21) is linearized to:

$$\frac{1}{q_e^A} = \frac{1}{k_A'} + \frac{K_B [B]}{k_A' K_A [A]} \tag{4.23}$$

Plotting $1 / q_e^A$ against $[B] / [A]$ leads to a straight line with a slope of $K_B / k_A' K_A$ and an intercept of $1 / k_A'$.

Similarly, for substance B, one may obtain:

$$\frac{1}{q_e^B} = \frac{1}{k_B'} + \frac{K_A [A]}{k_B' K_B [B]} \tag{4.24}$$

However, when substances A and B adsorb on two different active sites of the adsorbent surface, the competitive adsorption isotherm is not valid.

Figure 4.6 shows the competitive adsorption of mephobarbital by activated carbon in the presence of phenobarbital. It clearly illustrates that the extent of mephobarbital adsorption decreases in the presence of phenobarbital. This result shows that the two solutes are competing for the same adsorption sites on the activated carbon. The extent of mephobarbital adsorption in the presence of phenobarbital can be predicted by the competitive Langmuir adsorption isotherm.

Example 4.3

Fifty milligrams of activated carbon is mixed with 1 L of a mixture of drug compound A (25 mg) and excipient B (35 mg) until equilibrium is obtained. Calculate the equilibrium concentration of A and B. It was found that adsorption isotherms for A

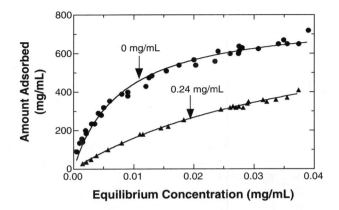

FIGURE 4.6 Adsorption of mephobarbital by activated carbon in the presence of phenobarbital. [Graph reconstructed from data by Wurster et al., *Pharmscitech,* 1(3), 25 (2000).]

and B follow the Langmuir equation. The following adsorption parameters for A and B were obtained:

$$k'_A = 0.05 \text{ g / g}, \quad k'_B = 0.1 \text{ g / g}, \quad K_A = 45,600 \text{ L / g}, \quad K_B = 8960 \text{ L / g}$$

Solution
From Equation (4.22)

$$q_e^A = \frac{k'_A K_A[A]}{1 + k'_A K_A[A] + k'_B K_B[B]}, \quad q_e^B = \frac{k'_B K_B[B]}{1 + k'_A K_A[A] + k'_B K_B[B]}$$

$$q_e^A = \frac{0.05 \times 4.56 \times 10^4[A]}{1 + 0.05 \times 4.56 \times 10^4[A] + 0.1 \times 8960[B]} = \frac{0.025 - [A]}{0.05} \tag{a}$$

$$q_e^B = \frac{0.1 \times 8960[B]}{1 + 0.05 \times 4.56 \times 10^4[A] + 0.1 \times 8960[B]} = \frac{0.035 - [B]}{0.05} \tag{b}$$

Dividing Equation (a) by Equation (b) yields:

$$\frac{2280[A]}{896[B]} = \frac{0.025 - [A]}{0.035 - [B]} \quad \text{or} \quad [A] = \frac{22.4[B]}{79.8 - 1384[B]} \tag{c}$$

Substituting Equation (c) into Equation (a) gives:

$$\frac{5107.2[B]}{79.8 + 56,838.08[B] - 1,240,064[B]^2} = \frac{1.995 - 57[B]}{0.05}$$

Then,

$$[B] = 0.03287 \text{ g} / \text{L} = 32.87 \text{ mg} / \text{L}$$

Substituting [B] into Equation (c) yields:

$$[A] = 0.02146 \text{ g} / \text{L} = 21.46 \text{ mg} / \text{L}$$

The adsorption phenomenon described so far deals with the adsorption of a molecule at an adsorbent surface site. It is possible for a molecule to be adsorbed at two or more sites. For example, in a molecule with two or more functional groups, each functional group may be adsorbed on one site. Suppose that a molecule is adsorbed at two different surface sites. The rate of adsorption is written as:

$$\text{Rate of adsorption} = k_a[A](1-\alpha)^2 \tag{4.25}$$

Desorption takes place from the two adsorbed sites and its rate is written as:

$$\text{Rate of desorption} = k_d\alpha^2 \tag{4.26}$$

Incorporating Equation (4.25) into Equation (4.26) at equilibrium leads to:

$$\alpha = \frac{(k_a / k_d)^{1/2}[A]^{1/2}}{1 + (k_a / k_d)^{1/2}[A]^{1/2}} \tag{4.27}$$

The amount of A adsorbed per unit weight of adsorbent is given by:

$$q_e = \frac{k'\alpha}{2} = \frac{k''(k_a / k_d)^{1/2}[A]^{1/2}}{1 + (k_a / k_d)^{1/2}[A]^{1/2}} \tag{4.28}$$

where $k'' = k' / 2$. The adsorption isotherm for this case is shown in Figure 4.7. If the concentration is very dilute, the denominator of Equation (4.28) gets closer to unity and Equation (4.28) becomes:

$$q_e = k''(k_a / k_d)^{1/2}[A]^{1/2} \tag{4.29}$$

At high concentrations, the denominator is much larger than 1, and Equation (4.28) yields:

$$q_e = k'' \tag{4.30}$$

As a result, adsorption is independent of the concentration at high concentrations.

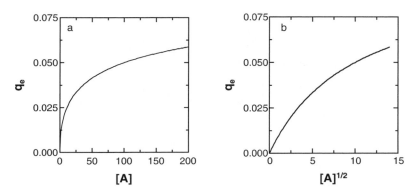

FIGURE 4.7 Adsoprtion isotherm with a binary site: (a) Langmuir and (b) adsorption with two sites.

4.1.3 Factors Affecting Adsorption

Several factors influence the extent of adsorption from solution; they will be briefly described in the sections that follow.

4.1.3.1 Nature of the Adsorbent

The physicochemical nature of the adsorbent can have decisive impacts on the rate and capacity for adsorption. Every solid material can be used as an adsorbent, but clay materials and activated carbon have been employed as particular adsorbents in pharmaceutical applications. Clays such as bentonite and kaolin have silicate groups on their surface and thus retain cation-exchange capacity. Positively charged compounds adsorb on such silicate materials by replacing similarly charged ions on the adsorbent surface (i.e., chemisorption or ion-exchange process). Inorganic adsorbents such as kaolin have different adsorption characteristics on different parts of the surface (anionic adsorbates on one part and cationic adsorbates on other parts). Due to the natural source of these clay adsorbents, the adsorption characteristics of a specific adsorbent are dependent on their origin and processing.

Activated carbon is commonly administered as an antidote to reduce poisoning by the adsorption mechanism. In addition, because drug adsorbs on activated carbon, a concentration gradient between the tissue and gastrointestinal fluids exists, and thus unwanted toxic substances diffuse out of the tissues (i.e., gastrointestinal dialysis). Ionic adsorbates adsorb much less to activated carbon due to the presence of electrostatic repulsion and polarity than their neutral counterpart molecules do.

Many commercial activated carbons have been prepared with various sources of raw materials and different processing conditions. As a result, the micropore structures and specific surface areas of activated carbons, which are the most profound influences on the extent of adsorption, vary, and in general, activated carbons have a surface area of up to 3000 m^2/g. The rate of adsorption increases with some function of the inverse of the radius of the activated carbon even though the adsorption capacity (i.e., equilibrium adsorption) is relatively independent of the particle diameter. However, for a highly porous adsorbent such as activated carbon, the

TABLE 4.2
Surface Areas of Various Activated Carbons and
Langmuir Constants of *p*-Nitrophenol

Carbon	Surface Area (m²/g)	Langmuir Constants K₁ (g/g)	K₂ (L/g)
BPL	1255	0.33	2.3
F400	853	0.30	6.2
FS100	751	0.28	5.6
WPLL	315	0.097	3.2
CBP	127	0.068	1.7

Source: Taken from Lynam et al., *J. Chem. Ed.,* 72, 80 (1995).

reduction of particle sizes may provide more open adsorption sites that were not available for adsorption in large particles or granules. Table 4.2 shows the effect of activated carbons on the Langmuir constants.

4.1.3.2 Nature of the Adsorbate

The solubility of the adsorbate is a controlling factor for adsorption with a given adsorbent. Its solubility in the solvent from which adsorption takes place has an inverse relationship with the extent of adsorption of an adsorbate (i.e., Lundelius' rule). It may be postulated that strong forces exist between the adsorbate and solvent, and the breakup of such forces should be needed before adsorption can occur. The higher the solubility of the adsorbate in a solvent, the greater the forces and the smaller the extent of adsorption.

For organic compounds consisting of hydrocarbon chains, solubility in water decreases with an increase in chain length of the homologous series (i.e., Traube's rule), because the compounds become more hydrophobic and nonpolar. More hydrophobic adsorbates are expelled from water and thus allow an increasing number of water–water bond to be reformed. A nonpolar adsorbate will be strongly adsorbed from a polar solvent by a nonpolar adsorbent but will not be adsorbed much on a polar adsorbent in a nonpolar solvent. Therefore, an increase in the polarity of an adsorbate decreases its adsorption on activated carbon, which is a relatively polar adsorbent, in water.

4.1.3.3 pH

The pH of a solution influences the extent of adsorption. The majority of pharmaceutically active drugs are weak acids or weak bases. The degree of ionization and solubility of the adsorbate drug molecule are dependent on pH. As described above, more ionized (i.e., polar) and soluble adsorbates adsorb much less than their un-ionized forms (i.e., lypophilic) do. For amphoteric adsorbates, a maximum adsorption capacity occurs at the isoelectric point (IEP), where the net charge of the adsorbate becomes zero, and at the lowest solubility. In general, pH and solubility

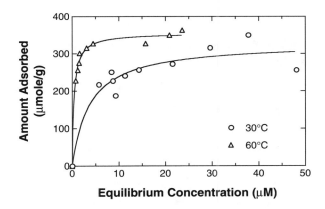

FIGURE 4.8 Adsorption isotherm of chlorhexidine on carbon black at two temperatures. [Graph reconstructed from data by Akaho and Fukumori, *J. Pharm. Sci.,* 90, 1288 (2001).]

influence adsorption jointly. However, solubility affects adsorption more profoundly. If a drug is un-ionized at the experimental pH and is freely soluble, the adsorbate is less adsorbed on an adsorbent than other, ionized drugs, which are much less soluble in water (e.g., hyoscine on magnesium silicate), would be.

4.1.3.4 Temperature

Adsorption is normally exothermic; thus a decrease in temperature will increase the extent of adsorption whereas an increase in temperature will increase the adsorption capacity for chemisorption (normally endothermic). The heat of adsorption, ΔH_{ads}, is defined as the total amount of heat evolved per a specific amount of adsorbate adsorbed on an adsorbent. Because adsorption from an aqueous solution occurs, ΔH_{ads} is small, and thus small changes in temperature do not alter the adsorption process much. The effect of temperature on adsorption can be expressed by:

$$\ln\left(\frac{q_1}{q_2}\right) = \pm\frac{\Delta H_{ads}}{R}\left(\frac{T_2 - T_1}{T_1 T_2}\right) \tag{4.31}$$

where q_1 and q_2 are the amounts adsorbed per gram of adsorbent at temperatures T_1 and T_2, respectively, and the sign is dependent on the endothermic (−) or exothermic (+) nature of the process. Figure 4.8 shows the temperature effect on the adsorption of chlorhexidine on carbon black.

4.2 LIQUID–LIQUID SYSTEMS (EMULSIONS)

An emulsion is a dispersed system where one liquid phase is finely subdivided as globules or droplets and uniformly distributed in the other liquid phase. The practical application of emulsions and their technology applies to pharmaceutical and cosmetic formulations. The usual globular or droplet sizes range from 0.1 to 10 μm.

TABLE 4.3
Surface Tensions (γ_s) and Interfacial Tensions (γ_I)
against Water at 20°C (mN/m)

Liquid	γ_s	γ_I	Liquid	γ_s	γ_I
Benzene	28.9	35.0	CCl_4	26.8	45.0
Chloroform	27.1	32.8	Ethanol	22.3	—
Ethyl ether	17.0	10.7	Glycerin	48.1	—
n-Hexane	18.4	51.1	Mercury	485	375
n-Octane	21.8	50.8	n-Octanol	26.5	8.51
Oleic acid	32.5	15.6	Water	72.9	—

Source: Taken from P. Becher, *Emulsion: Principles and Practices,*
2nd Ed., Reinhold, New York, 1962.

Emulsifying agents should be present in the dispersed system to produce stable emulsions. Liquid–liquid interfacial phenomena and emulsion stability will be discussed.

4.2.1 Liquid–Liquid Interfacial Tension

At the liquid–liquid interface between a hydrocarbon oil and water under mixing, the molecules encounter unbalanced attraction forces, pull inwardly, and contract as other molecules leave the interface for the interior of the bulk liquid. As a result, spherical droplets are formed. Customarily, the boundaries between a liquid and gas and between two liquids are the surface and the interface, respectively. The interfacial tension (or interfacial free energy) is defined as the work required to increase the interfacial area of one liquid phase over the other liquid phase isothermally and reversibly. Moving molecules away from the bulk to the surface or interfacial surface requires work (i.e., an increase in free energy). Water molecules and hydrocarbon oil molecules at the interface are attracted to the bulk water phase as a result of water–water interaction forces (i.e., van der Waals dispersion γ_w^d and hydrogen bonding γ_w^h), to the bulk oil phase due to the oil–oil dispersion forces, γ_o^d, and to the oil–water phase by oil–water interactions, γ_{ow}^d (i.e., dispersion forces). As mentioned in Chapter 3, the oil–water dispersion interactions are related to the geometric mean of the water–water and oil–oil dispersion interactions. The interfacial tension is written as:

$$\gamma_{OW} = \gamma_O^d + \gamma_W^d + \gamma_W^h - 2\gamma_{OW}^d = \gamma_O^d + \gamma_W^d + \gamma_W^h - 2 \times \left(\gamma_O^d \times \gamma_W^d\right)^{1/2} \qquad (4.32)$$

Table 4.3 shows the surface tensions and the interfacial tensions against water at 20°C. Based on the interfacial tension or surface tension measurement, it is possible to calculate the water–water dispersion and hydrogen bonding forces. The value of the surface tension is the sum of the combined dispersion and the hydrogen bonding forces. For example, for the water–n-octane system,

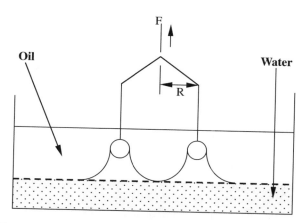

FIGURE 4.9 The ring method for the measurement of interfacial tension.

$$50.8 = 21.8 + 72.8 - 2 \times (\gamma_w^d \times 21.8)^{1/2}$$

$$\gamma_w^d = 22.0 \ \text{mN} / \text{m} \quad \text{and} \quad \gamma_w^h = 72.8 - 22.0 = 50.8 \ \text{mN} / \text{m}$$

The ring method (du Nuoy tensiometer) can be used to measure the interfacial tension as shown in Figure 4.9. The method measures the force required to detach a platinum wire ring from the interface by pulling on the ring. The mathematical relationship between the pulling force and interfacial tension is given by:

$$\gamma_{ow} = \frac{\beta \, F}{4 \, \pi R} \tag{4.33}$$

where F is the pulling force, R is the mean radius of the inner and outer radii of the ring, and β is a correction factor. The correction factor is added to Equation (4.33) to account for the shape of the liquid held up by the ring at the detachment point, which results in nonvertical interfacial tension forces. The contact angle between the ring and the lower liquid must be zero. This can be achieved by careful cleansing and flaming of the ring. The ring should be horizontally balanced on a surface.

The Wilhelmy plate method, as shown in Figure 4.10, is similar to du Nouy's ring method, but it uses a thin mica plate or microscope slide. The plate is suspended from a balance and dips into the liquid. The force, F, required to detach the liquid meniscus surrounding the plate depends on the surface tension or interfacial tension by:

$$F = W_{det} - W = 2 \, (x + y) \, \gamma \cos \theta \tag{4.34a}$$

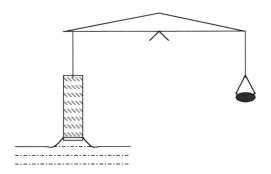

FIGURE 4.10 Wilhelmy plate method.

where W_{det} and W are the weight on the balance at the point of detachment and the weight of the plate, respectively, x and y are the length and thickness of the plate, respectively, and θ is the contact angle. In general, $\theta = 0$ and $x \gg y$. Then Equation (4.34a) becomes:

$$F = 2 \times x \times \gamma \quad \text{or} \quad \gamma = \frac{F}{2\,x} \tag{4.34b}$$

4.2.2 ADSORPTION OF SURFACTANTS AT INTERFACES

Substances having both polar [e.g., $-COO-$, $-SO_4^-$, $-(CH_2CH_2O)_nOH$, or $-OH$] and nonpolar (e.g., $-CH_2-$) regions in their molecular structures are called surface active agents or surfactants. These materials are soluble in both water and hydrocarbon oils. Upon addition of the surfactants into the dispersed system, the polar and nonpolar groups orient themselves in a monomolecular layer facing the polar (i.e., water) and nonpolar solvents (i.e., hydrocarbon oils), respectively. Surfactants diffuse from the solution onto the interface where adsorption and accumulation take place. The interfacial tension must be lowered for the interface to expand. This concept is balanced against the propensity of the bulk phase for complete mixing due to thermal motion. If the interfacial tension is decreased sufficiently, the dispersed system will readily be emulsified.

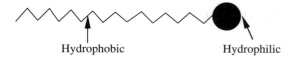

Hydrophobic   Hydrophilic

Surface–active agent

In some instances, it has been observed that the addition of electrolyte and sugars into water increases the interface tension. The adsorbed surfactants migrate away from the interface into the bulk phase (i.e., negative adsorption).

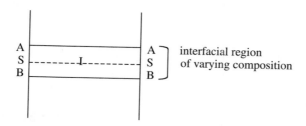

interfacial region
of varying composition

FIGURE 4.11 An interface between two liquid phases in the presence of an adsorbed layer.

As the amount of the surfactant in water is increased, the interface saturates to a point beyond which no further decrease in the interfacial tension occurs. At this concentration, the surfactant molecules start forming micelles (see Section 4.2.6). The inflection point of the interfacial tension vs. concentration curve is called the critical micelle concentration.

Measurement of the interfacial tension can estimate the amount of surfactant present at the interface, called the surface excess. If the bulk liquids (A and B) extend to the interface SS with no compositional change (Figure 4.11), surface excess is present. The total thermodynamic energies of a system and the interface layer I for an open system are given by Equation (4.35a) and Equation (4.35b), respectively:

$$E = TS - PV + \sum n_i \mu_i \qquad (4.35a)$$

$$E^I = TS^I - PV^I + \gamma A + \sum n_i^I \mu_i \qquad (4.35b)$$

where A is the interfacial surface area. Differentiating Equation (4.35b) yields:

$$dE^I = TdS^I + S^I dT - PdV^I - V^I dP + \gamma dA + Ad\gamma + \sum \mu_i dn_i^I + \sum n_i^I d\mu_i \qquad (4.36)$$

From the first and second laws of thermodynamics for an interfacial layer,

$$dE^I = TdS^I - PdV^I + \gamma dA + \sum \mu_i dn_i^I \qquad (4.37)$$

Substituting Equation (4.36) into Equation (4.37) gives:

$$S^I dT - V^I dP + Ad\gamma + \sum n_i^I d\mu_i = 0 \qquad (4.38)$$

At constant temperature and pressure, Equation (4.38) becomes:

$$d\gamma = -\sum \frac{n_i^I}{A} d\mu_i = -\sum \Gamma_i d\mu_i \qquad (4.39)$$

where $\Gamma_i = n_i^l / A$ is the surface excess concentration of the component i in the interface.

For a two-component system (i.e., water and surfactant), Equation (4.39) yields:

$$d\gamma = -\Gamma_w d\mu_w - \Gamma_s d\mu_s \qquad (4.40)$$

where the subscripts w and s denote water and the surfactant, respectively. After careful consideration of the interfacial layer of the adsorbed surfactant, the location of SS for the surface excess concentrations is arbitrarily chosen to be at $\Gamma_w = 0$. Then Equation (4.40) becomes:

$$d\gamma = -\Gamma_s d\mu_s \qquad (4.41)$$

The infinitesimal chemical potential change of the surfactant is given by:

$$d\mu_s = RTd\ln a_s \qquad (4.42)$$

Substituting Equation (4.42) into Equation (4.41) gives:

$$\Gamma_s = -\frac{1}{RT}\frac{d\gamma}{d\ln a_s} = -\frac{a_s}{RT}\frac{d\gamma}{da_s} \qquad (4.43)$$

For dilute solutions, activity a_s may be replaced by the concentration c_s:

$$\Gamma_s = -\frac{c_s}{RT}\frac{d\gamma}{dc_s} \qquad (4.44)$$

Equation (4.44) is the Gibbs energy for the adsorption of surfactant at the interface. Equation (4.44) is applied to systems containing a nonionic surfactant as well as generalized for the consideration of adsorption of ionic substances in order to maintain electroneutrality at the interface:

$$\Gamma_s = -\frac{c_s}{jRT}\frac{d\gamma}{dc_s} \qquad (4.45)$$

where $j = 1$ for nonionic surfactants, ionic surfactants in dilute solutions, and excess inert electrolyte influenced by the electrical shield effect, and $j = 2$ for ionic surfactants in concentrated solutions.

As the concentration of surfactant in an aqueous solution is increased, the surface tension is appreciably lowered even at low concentrations. Further addition leads to a saturated level at the surface where the surfactant molecules are closely packed. Beyond saturation the excess surfactants form micelles within the aqueous solution and there is no longer a change in the surface tension, as illustrated in Figure 4.12.

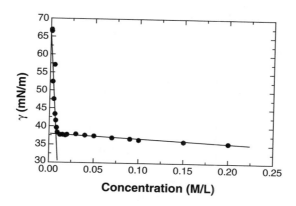

FIGURE 4.12 Plot of surface tension vs. log concentration of sodium lauryl sulfate. [Graph reconstructed from data by Castro et al., *J. Chem. Ed.*, 14, 78, 347 (2001).]

Micelles are formed in order to protect the hydrophobic regions of the amphiphilic surfactant from the aqueous solution. The surface area S occupied by the surfactant molecule can be determined by:

$$S = \frac{1}{N_A \Gamma_s} \qquad (4.46)$$

where N_A is Avogadro's number. Substituting Equation (4.43) into Equation (4.46) yields:

$$S = -\frac{RT}{N_A} \left(\frac{d\gamma}{d\ln c_s} \right)^{-1} \qquad (4.47)$$

Example 4.4

The surface tension vs. concentration of sodium lauryl sulfate is plotted in Figure 4.12. Calculate the area per molecule occupied by the surfactant at the air–water interface at 25°C.

Solution

Solution: From Figure 4.12, the slope ($= d\gamma / \ln c_S$) can be determined:

$$\frac{d\gamma}{d\ln c_s} = \frac{35.52 - 39.66}{(-1.609) - (-4.828)} = -1.286$$

$$S = -\frac{8.314 \times 298}{-1.286 \times 6.023 \times 10^{23}} = 3.195 \times 10^{-21} \quad m^2$$

The surface activity of the surfactant is related to its amphiphilic properties. The longer the hydrocarbon chain of a homologous series of surfactants, the greater the surface activity. On the other hand, the increase in the length of the hydrophilic chain [i.e., $-(CH_2CH_2O)_nOH$] results in a reduced surface activity and hence, increases the surface tension and the critical micelle concentration. Traube's rule states that the addition of a CH_2 group to a homologous series of surfactants lowers the surfactant concentration for the surface tension in dilute aqueous solution and the interfacial tension at the oil–water interface threefold.

4.2.3 SURFACTANTS AND THEORY OF EMULSIFICATION

To prepare homogeneous and stable emulsions from two pure liquids without a continuous mixing, a third material (i.e., emulsifying agent or emulgent) must be incorporated into the system. The materials commonly used as emulsifying agents can be divided into three categories: surface-active, naturally occurring and semi-synthetic, and finely divided solids. In each category, different stabilizing mechanisms are taken advantage of in order to achieve a stable system.

4.2.3.1 Surface-Active Materials

As discussed before, there are two regions (i.e., hydrophilic and hydrophobic) in the surfactant molecules. These surfactants are classified into four main categories depending on the nature of the charge carried by the hydrophilic part of the surfactant: anionic, cationic, nonionic, and ampholytic surfactants. Some common examples of surfactants are listed in Table 4.4.

Anionic surfactants are negatively charged in an aqueous solution (i.e., $-COO^-$, $-OSO_3^-$), and widely used because of their cost and performance. Sodium lauryl sulfate, the main component of which is sodium dodecyl sulfate, is highly soluble in water and commonly used to form oil-in-water (O/W) emulsions. Reacting an alkali hydroxide with a fatty acid (e.g., oleic acid) can produce alkali metal soaps (e.g., sodium oleate). Careful attention must be paid to the pH of the dispersion medium and the presence of multivalent metals (see Section 4.2.5). Alkali earth metal soaps (e.g., calcium oleate) produce stable water-in-oil (W/O) emulsions because of their low water solubility and are produced by reacting oleic acid with calcium hydroxide. Triethanolamine stearate produces stable O/W emulsions *in situ* by reacting triethanolamine in aqueous solution with melted stearic acid at approximately 65°C (e.g., vanishing cream).

Cationic surfactants are positively charged in an aqueous solution (e.g., quaternary ammonium and pyridinium), and expensive. Because of their bactericidal action, they are widely used for other applications such as preservatives, sterilizing contaminated surfaces, and emulsions.

Nonionic surfactants consist of a $-(CH_2CH_2O)_nOH$ or $-OH$ as the hydrophilic group and exhibit a variety of hydrophile–lipophile balances (HLB) which stabilize O/W or W/O emulsions. Unlike anionic and cationic surfactants, nonionic surfactants are useful for oral and parenteral formulations because of their low irritation and toxicity. Based on their neutral nature, they are much less sensitive to changes in the pH of the medium and the presence of electrolytes. The best use of nonionic surfactants is to produce an equally balanced HLB of two nonionic surfactants: one

TABLE 4.4
Surface-Active Agents

Name	Hydrophobic	Hydrophilic

Anionic

Sodium oleate $\qquad CH_3(CH_2)_7CH=CH(CH_2)_7COO^-Na^+$

Sodium palmitate $\qquad CH_3(CH_2)_{14}COO^-Na^+$

Sodium lauryl sulfate $\qquad CH_3(CH_2)_{11}SO_4^-Na^+$

Sodium dioctyl sulfosuccinate

$$CH_3(CH_2)_7O_2CCH_2CH$$
$$\overset{\|}{CH_3(CH_2)_7O_2CSO_3^-Na^+}$$

Cationic

Cetylpyridinium chloride $\qquad CH_3(CH_2)_{14}CH_2N^+C_5H_5Cl^-$

Bezalkonium chloride $\qquad C_8H_{17}(\text{to } C_{18}H_{37})N^+(CH_3)_2Cl^- - CH_2 - C_6H_5$

Hexadecyltrimethyl ammonium chloride $\qquad CH_3(CH_2)_{15} - N^+(CH_3)_3Cl^-$

Nonionic

Polyoxyl 8 dodecyl ether $\qquad C_{12}H_{25} - (OCH_2CH_2)_8OH$

Sorbitan monostearate
(Span 60)

Polyoxyethylene sorbitan monolaurate
(Polysorbate 20 or Tween 20)

sum of w+x+y=20

Ampholytic

n-Dodecyldimethylbetaine $\qquad C_{12}H_{25} - N^+(CH_3)_2 - CH_2COO^-$

Lecithin

$$CH_2 - CO_2 - R_1$$
$$CH_2 - CO_2 - R_2$$
$$CH_2PO_4^- - CH_2CH_2N^+(CH_3)_3$$

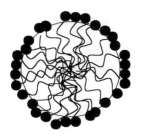

FIGURE 4.13 Monolayer surfactant film.

hydrophilic and one hydrophobic (see Section 4.2.4). Sorbitan esters (Spans) are the products of the esterification of a sorbitan with a fatty acid. Their hydrophilicity comes from the hydroxyl groups of the saturated cyclic ring. They are not soluble in water and used for W/O-type emulsions. Polysorbates (Tweens), on the other hand, are soluble in water since a number of ethylene oxides are adducted by the hydroxyl groups of the sorbitan esters. They are hence used as emulsifying agents for O/W emulsions. In general, both sorbitan esters and polysorbates are used in conjunction to produce a wide range of emulsions (see Section 4.2.4). Fatty alcohol polyoxyethylene ethers are condensation products of fatty alcohols with polyethylene glycol, while fatty acid polyoxyethylene esters are esterification products of fatty acids with polyethylene glycol. They are soluble in water and used in conjunction with auxiliary emulsifying agents (e.g., cetyl and stearyl alcohols) to give O/W emulsions.

Ampholytic surfactants possess both cationic and anionic groups in the same molecule and are dependent on the pH of the medium. Lecithin is used for parenteral emulsions.

Upon mixing two immiscible liquids, one of the two liquids (i.e., the dispersed phase) is subdivided into smaller droplets. The surface area and the interfacial free energy increase, and the system is then thermodynamically unstable. Without continuous mixing, the droplets will be stabilized throughout the dispersion medium by dissolving the surface-active agent. There are several theories for the stabilization of emulsions but a single theory cannot account for the stabilization of all emulsions.

In the *interfacial tension theory,* the adsorption of a surfactant lowers the interfacial tension between two liquids. A reduction in attractive forces of dispersed liquid for its own molecules lowers the interfacial free energy of the system and prevents the coalescence of the droplets or phase separation. Therefore the surfactant facilitates the stable emulsion system of the large interfacial area by breaking up the liquid into smaller droplets. However, the emulsions prepared with sodium dodecyl (lauryl) sulfate separate into two liquids upon standing even though the interfacial tension is reduced. The lowering of the interfacial tension in the stabilization of emulsions is not the only factor we should consider.

The *interfacial film theory* is an extended interfacial tension theory, in which the adsorbed surfactant at the interface surrounds the dispersed droplets forming a coherent thin monolayer film (Figure 4.13). As the droplets approach each other, coalescence is prevented. The stability of the emulsions depends on the characteristics of the monolayer film formed at the interface. Monolayer films are classified as gaseous, condensed, and expanded films.

In *gaseous films,* the adsorbed surfactant molecules separate, do not adhere to each other laterally, and move freely around the interface. Upon collision, the surface pressure, which is the expanding pressure pressed by the monolayer, approaches zero in the form of a rectangular hyperbola when compared to other hard films. One example of a gaseous film is that of sodium dodecyl sulfate. The surfactant is anionic. The charged sulfate head groups repel one another in the aqueous solution as the droplet covered with the film moves closer to another. When the charged film is strongly anchored to the dispersed phase, the emulsion is stable. In the case of sodium dodecyl sulfate, the monolayer film is loosely fixed. The adsorbed molecules move away from the interface and coalescence occurs.

On the other hand, long straight-chain fatty acids, such as palmitic and stearic acids, form a *condensed film.* The molecules of the fatty acid are more tightly packed and the film steeply rises from the compression. The hydrocarbon chains are adjacent to and in cohesive contact with one another. They are able to hold the adsorbed molecules when the chains interlock, where the molecules do not freely move in the interface, leading to a stable emulsion. Similar condensed monolayer films can be formed with cholesterol. *Expanded films* are the intermediate physical states of the monolayer films in the condensed and gaseous films. For example, oleic acid forms a more expanded film than palmitic and stearic acids do. The hydrocarbon chains in oleic acid are less cohesive and less orderly packed in the liquid than those in stearic acid. The unsaturated double bond is polar and has a greater affinity for water. The attractive force between the polar group (i.e., double bond) and water is overcome. In surfactants, the presence of bulky head groups, bulky branched hydrocarbon chains, multiple polar groups, and bent-shaped hydrocarbon chains causes lateral cohesion to be reduced and expanded films to form.

Nonionic surfactants produce the same interfacial films in the interface in a similar fashion as that mentioned above. As expected, there is no charge repulsion contribution to the stability of the emulsion. However, the polar groups of the surfactants (i.e., polyoxyethylene) are hydrated and bulky, causing steric hindrance among droplets and preventing coalescence.

Combinations of surfactants are often used rather than a single surfactant in order to improve emulsion stability. When a water-soluble surfactant (dissolved in an aqueous phase) that produces a gaseous film, such as sodium cetyl sulfate, is mixed with an oil-soluble auxiliary surfactant (dissolved in oil phase), such as cholesterol, a stable *interfacial complex condensed film* will be formed in the interface. This film is flexible, highly viscous, coherent, elastic, and resistant to rupture since the molecules are efficiently packed between each other (Figure 4.14). It produces an interfacial tension much lower than that of the pure component alone. An additional factor contributing to the stability of the emulsion arises from the presence of a surface charge head group, which is responsible for the repulsion among the droplets. When oleyl alcohol replaces cholesterol, sodium cetyl sulfate does not stabilize the emulsion because its *cis* configuration interferes with the formation of the condensed film. Other examples are sodium lauryl sulfate/glycerol monostearate, sodium stearate/cholesterol, and sodium oleate/cetyl alcohol. This approach is also applied to mixed nonionic surfactants. When a mixture of Tween 40 (polyoxyethylene sorbitan monopalmitate) and Span 80 (sorbitan monooleate) is

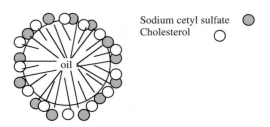

FIGURE 4.14 Interfacial condensed film of two surfactants at the oil–water interface.

used in O/W-type emulsions, the hydrocarbon chains of Tween 40 are positioned in between those of Span 80, leading to an effective van der Waals attraction between the hydrocarbon chains. As mentioned before, steric hindrance, caused by the sorbitan ring and the bulky hydrated polyoxyethylene chains, stabilizes the emulsions.

4.2.3.2 Naturally Occurring and Semisynthetic Materials

Naturally occurring materials, called hydrophilic colloids, are used to stabilize emulsions and form O/W-type emulsions. They include polysaccharides (e.g., acacia, tragacanth, agar, pectin, and alginates) and proteins (e.g., gelatin and casein). The major problems in using polysaccharides are their susceptibility to bacterial or mold growth because of their natural origins and the batch-to-batch (i.e., year-to-year, source-to-source) variation in the quality of the product. Therefore, these materials are frequently used in extemporaneous emulsions. The most commonly used emulsifying agent of this kind is acacia. Unlike other polysaccharides, acacia has low viscosity and creaming is likely to occur. The creaming can be retarded by homogenizing the emulsion. For this reason, a suspending agent (e.g., alginate) is incorporated to retard the rising droplets and provide stability to the emulsion. To counteract the problem of batch-to-batch variation, semisynthetic materials, produced from cellulose (e.g., methylcellulose and sodium carboxymethylcellulose), are used. Because a number of chemical processes have been used to produce these semisynthetic materials, they are not susceptible to bacterial contamination.

Unlike simple synthetic surfactants, these materials do not lower appreciably the interfacial tension but form a *multimolecular layer film* at the oil–water interface (Figure 4.15), in the same manner as particle dispersion (see Section 4.3.1). The multilayer films are strong and elastic and give mechanical protection to coalescence. Both the carboxylic acid groups in the polymer chain of polysaccharides and the amino acid groups in proteins are ionized at a particular pH range, thus creating an electrostatic charge repulsion that further stabilizes emulsions. Emulsions prepared from proteins (e.g., gelatin) often have a watery consistency. Emulsions can also be prepared from a mixture of a surfactant with a natural emulsifying agent, such as tragacanth and Spans and acacia and Tweens.

4.2.3.3 Finely Divided Solids

Finely divided solid particles produce stable emulsions by preferentially wetting one of the phases (Figure 4.16). As more solid particles are lodged at the interface, they

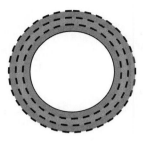

FIGURE 4.15 Multilayer films.

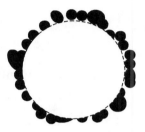

FIGURE 4.16 Adsorption of finely divided particles on liquid droplets.

adhere strongly to each other, forming a stable film at the surface. Examples include clays (e.g., bentonite and magnesium aluminum silicate), colloidal silicone dioxide, aluminum hydroxide, magnesium hydroxide, and carbon black. When clays and aluminum and magnesium hydroxides are preferentially wetted by water, the contact angle is less than 90°, and O/W-type emulsions are formed. The most effective wetting liquid makes up the continuous phase, which is dependent on the volume ratio of the two liquids. For example, bentonite forms W/O-type emulsions when the oil phase volume is much greater than the aqueous phase. One nonpharmaceutical application of finely divided particles is the production of spherical solid beads from organic monomer liquid via the suspension polymerization process in which gelatinous magnesium hydroxide is used to coat the organic droplets to protect them from being agglomerated.

4.2.4 TYPE OF EMULSION AND HLB SYSTEM

The type of emulsion produced when an oil and water are mixed together is determined by:

1. The phase volume ratio present in the emulsion
2. The characteristics of the surfactant

The continuous phase is usually present in the phase with the larger amount of volume. However, even though a phase has a higher volume (over 50%), it can be the dispersed phase. Theoretically, 74% of the total volume can be occupied by the

TABLE 4.5
Classification of Surfactants

HLB	Applications	HLB	Dispersibility in Water
1–3	Antifoaming agents	1–4	Nil
3–6	W/O emulsifying agents	3–6	Poor
7–9	Wetting agents	6–8	Unstable milky dispersion
8–16	O/W emulsifying agents	8–10	Stable milky dispersion
13–15	Detergents	10–13	Translucent dispersion
15–18	Solubilizing agents	13–	Clear solution

TABLE 4.6
HLB Values for Selected Emulsifying Agents

Surfactants	HLB	Surfactants	HLB
Ethyleneglycol distearate	1.5	Propyleneglycol monostearate	3.4
Span 80	4.3	Span 60	4.7
Span 40	6.7	Acacia	8.0
Methyl cellulose	10.5	Triethanolamine oleate	12.0
Triton X-100	13.5	Tween 60	14.9
Tween 80	15.0	Na oleate	18.0
K oleate	20.0	Na lauryl sulfate	40.0

dispersed phase, which is tightly packed with monodispersed spherical droplets. The nature of the surfactant used in the emulsion is important for the type of emulsion. As mentioned in Section 4.2.3, the preferential wetting theory can be applied to other surfactants. The characteristics of both the polar (hydrophilic) and nonpolar (hydrophobic) groups present in the surfactant determine the type of emulsion. When the surfactants are more hydrophilic and polar (e.g., sodium oleate), they form O/W-type emulsions. When they are more hydrophobic and nonpolar (e.g., calcium oleate), they form W/O-type emulsions. Bancroft's rule states that the liquid phase, in which the surfactant is more soluble, forms the continuous phase. This rule can be applied to nonionic surfactants. For example, sorbitan esters (i.e., the Span series), which are soluble in oil, form W/O-type emulsions while polyoxyethylene sorbitan esters (i.e., the polysorbate or Tween series) form O/W-type emulsions.

The hydrophile–lipophile balance (HLB) system is the measure of the surfactant's polarity as well as other physical properties of surfactants and the emulsifying materials. The more lipophilic the surfactant is, the lower the HLB values will be. Table 4.5 empirically classifies and compares surfactants according to their optimum use. Table 4.6 shows the HLB values for a selected group of surfactants. The HLB value of the surfactant or surfactant mixture should be matched with that of the oil or the mixture of oils to ensure a stable emulsion. The required HLB values of a

TABLE 4.7
Required HLB Values for Selected Oils and Waxes

Oils or Waxes	O/W Emulsion	W/O Emulsion
Cottonseed oil	6–7	
Petrolatum	8	
Beeswax	9–11	5
Mineral oil	10–12	5–6
Lanolin, anhydrous	12–14	8
Cetyl alcohol	13–16	

variety of oils can be determined experimentally by evaluating the system with minimum separation (or creaming) phases. The required HLB values of oils for both O/W and W/O emulsions are given in Table 4.7.

There are several empirical expressions to calculate the HLB values based on the chemical structures present. If the hydrophilic region is polyoxyethylene, the HLB value is calculated by:

$$HLB = E / 5 \qquad (4.48)$$

where E is the weight percent of oxyethylene chains in the surfactant. The HLB values of the surfactants based on polyhydric alcohol fatty acid esters may be estimated by:

$$HLB = 20\left(1 - \frac{S}{A}\right) \qquad (4.49)$$

where S is the saponification number of the ester and A is the acid number of the fatty acid. If one cannot obtain the saponification numbers (e.g., beeswax and lanolin derivatives), their HLB values may be calculated by:

$$HLB = (E + P) / 5 \qquad (4.50)$$

where P is the weight percent of the polyhydric alcohol groups (e.g., glycerol or sorbitol) in the material.

It is not easy to match the required HLB value of the oil or the oil mixture with that of a single surfactant to form the most stable emulsion. The appropriate combination of surfactants (usually a binary system) should be chosen. The HLB value of the binary mixture of surfactants A (HLB_A) and B (HLB_B) is calculated by:

$$HLB_{mixture} = f_A \times HLB_A + (1 - f_A) \times HLB_B \qquad (4.51)$$

where f_A is the weight fraction of surfactant A in the mixture.

The selection of the mixture of surfactants should be made after the careful consideration of the interfacial film, as described in Section 4.2.3. In most cases, the most stable emulsions are made from surfactants that contain the same number of hydrocarbon chains (e.g., sorbitan monooleate and polyoxyethylene sorbitan monooleate). The optimum HLB value of the surfactants in the emulsion predicts the smallest mean droplet size that produces a stable emulsion.

Example 4.5

Calculate the amount of emulsifiers to prepare a stable 250 g O/W emulsion of the compositions given below. Two surfactants are used: Span 80 and Tween 60.

Ingredients	Percent	Required HLB
Beeswax	24	9
Mineral oil	14	11
Cetyl alcohol	5	14
Emulsifiers	5	
Purified water q.s.	100	

Solution

First, the required HLB value of the oil phase mixture must be calculated. The total weight percent of the oil phase is 43%. The weight fractions of each oil in the oil phase are 24/43, 14/43, and 5/43 for beeswax, mineral oil, and cetyl alcohol, respectively. The HLB value of the oil mixture is given by:

$$HLB_{oil} = 9 \times \frac{24}{43} + 11 \times \frac{14}{43} + 14 \times \frac{5}{43} = 10.23$$

The HLB_{oil} should be matched with the HLB value of the mixture of two surfactants.

$$HLB_{oil} = HLB_{emulsifiers} = f_A \times HLB_A(\text{Span 80}) + (1 - f_A) \times HLB_B(\text{Tween 60})$$

$$10.23 = f_A \times 4.3 + (1 - f_A) \times 14.9 \qquad f_A = 0.44$$

The amount of Span 80 is: $250 \text{ g} \times 0.05 \times 0.44 = 5.5 \text{ g}$

The amount of Tween 60 is: $250 \text{ g} \times 0.05 \times 0.56 = 7.0 \text{ g}$

Another quantitative expression can be used to account for the contributions of the hydrophilic and hydrophobic groups to the HLB value of surfactant:

$$HLB = \sum(\text{hydrophilic group number}) - \sum(\text{hydrophobic group number}) + 7 \quad (4.52)$$

TABLE 4.8
Group Contributions to HLB Values

Hydrophilic Groups	Group Number	Hydrophobic Groups	Group Number
$-SO_4^-Na^+$	38.7	$-CH-$	
$-COO^-K^+$	21.1	$-CH_2-$	-0.475
$-COO^-Na^+$	19.1	$-CH_3$	
Tertiary amine N	9.4	$=CH-$	
Ester (sorbitan)	6.8		
$-COOH$	2.1		
Hydroxyl	1.9		
Hydroxyl (sorbitan)	0.5		

Source: Taken from Davies and Rideal, *Interfacial Phenomena,* Academic Press, New York, 1961, pp. 371–378.

Table 4.8 gives the group numbers. However, Equation (4.52) is not self-consistent and does not predict the HLB of nonionic surfactants containing polyoxyethylene fatty alcohol.

The properties and uses of surfactants are strongly dependent on the HLB (as described above), the oil-water partition coefficient (K_{ow}), and the solubility parameter. The relationship between HLB and K_{ow} of nonionic surfactants has been examined and is expressed by:

$$HLB = a + b \log K_{ow} \tag{4.53}$$

where a and b are the constants. Figure 4.17 shows that a change in the hydrocarbon moiety (e.g., octoxynol vs. nonoxynol) affects the relationship between the HLB and K_{ow} far more than a change in the number of oxyethylene units in the homologue series. However, different surfactant categories show different lines that are far apart.

Similarly, a linear relationship between the HLB and the overall solubility parameter (δ_o) has been investigated by:

$$HLB = a + b\,\delta_o \tag{4.54}$$

As observed in the relation between the HLB and K_{ow}, there is an excellent linear relation within the same homologous series, but different categories of surfactants give different lines with surprisingly similar slopes (Figure 4.18).

After choosing the combination of surfactants, it is up to the formulator to determine the specific amounts of surfactants needed in the mixture. Based on creaming or phase separation through a series of trial and error, the surfactant

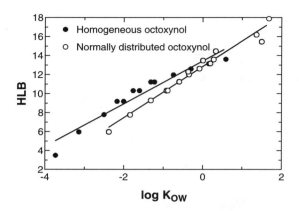

FIGURE 4.17 Relationship between the HLB and K_{OW}. [Graph reconstructed from data by H. Schot, *J. Pharm. Sci.*, 84, 1215 (1995)]

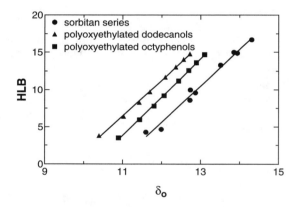

FIGURE 4.18 Relation between the HLB and the overall solubility parameter (δ_o). [Graph reconstructed from H. Scott, *J. Pharm. Sci.*, 73, 790 (1984).]

concentration is adjusted to produce a stable emulsion system. The quantity of surfactant in the mixture, M_S, is calculated by:

$$M_S = \frac{6(\rho_s / \rho)}{10 - 0.5 \, RHLB} + \frac{4Q}{1000} \tag{4.55}$$

where ρ and ρ_S are the density of the dispersed phase and the surfactant mixture, respectively, and Q is the percent of the continuous phase.

The HLB system used above does not take into consideration the temperature effects. Upon heating, an O/W emulsion prepared with nonionic surfactants inverts to a W/O emulsion because the hydrogen bondings in the polyoxyethylene groups are broken, and the HLB value of the surfactant becomes smaller. The higher the phase inversion temperature (PIT), the slower the rate of globule coalescence and the more stable the emulsion.

4.2.5 INSTABILITY OF EMULSIONS

Stable emulsions maintain the initial characteristics of the droplets. With the aid of emulsifying agents, they are uniformly distributed throughout the dispersed phase. However, they can be destabilized by various factors.

Upon standing, an emulsion may cream up or settle down, according to Stoke's law (Section 4.3.3.), into two layers. One layer has a more concentrated disperse phase than the other. Even though *creaming* or *settling* does not lead to serious instability, the creamed or settled emulsion product is not pharmaceutically or cosmetically elegant, and the patient may get an inadequate dose. In addition, flocculation and/or coalescence can occur because the concentrated droplets are too close to each other. The creaming or settling is decreased by reducing the droplet size and increasing the viscosity of the dispersion. When the emulsion is homogenized, the droplet size decreases and the number of droplets and viscosity of the emulsion increase. The addition of hydrocolloids increases the viscosity of the disperse phase, forming a viscous barrier network around the droplets. Thus, it is possible to obtain stable emulsions well below the optimum HLB value when using very small droplets and thickening agents. The creamed or settled emulsion is easily redispersed by simple shaking.

Flocculation of droplets occurs in the secondary minimum according to the DLVO (Deryagin, Landau, Verwey and Overbeek) theory (see Section 4.3.3). The flocs maintain their own individual identity and act together in conjunction, increasing the rate of creaming or sedimentation. The flocculated emulsion is again easily redispersed by shaking. As mentioned before, flocculation may lead to coalescence. When there is a high charge density on the droplets, the degree of flocculation is reduced.

The *coalescence* or complete separation of an emulsion occurs when two particles approach each other and no barrier exists between them. This process is avoided by producing a strong condensed mixed monolayer film or a multilayer coating around the droplets. A stable W/O emulsion is produced from surfactants or a mixture of surfactants that have very long hydrocarbon chains.

Addition of chemicals without careful consideration may break an emulsion. An emulsion prepared with ionic surfactants should not be mixed with chemically incompatible materials of opposite charge. The pH of the emulsion should be alkaline if the emulsion is made with alkali soaps. At an acidic pH, the carboxylate ion of the soap is converted to the carboxylic acid, which is not water-soluble and an emulsifying agent. An alkali-soap stabilized O/W-type emulsion may be inverted to a W/O-type emulsion by adding a divalent electrolyte. The carboxylate ion reacts with the divalent electrolyte to form an alkali earth soap that is an oil-soluble surfactant. Addition of a common electrolyte to an emulsion prepared with ionic surfactants suppresses the ionization according to the Le Chatelier rule (e.g., ammonium oleate and ammonium chloride). The presence of noninteractive electrolytes in the emulsions alters the polar nature of the interfacial film. For example, the

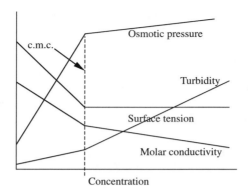

FIGURE 4.19 Physicochemical characteristics of surfactant solutions.

addition of NaCl to an O/W emulsion may dehydrate (or salt out) the monolayer film concentration lowering the HLB value of the surfactant and precipitating the surfactant.

4.2.6 MICELLIZATION AND SOLUBILIZATION

In dilute aqueous solutions, surfactants have normal electrolyte or solute characteristics and are formed at the interface. As the surfactant concentration increases beyond the well-defined concentrations (i.e., critical micelle concentration, c.m.c.), the surfactant molecules become more organized aggregates and form micelles. At the c.m.c., the physicochemical characteristics of the system (osmotic pressure, turbidity, surface tension, and electrical conductivity) are suddenly changed, as shown in Figure 4.19.

This behavior is expected since the hydrophobic chains move away from the water and orient themselves towards the core of the micelle. This increases the movement of the hydrocarbon chains within the core. As a result, the minimum free energy is achieved from the intermolecular attraction between the lipophilic chains. Ionic or polar groups sufficiently compensate for the disturbance of the water–water hydrogen bondings with water–solute hydrogen bondings. Water molecules structurally surround the hydrophobic region of the surfactant molecule, causing a large decrease in the entropy change. Meanwhile the polar hydrophilic groups form hydrogen bondings. This withdrawal of the lipophilic groups from the aqueous phase is due to strong attractive water–water interactions as a result of hydrogen bonding. It is often known as the *hydrophobic effect*.

As the length of the hydrocarbon chain increases, it is thermodynamically more favorable, and the molecule forms a micelle. As the length of the hydrophobic chain increases by an additional CH_2 group, the c.m.c. of the ionic surfactants is reduced to less than half. Nonionic surfactants are able to form micelles at much lower concentrations than ionic surfactants do because of the absence of the electrostatic repulsion between ionic head groups. Likewise, the addition of a simple electrolyte lowers the electrostatic repulsion between the ionic head groups, and micelle formation occurs at

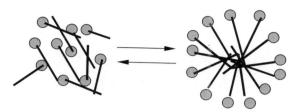

FIGURE 4.20 Equilibrium between dissociated monomers and a micelle.

lower concentrations. An increase in the length of the hydrophilic chain length [e.g., $-OCH_2CH_2-$] increases the c.m.c. due to the greater hydrophilicity of the surfactant. As organic molecules are added to the micelle solution, the outer region of the micelle is altered, depending on the organic materials. Medium chain-length alcohols, which have a polar nature, situate around the shell of the micelle lowering the electrostatic repulsion and steric hindrance, as well as the c.m.c.

Two current approaches to explain the process of micellization are: law of mass action and phase separation. In the law of mass action, micellization is treated as an equilibrium process between the progressive association and dissociation of the monomers (Figure 4.20). In phase separation, two phases (i.e., surfactant monomers in aqueous phase and micelles) are in equilibrium above the c.m.c. In this model, micellization takes place as a one-step process.

Micellization using an anionic surfactant (e.g., M^+R^-) may be described as:

$$aM^+ + bR^- \rightleftharpoons [M_aR_b]^n \qquad (4.56)$$

where a and b are the numbers of the surfactant ions and their counterions, respectively, to form a negatively charged micelle, and n is the net charge ($= a - b$). From the law of mass–action, the equilibrium constant, $K_{micelle}$, is defined as:

$$K_{micelle} = \frac{[M_aR_b]^n}{[M^+]^a[R^-]^b} \qquad (4.57)$$

The standard state of free energy change of micellization, $\Delta G^\circ_{micelle}$, is the standard free energy change per one mole of surfactant.

$$\Delta G^\circ_{micelle} = \frac{\Delta G^\circ}{b} = -\frac{RT}{b} \ln K_{micelle} \qquad (4.58)$$

Substituting Equation (4.57) into Equation (4.58) yields:

$$\Delta G^\circ_{micelle} = -\frac{RT}{b} \ln \frac{[M_aR_b]^n}{[M^+]^a[R^-]^b} = -\frac{RT}{b} \left[n \ln[M_aR_b] - a \ln[M^+] - b \ln[R^-] \right] \qquad (4.59)$$

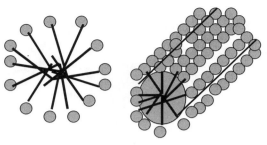

Spherical micelle   Cylindrical micelle

FIGURE 4.21 Micellar structures.

At the c.m.c., $[M^+] = [R^-]$ and applying the phase-separation theory, in which micellization is an abrupt process, gives $n \ln[M_a R_b] = 0$. Then,

$$\Delta G^o_{micelle} = RT\left(1 + \frac{a}{b}\right) \ln(c.m.c.) \qquad (4.60)$$

For nonionic surfactants, $a = 0$ and Equation (4.60) becomes:

$$\Delta G^o_{micelle} = RT \ln(c.m.c.) \qquad (4.61)$$

According to the Maxwell relationship [Equation (1.105)],

$$\Delta S^o_{micelle} = -\frac{\partial \Delta G^o_{micelle}}{\partial T} = -RT \frac{d \ln(c.m.c.)}{dT} - R \ln(c.m.c.) \qquad (4.62)$$

and $\qquad \Delta H^o_{micelle} = \Delta G^o_{micelle} + T\Delta S^o_{micelle} = -RT^2 \frac{d \ln(c.m.c.)}{dT} \qquad (4.63)$

The increase in temperature increases the thermal motion of the surfactants, and micelles are formed at higher concentrations, even though this is not always the case. As a result, $d \ln(c.m.c.)/dT > 0$; the entropy change in Equation (4.62) has a negative value. During the micellization process, a negative entropy change is expected to occur as the water molecules form structured clusters around the hydrophobic parts. As indicated in Equation (4.63), the micellization process is exothermic, even though this is not universal.

The exact shapes of the micelles are unknown, and this subject is open for discussion. Possible micellar structures could be spherical or nearly spherical over a wide range of concentrations not too far from the c.m.c. In a highly concentrated solution, the micellar shape is elongated and forms larger, nonspherical (i.e., cylindrical or lamellar) liquid structures, as illustrated in Figure 4.21. The size of a spherical micelle is determined by the length of the hydrocarbon chain in the

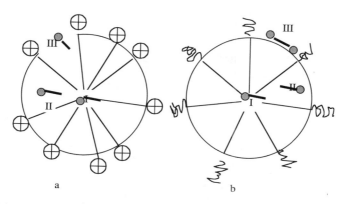

FIGURE 4.22 Sites of solubilization in (a) ionic and (b) nonionic micelles.

surfactant. When micelles are approximately monodispersed, monodispersed latex particles result from the emulsion polymerization. Water may be bound if it penetrates into a few CH_2 groups located along the hydrocarbon chains on the surface of the micelle. For example, a micelle surface prepared with dodecyl sulfate consists of 1/3 polar sulfate groups and 2/3 hydrocarbons. This arrangement of micellar structure (interior and outer regions) may influence the solubilization of otherwise insoluble compounds.

The micellar core is essentially similar to liquid paraffin, which is capable of solubilizing otherwise insoluble organic compounds by bringing them into the interior of the micelles. For example, phenol, whose solubility in water is about 2%, can be dissolved more than 20% in a micellar solution prepared with sodium oleate. The site of solubilization within the micelle extends from the outer surface up to the deep core and results from the balance of polar and nonpolar interactions between the surfactant and the solubilisate. Figure 4.22 shows a schematic representation of the solubilization sites in ionic and nonionic micelles. Nonpolar substances (e.g., aliphatic hydrocarbons) are easily solubilized in the lipophilic deep center of the micelle (I in Figure 4.22a). In this case, the solubilization capacity of the substances increases with increasing alkyl chain length. If water-insoluble substances have polar groups, the location of the molecule depends on the strength of the polar group. As already mentioned, a water-insoluble material with intermediate polar groups can be positioned in the vicinity of the shell side of the micelle or deep inside the micelle if there is bound water within a few CH_2 groups in the hydrocarbon chains on the surface (III in Figure 4.22a). Polar materials are solubilized in the polyoxyethylene shell (known as the palisade layer) of the nonionic surfactants (III in Figure 4.22b). An increase in the polyoxyethylene chain length of a nonionic surfactant leads to the solubilization of fewer molecules per micelle and increases the total amount solubilized per mole of surfactant.

The major benefit of the solubilization principle is the increased water solubility of water-insoluble drugs such as phenolic compounds, iodine, steroids, and vitamins. The solubilization of water-insoluble materials in micelles may have some effects on drug activity and absorption. In addition, drugs in the micelles may prefer to stay

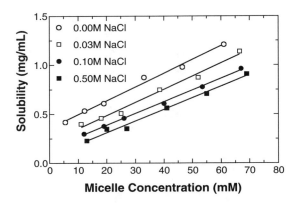

FIGURE 4.23 The effect of NaCl and micelle concentrations on the solubilization of gliclazide by sodium dodecyl sulfate. [Graph reconstructed from data by Alkhamis et al., *J. Pharm. Sci.*, 92, 839 (2003).]

inside the micelles rather than be absorbed in the mucous membranes. Figure 4.23 shows the effect of micellar concentration on the solubilization of gliclazide by sodium dodecyl sulfate (SDS).

Solubilization of hydrolyzable drugs in micelles retards the rate of hydrolysis since the nonpolar chains, containing the hydrolyzable bonds, are situated in the deep core of a micelle. Anionic micelles repel the incoming OH^- and hold the H^+ in the vicinity of the surface avoiding further penetration of H^+ into the micelle. If micelles are formed by self-emulsifying drugs such as penicillin G, they are reportedly more stable than their simple solutions under the same conditions of pH and ionic strength.

The maximum additive concentration (MAC) is defined as the maximum amount of solubilisate, at a given concentration of surfactant, that produces a clear solution. Different amounts of solubilisates, in ascending order, are added to a series of vials containing the known concentration of surfactant and mixed until equilibrium is reached. The maximum concentration of solubilisate that forms a clear solution is then determined visually. This same procedure can be repeated for the different concentrations of surfactant in a known amount of solubilisate in order to determine the optimum concentration of surfactant (Figure 4.24). Based on this information, one can construct a ternary phase diagram that describes the effects of three constituents (i.e., solubilisate, surfactant, and water) on the micelle system. Note that unwanted phase transitions can be avoided by ignoring the formulation compositions near the boundary. In general, the MAC increases with an increase in temperature. This may be due to the combination of the increase of solubilisate solubility in the aqueous phase and the micellar phase rather than an increased solubilization by the micelles alone.

4.2.7 MICROEMULSIONS

When two immiscible liquids are brought into contact, emulsification or solubilization can occur depending on the relative proportion of oil to surfactant. A lower

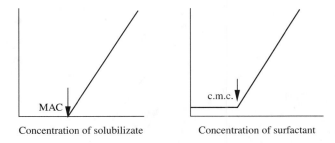

FIGURE 4.24 Determination of the maximum additive concentration.

proportion of surfactant is required for emulsification (i.e., O/W), higher for solu-bilization. When the aggregated size of droplets is below 7.5 nm, micelles form because dispersed molecules outnumber surfactant molecules in the aggregated structure of droplets in the interface. When the ratio of surfactant to dispersed phase decreases, in the droplet size of 10 to 200 nm, the surfactant molecules outnumber the dispersed phase and microemulsions are likely to form. A microemulsion is a stable, transparent, and monodisperse system in which the volume fraction of the dispersed phase ranges from 20 to 80%. Microemulsions are also known as swollen micellar systems. Microemulsions are a transition state between micelles and ordi-nary emulsions (macroemulsions). However, the distinction between swollen micelles and small-droplet emulsions is debatable. A microemulsion consists of four components: oil, water, surfactant, and a cosurfactant. All single ionic surfactants and most single nonionic surfactants cannot lower the interfacial tension between oil and water to zero. As a result, a cosurfactant is required. Normally, O/W micro-emulsions require less amount of cosurfactant than W/O microemulsions do. Typi-cally, microemulsions are produced by 10 to 70% water, 10 to 70% oil, and 5 to 40% surfactant including a cosurfactant. Figure 4.25 shows the pseudo-ternary phase diagram of oil, water, and the mixture of surfactants and cosurfactant.

4.3 SOLID–LIQUID SYSTEMS (SUSPENSIONS)

Suspensions are coarse dispersions of finely divided solids in a liquid. The solid particles have a mean particle size greater than 0.1 μm in diameter. Pharmaceutical suspensions are administered orally, topically, and parenterally and should avoid the following problems: sedimentation, caking, flocculation, and particle growth. Phys-icochemical principles in the solid/liquid interface will be discussed in this section as they pertain to the preparation of good pharmaceutical suspensions.

4.3.1 WETTING AND WETTING AGENTS

One of the problems faced in formulating suspensions is that finely divided particles are not easily wetted in water. This may be the result of the hydrophobic nature of the drugs and/or entrapped gases (i.e., air). The wetting process is the displacement of one fluid by another from the solid surface. When wetting solids, the entrapped

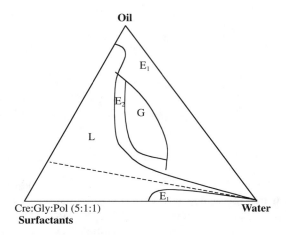

FIGURE 4.25 Three-component phase diagram for the solubilization. Cre, Cremophor RH 40; Gly, glyceride; Pol, poloxamer 124; L, isotropic microemulsion; G, gel; E_1, crude O/W emulsion; E_2, W/O emulsion. [Graph reconstructed from data by Kim et al. *Pharm. Res.,* 18, 454 (2002).]

air is displaced by water at the particle surfaces. The wettability of the particle is measured by the contact angle of the particle with water.

Suppose that water is not originally in contact with the solid surface and adheres to it (i.e., adhesional wetting). When the drop of water is laid on a flat, smooth, solid surface, three forces are at work: surface tension between the solid and air, γ_{SA}; interfacial tension between the solid and water, γ_{SW}; and surface tension between water and air, γ_{WA}. Incorporating only the horizontal components of these forces leads to:

$$\gamma_{SA} = \gamma_{SW} + \gamma_{WA}\cos\theta \qquad (4.64)$$

where θ is called the contact angle. Equation (4.64) is called Young's equation. Figure 4.26 shows the water drop in contact with a solid surface.

The adhesion work, W^a_{SW}, is the work required to separate a liquid/solid interface into a solid/air and a liquid/air interface. It is also known as the Dupre equation:

$$W^a_{SW} = -\Delta G_{adhesion} / A = \gamma_{SA} + \gamma_{WA} - \gamma_{SW} \qquad (4.65)$$

where A is the solid surface area. Substituting Equation (4.64) into Equation (4.65) yields the Young–Dupre equation:

$$W^a_{SW} = \gamma_{WA}(1+\cos\theta) \qquad (4.66)$$

When the attractive forces between the solid and water are equal to or greater than the forces between water molecules, θ is equal to 0°, $W^a_{SW} = 2\gamma_{WA}$, and the

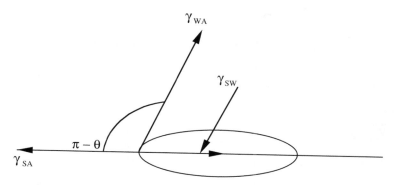

FIGURE 4.26 Water drops on a solid surface.

water drop will be completely spread or wetted on the solid surface. If θ is equal to 180°, no wetting occurs on the solid surface. The solid surface is partially wetted at $0° < \theta < 180°$, and water coheres to other water molecules rather than adhering to the solid.

Suppose that the solid is originally not in contact with water but is immersed completely (i.e., immersional wetting). In this case, the water penetrates the capillaries in the solid. The energy change for immersional wetting, called the adhesion tension, is given by:

$$W_{SW}^{i} = -\Delta G_{immersion} / A = \gamma_{SA} - \gamma_{SW} \tag{4.67}$$

Substituting Equation (4.64) into Equation (4.67) gives:

$$W_{SW}^{i} = \gamma_{WA} \cos \theta \tag{4.68}$$

When $\theta < 90°$, the adhesion tension is positive, and the penetration of water into the capillaries under no applied pressure becomes spontaneous. However, if $\theta > 90°$, work would be needed in order to immerse the solid in water.

Once the solid is immersed in water, the process of spreading water over the surface of the solid (i.e., spreading wetting) is an important one. The water already in contact with the solid surface spreads so that the interfacial area between the solid and water increases and that between the solid and air decreases. The energy change for a spreading wetting is often called the spreading coefficient and given by:

$$W_{SW}^{s} = -\Delta G_{spreading} / A = \gamma_{SA} - (\gamma_{SW} + \gamma_{WA}) \tag{4.69}$$

Substituting Equation (4.64) into Equation (4.69) leads to:

$$W_{SW}^{s} = \gamma_{WA} (\cos \theta - 1) \tag{4.70}$$

TABLE 4.9
Contact Angles of Selected Pharmaceutical Powders

Material	Contact Angle (degrees)	Material	Contact Angle (degrees)
Acetaminophen	59	Aspirin	77
Caffeine	43	Chloramphenicol	59
Lactose	30	Mg stearate	121
Phenacetin	78	Phenobarbital	86
Prednisolone	43	Prednisone	63
Salicylic acid	103	Sodium chloride	28
Sodium stearate	84	Stearic acid	98
Sulfadiazine	71	Sulfathiazole	53
Theophylline	48	Vinylbarbital	71

Source: C. F. Lerk et al., *J. Pharm. Sci.,* 65, 843 (1976) and 66, 1480 (1977).

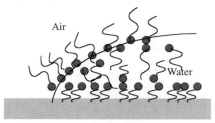

Hydrophobic Surface

FIGURE 4.27 Wetting a hydrophobic solid surface with the aid of a wetting agent.

   In Equation (4.70), the spreading of water over a smooth solid surface is spontaneous only for $\theta = 0°$. However, when the solid surface is rough, even for small contact angles (i.e., $\theta > 0°$), the spreading may occur.
   Table 4.9 shows the contact angles of various pharmaceutical materials in water. Some powders, such as chloramphenicol palmitate, magnesium stearate, phenylbutazone, and salicylic acid, are thermodynamically unfavorable for wetting. As shown in Equation (4.70), the contact angle must be close to 0°C for water to wet a solid powder. One approach to enhance the wettability of a solid in water is the use of surface-active agents (or surfactants), also known as wetting agents, in suspensions. Surfactants decrease the water/air surface tension (γ_{WA}) and adsorb on the solid surface, lowering the solid/water interfacial tension (γ_{SW}), as shown in Figure 4.27. Both effects either increase the value of $\cos\theta$ or lower the contact angle and thus improve the dispersion of the solid powder. The most widely used wetting agents are surfactants, hydrophilic colloids, and solvents.

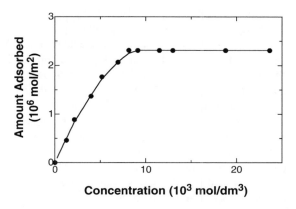

FIGURE 4.28 Typical adsorption isotherms of ionic surfactants on a solid surface. [Graph reconstructed from data by Day et al., *Adv. Chem. Ser.,* 79, 135 (1968).]

4.3.1.1 Surfactants

Surfactants have the property of adsorbing strongly on hydrophobic particle surfaces. They consist of a hydrophilic polar head such as $-(CH_2CH_2O)_nOH$, $-OSO_2^-Na^+$, $-N^+(CH_3)_2(CH_2)_2SO_3^-$ and a hydrophobic tail (i.e., linear or branched hydrocarbon chain). The hydrophobic tail adsorbs on the hydrophobic particle surfaces while the hydrophilic head sticks out toward water. The particles are thus hydrated. Surfactants with a hydrophilic/lipophilic balance (HLB) (see Section 4.2) value close to 7 to 9 are well suited as wetting agents. These surfactants form monolayers on the solid surface.

The characteristics of the solid surface play an important role in the adsorption of surfactants in the solid/water interface. The surfaces are either hydrophilic or hydrophobic. At low coverage, attractive interactions may occur between hydrophobic solid surfaces and hydrophobic surfactant chains, resulting in enhanced adsorption. In high surfactant-adsorbed layers, the hydrophobic chains of the surfactant are adjacent to each other and may cluster together due to the hydrophobic interactions (among surfactants), resulting in enhanced adsorption. The surface charge of the solid is also an important parameter since the adsorption of ionic surfactants is highly dependent on the nature of the charge, the degree of the charge density, and the concentrations. In this case, chemisorption may occur. For instance, the anionic groups in the surfactants may be exchanged with the anionic ions on the solid surface and then be able to form chemical linkages with the cationic groups on the solid surface.

In general, the adsorption of ionic surfactants follows the Langmuir isotherm, as discussed in Section 4.1. The adsorption of the surfactants onto the solid surfaces is dependent on the orientation and the packing efficiency of the solid surfaces. The onset of the adsorption plateau may occur at the critical micelle concentration (c.m.c.) of the surfactant in water, as shown in Figure 4.28. If the adsorption isotherm has a steep inflection point, two stages of adsorption processes may be considered. At low coverage, the hydrophobic chain and the hydrophobic surface interact and thus parallel adsorption of the surfactant on the surface takes place. At high coverage, only the hydrophobic chain interactions may be dominant, and thus a vertical arrangement of the surfactants on the surface may be seen. However, if the surfactants are ionic, the presence of salts (e.g., NaCl) in water may alter the adsorption isotherm. For example, the anionic surfactants (e.g., sodium lauryl sulfate, SLS) reach the equilibrium adsorption at a much smaller concentration because the presence of the electrolyte changes the c.m.c. of the ionic surfactants. When the surfactants have opposite charges on the solid surfaces, low coverage adsorption may take place by a simple exchange of the surfactant ions with the mobile ions of the solid surface. As the coverage increases, the hydrophobic chain interactions increase and thus enhance the adsorption process. In this case, the length of the hydrophobic chain of the surfactants is longer, causing the adsorption of the surfactants to be higher. When the solid surface is fully occupied with ionic surfactants, the total net charge on the solid surface will be zero. Beyond this, adsorption is hindered by the Coulombic forces imposed on the adsorbed ionic surfactants and the surfactants waiting to be adsorbed. Adsorption of such ionic surfactants onto the solid surface alters the charge property of the solid surface; this should be considered when dealing with a controlled flocculation process (see Section 4.3.2).

No Coulombic forces are present between the solid surfaces and the nonionic surfactants. Adsorption of the nonionic surfactants onto the solid surface may depend on the nature of the surface — polar vs. nonpolar. If the solid surface is nonpolar, the adsorption isotherm is illustrated in Figure 4.29. At low concentrations, nonionic surfactants may adsorb parallel to the solid surface (A) until a saturated monolayer (B) is formed. Up to this point, the Langmuir isotherm is satisfied. If there is more adsorption beyond this point, the polar head groups start to depart from the hydrophobic surface (C). At higher concentrations, the hydrophobic chain stands vertically on the hydrophobic surface while the polar head groups are projected towards the water (D). When the solid surface is polar, the polar head groups of the surfactants start to orient themselves towards the polar surfaces. At higher surfactant concentrations, the surfactants align themselves vertically with the hydrophobic tail groups projecting towards water. A further increase in the surfactant concentrations intensifies the vertically aligned hydrophobic chain interactions, and this leads to enhanced adsorption (E). In this case, adsorption beyond a monolayer may be possible. One may observe a sharp increase in the adsorption near the c.m.c. In practice, the adsorption of nonionic surfactants is not well understood, and many ambiguities exist. A number of surfactants (e.g., ionic and nonionic) are described in Section 4.2.3.

4.3.1.2 Hydrocolloids

Water-soluble polymers coat hydrophobic solid surfaces with multilayers and thus render the solid hydrophilic (i.e., wetting). The number of adsorbed chains (or the amount of polymer adsorbed) per surface site (or unit weight of adsorbent) is related to the volume fraction of segments in each layer. As the length of the chains increases,

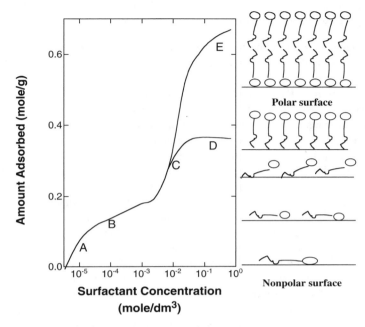

FIGURE 4.29 Adsorption isotherms of nonionic surfactants on the polar and nonpolar solid surfaces. [Graph reconstructed from data by T. F. Tadros, *Solid/Liquid Dispersions,* Academic Press, New York, 1987.]

the adsorbed amount increases (i.e., high affinity). The adsorbed amount may be indicative of the extent of the adsorbed layer even though it is not possible to directly verify the thickness of the adsorbed layer. The thickness varies with the amount adsorbed and the molecular weight of the polymer. The thickness of the adsorbed layer is not dependent on the molecular weight of polymer if the amount adsorbed is less than 0.7 mg/m^2. If the amount adsorbed is greater than 0.8 mg/m^2, the thickness will increase as the amount adsorbed and the molecular weight increase. The dependence of the thickness on the molecular weight is proportional to $r^{0.8}$, where r is the length of the chains. When ionic polymers are used to wet the hydrophobic solid surface, the increase in the ionic strength of water enhances the adsorption due to a decrease in the electrostatic repulsions of the ionic chains. In addition, the layer may be dense and compressed by the charged hydrocolloids. A number of hydrocolloids used as wetting agents as well as suspending agents are listed in Section 4.2.3.

4.3.1.3 Solvents

Solid particles are not readily wettable when air is entrapped because the contact angle widens. Hydroscopic (or water-miscible) materials such as glycerin, alcohol, and glycol penetrate the spaces occupied by air and displace it. During the dispersion process, the hydroscopic materials separate the agglomerates and coat the particles so that water can flow into and wet the particles.

4.3.2 ELECTRICAL DOUBLE LAYER AND STABILIZATION OF COLLOIDAL PARTICLES

Upon contact with an aqueous medium, most materials acquire a surface electric charge. A variety of processes have charging mechanisms, including ion adsorption, ionization, and ion dissolution.

Ion adsorption: Positively or negatively charged ions can be adsorbed on the solid surface. Most surfaces are negatively charged because positive ions are more hydrated than negative ones and thus stay in the bulk aqueous medium. Therefore, the negative ions, which are less hydrated and more polarized, have a tendency to be adsorbed. In the case of pure water, hydroxyl ions are preferentially adsorbed. When negatively charged ions are adsorbed and the suspended particles are subjected to an electrical field, the particles move toward the positively charged electrode. Thus, the negatively charged ions are adsorbed onto the particles. Surfactants can be used to wet the particles. In this case, the ionic nature of the surfactants will determine the net surface charge as they are adsorbed. Hydrophobic surfaces adsorb more readily than hydrated ones. When the surfaces are charged, counter ions are preferentially adsorbed, and this may lead to a charge reversal if the amount of adsorbed counter ions is more than the amount required to neutralize the charge.

Ionization: Charges on the particles of acidic and basic drugs, proteins and amino acids can be acquired by the ionization of the carboxylic acid and amine groups to give $-COO^-$ and $-NH_3^+$, respectively. In these cases, the net charge depends on the pH of the solution and the pK_a of the chemical groups in the particle. At pH $<< pK_a$, acidic drugs are neutrally charged because of the unionization of the drugs while basic drugs are fully positively charged. Proteins consisting of both acidic and basic groups are ionized at a specific pH. When the net charge is zero, this pH is called the isoelectric point, and a zwitterion forms. At the isoelectric point, proteins are least soluble in water and are easily precipitated by the presence of water-soluble salts.

Ion dissolution: This is less common for pharmaceutical cases. Ionic charges are acquired by the unequal dissolution of the oppositely charged ions due to the excessive presence of ions in a solution. The concentrations of the excessive ions determine the electrical potential at the surface (i.e., potential determining ions).

4.3.2.1 The Electrical Double Layer

Suppose a negatively charged solid particle is in contact with water containing electrolytes. The negative charge of the particle surface affects the distribution of ions in an aqueous solution. Opposite charge ions (i.e., positive ions in this case) to the surface charge are attracted to and held firmly by the negatively charged surface. Since the electric forces are strong enough to overcome the thermal motion, negatively charged ions are repelled from the charged surface. The remaining ions in solution move freely as a result of thermal motion. The resultant charge distribution (i.e., electric double layer), as shown in Figure 4.30, consists of the fixed charged surface and the diffuse layer that has a net charge equal to that of the fixed layer but of opposite sign.

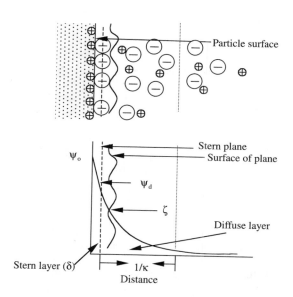

FIGURE 4.30 Schematic representation of the electrical double layer with a potential change in the distance from a solid surface.

Quantitative treatment of the electrical double layer is rather complicated and poses unresolved problems. According to the theory of Gouy, Chapman, and Stern, the two parts of the electrical double layer are separated by a plane (i.e., Stern plane) that is located on the center of the hydrated ions at the surface. There is a difference in potential within the double layer due to the electrical charges. The potential changes from the surface potential, ψ_o, to the Stern potential, ψ_d, and decays gradually from ψ_d to zero in the diffuse double layer. A plane of shear is also present between the fixed ions and the electrolyte solution. The location of the plane of shear cannot be singled out since a certain amount of solvent will be bound to the charged surface and the ions and become an integral part of the electrokinetic unit. However, the surface of shear may be found at a small distance away from the Stern plane. The potential between the surface of shear and the charged surface is called the zeta (ζ) potential and is slightly smaller than ψ_d.

The inner part of the double layer may include specifically adsorbed ions. In this case, the center of the specifically adsorbed ions is located between the surface and the Stern plane. Specifically adsorbed ions (e.g., surfactants) either lower or elevate the Stern potential and the zeta potential as shown in Figure 4.31. When the specific adsorption of the surface-active or polyvalent counter ions is strong, the charge sign of the Stern potential will be reversed. The Stern potential can be greater than the surface potential if the surface-active co-ions are adsorbed. The adsorption of nonionic surfactants causes the surface of shear to be moved to a much longer distance from the Stern plane. As a result, the zeta potential will be much lower than the Stern potential.

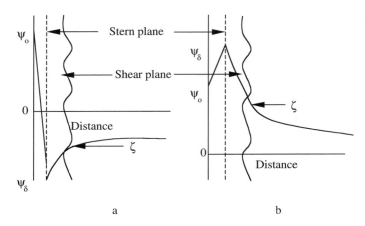

FIGURE 4.31 Changes in potential with distance: (a) charge reversal due to the adsorption of surface-active or polyvalent counterions; (b) adsorption of surface-active co-ions.

The potential in the diffuse layer decreases exponentially with the distance to zero (from the Stern plane). The potential changes are affected by the characteristics of the diffuse layer and particularly by the type and number of ions in the bulk solution. In many systems, the electrical double layer originates from the adsorption of potential-determining ions such as surface-active ions. The addition of an inert electrolyte decreases the thickness of the electrical double layer (i.e., compressing the double layer) and thus the potential decays to zero in a short distance. As the surface potential remains constant upon addition of an inert electrolyte, the zeta potential decreases. When two similarly charged particles approach each other, the two particles are repelled due to their electrostatic interactions. The increase in the electrolyte concentration in a bulk solution helps to lower this repulsive interaction. This principle is widely used to destabilize many colloidal systems.

4.3.2.2 The Stabilization and Destabilization of Colloid Systems

The fine particles dispersed in a liquid first collide with each other and then have a tendency to aggregate. The stability of the dispersion depends on the interaction forces between the particles during these collisions. Five such forces are:

1. Van der Waals attractive forces
2. Electrostatic repulsive forces
3. Solvation forces
4. Compression of the electrical double layer
5. Polymeric interparticle bridging

Electrical double layer compression. Addition of small amounts of electrolyte to dispersed colloidal particles causes them to coagulate. In coagulation, the particles are closely clustered together and hard to disperse again. The addition of an electrolyte causes the compression of the diffuse layer in the double layer surrounding the particles. Increasing the electrolyte concentration in the solution lowers the volume of the diffuse layer required to maintain electroneutrality, and thus causes a reduction in the thickness of the diffuse layer. When the repulsive interaction forces between two similarly charged particles are reduced and the van der Waals attractive forces are increased, the particles come closer together and coagulate. The effectiveness of the electrolyte on the destabilization of the particles depends markedly on the number of charged counterions in the primary charge of the particles. It is independent of the number of charged co-ions, the specific properties of the counterions, and the concentration of the particles. It has been observed that the concentrations of mono-valent, divalent, and trivalent counterions required to destabilize or coagulate a charged colloid are approximately in the ratio of $1^{-6}: 2^{-6}: 3^{-6}$, respectively. This is known as the Schulze–Hardy rule.

A quantitative treatment of the effects of electrolytes on colloid stability has been independently developed by Deryagen and Landau and by Verwey and Over-beek (DLVO), who considered the additive of the interaction forces, mainly *electrostatic repulsive* and *van der Waals attractive* forces as the particles approach each other. Repulsive forces between particles arise from the overlapping of the diffuse layer in the electrical double layer of two approaching particles. No simple analytical expression can be given for these repulsive interaction forces. Under certain assumptions, the surface potential is small and remains constant; the thickness of the double layer is large; and the overlap of the electrical double layer is small. The repulsive energy (V_R) between two spherical particles of equal size can be calculated by:

$$V_R = \frac{32 \pi a \varepsilon k^2 T^2 \gamma^2}{z^2 e^2} \exp(-\kappa H) \tag{4.71}$$

where ε is the permittivity of the polar disperse phase, a is the particle radius, κ is the reciprocal of the thickness of the double layer (i.e., Debye–Hückel length), and H is the distance between the Stern layers of two particles. The repulsive energy decays exponentially with the distance between two particles and decreases as the Debye–Hückel length (i.e., $1/\kappa$) decreases. In other words, increasing the electrolyte concentration and/or the number of charged counterions results in a decrease in the thickness of the double layer and hence lowers the repulsive energy.

The attractive energy between two particles of the same kind arises from van der Waals attractive forces (i.e., dispersion forces) due to the electromagnetic attractions. An exception is highly polar substances. In an assembly of molecules, the van der Waals forces of attraction are additive. Therefore, the attractive energies between two particles can be calculated from the addition of all the attractions between a pair of atoms or molecules on neighboring molecules. The dispersion force between two molecules varies with the inverse sixth power of the intermolecular distance. The energy of attraction (V_A) for two particles of equal size a , at a distance of separation H , (for a $\gg$ H) is given by:

$$V_A = -\frac{Aa}{12H} \tag{4.72}$$

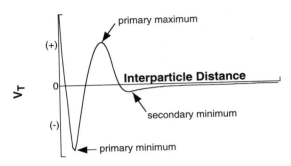

FIGURE 4.32 Schematic form of the total potential energy–distance curves.

where A is the Hamaker constant. The energy of attraction is inversly proportional to the distance between the two particles.

The total energy of interaction (V_T) is obtained from the summation between the electrostatic repulsive energy (i.e., the electrical double layer) and the attractive energy (i.e., van der Waals forces):

$$V_T = V_R + V_A \qquad (4.73)$$

Figure 4.32 illustrates the potential energy–distance curve with respect to the distance of separation H. It shows the general characteristics of the maximum and minimum energy levels in the curve. As predicted by Equation (4.71) and Equation (4.72), the double-layer repulsive forces decay exponentially while the van der Waals attractive forces are linearly inverse. As a result, the van der Waals energy predominates at small and large interparticle distances. At intermediate distances, the double-layer repulsive forces are predominant. Consequently, there will be a primary minimum at small distances followed by a primary maximum at intermediate distances. However, the energy curves are dependent on the actual values of the two forces. When the double-layer repulsion is less than van der Waals attraction at any interparticle distance, the maximum will be small and flat. At a primary minimum, the two interacting particles cannot be escapable, and irreversible changes between these particles may occur, such as crystallization. If the primary maximum is sufficiently high compared to the thermal energy (kT) of the particles, the two particles will not reach a state of close approach and thus are dispersed. The potential energy–distance curve also has a secondary minimum at relatively large distances. If the secondary minimum is small compared to the thermal energy, the particles will always repel one another and will not aggregate. Otherwise, the secondary minimum can trap particles to give a loose, easily reversible assembly of particles (i.e., flocculation). The magnitude of the secondary minimum depends on the particle size. For a small particle, when the primary maximum is so large, the coagulation of the particles into the primary minimum is prevented, and a secondary minimum will not appear. For flocculation to occur, the particle must be 1 μm or greater in radius.

Adding electrolytes to the stable colloidal particle solution compresses the electrical double layer and consequently $1/\kappa$ decreases. The transition from stability to coagulation may occur. The critical coagulation concentration (c.c.c) is the concentration of the electrolyte that is just enough to coagulate a colloidal particle. A mathematical equation for the c.c.c. of an electrolyte can be derived from the substitution of Equation (4.71) and Equation (4.72) into Equation (4.73):

$$V_T = \frac{32\pi\varepsilon a k^2 T^2 \gamma^2}{e^2 z^2} \exp(-\kappa H) - \frac{Aa}{12H} \tag{4.74}$$

The c.c.c occurs under certain conditions: $V_T = 0$ and $dV_T / dH = 0$ for the same value of H.

Taking the derivative of Equation (4.74) gives:

$$\frac{dV_T}{dH} = -\kappa V_R - \frac{V_A}{H} = 0 \tag{4.75}$$

and

$$V_T = V_R + V_A = 0 \tag{4.76}$$

Substituting Equation (4.75) into Equation (4.76) leads to $\kappa H = 1$, and substituting it into Equation (4.76) yields:

$$\kappa = \frac{443.8\varepsilon \, \pi^2 T^2 \gamma^2}{A e^2 z^2} \tag{4.77}$$

However, the inverse thickness of the double layer is given by:

$$\kappa = \left(\frac{2e^2 N_A c z^2}{\varepsilon k T} \right)^{1/2} \tag{4.78}$$

where N_A is the Avogadro number and z is the charge number of the ions.

Substituting Equation (4.78) into Equation (4.77) for an aqueous dispersion at 25°C gives:

$$c.c.c. = \frac{3.84 \times 10^{-39} \gamma^4}{A^2 z^6} \, mol / dm^3 \tag{4.79}$$

Equation (4.79) predicts that c.c.c. is inversely proportional to z^6. The c.c.c. is determined experimentally and tends to show a much stronger dependence on the number of charged ions than the one predicted by Equation (4.79). Equation (4.79) is used for the ideal situation even though the mathematical expressions become complicated when specific ion adsorption and solvation are taken into account.

Addition of soluble macromolecules (polymers) in the colloidal dispersion can stabilize the colloidal particles due to the adsorption of the polymers to the particle surfaces. The soluble polymers are often called protective agents or colloids. If the protective agents are ionic and have the same charge as the particles, the electrical double-layer repulsive forces will be increased and thus the stability of the colloidal particles will be enhanced. In addition, the adsorbed polymers may help weaken the van der Waals attraction forces among particles. However, the double-layer repulsion and the van der Waals attraction cannot account for the entire stabilization of the particle dispersions.

The term *steric stabilization* is used to describe possible stabilizing mechanisms attributable to the adsorbed polymers. When the particles of the adsorbed hydrated polymers collide, desorption of the protective colloids could occur at a point of contact. The free energy of desorption is positive, and the repulsion or stability between particles is enhanced. The time needed for the adsorption/desorption of the protective agents to occur is longer than that of the collision to reach a primary minimum coagulation. Therefore, coagulation does not occur. When the particles collide, the adsorbed hydrated layers are forced together but cannot interpenetrate each other, especially if the dispersion medium is a good solvent for the adsorbed polymer. This reduces the number of configurations available to the adsorbed polymers, resulting in a negative entropy change and an increase in free energy. Interparticle repulsion and stability are enhanced by this elastic effect. On the other hand, if the dispersion medium is a poor solvent, the adsorbed layers between the particles may interpenetrate each other, and an attraction results. However, whether the repulsion or attraction will take place depends entirely upon polymer–polymer and polymer–dispersion medium interactions.

The interpenetration of the polymer chains occurs at a point in which the elastic repulsion hinders further interpenetration, thus causing changes in enthalpy and entropy. Thermodynamically steric stabilization can be explained by Gibbs free energy (i.e., $\Delta G = \Delta H - T\Delta S$). It is necessary to have a positive ΔG for dispersion stabilization and a negative ΔG for particle aggregation. The dispersion stability is obtained from a positive ΔH and/or a negative ΔS. When the particles interpenetrate, the probability of contact between adsorbed macromolecules is increased. As a result, some of the bound water molecules are released. The bound water molecules have lesser degrees of freedom than the free water molecules do. In this process, energy must be supplied (i.e., heat absorption), so that a positive enthalpy change ($+\Delta H$) can be obtained. A decrease in entropy is expected at the interaction contact zone but it is subdued by the positive entropy change in the free water molecules. When the polymer chains interpenetrate, conformational freedom is lost and a negative entropy change results. The colloidal dispersion at any temperature will then be stable. The stability of the colloidal dispersion is dependent on the θ–temperature, at which the free energy change is equal to zero, unless ΔH is positive and ΔS is negative. If both ΔH and ΔS are positive, upon heating, the dispersion above the θ–temperature would aggregate, resulting from $\Delta H < T\Delta S$ (i.e., enthalpic stabilization). If both ΔH and ΔS are negative, upon cooling, the dispersion below the θ–temperature would aggregate resulting from $\Delta H > T\Delta S$ (i.e., entropic stabilization). Figure 4.33 shows the enthalpic stabilization process.

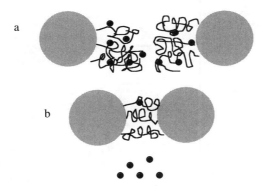

FIGURE 4.33 Enthalpic stabilization: (a) particles with hydrated stabilizing polymer chains; (b) overlapping stabilizing chains with released water molecules.

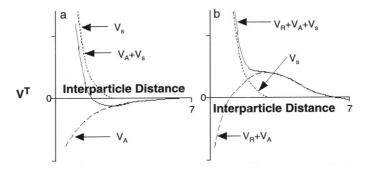

FIGURE 4.34 Schematic energy interaction diagrams for two sterically stabilized particles: (a) without electrical double-layer repulsion; (b) with electrical double-layer repulsion.

In a sterically stabilized dispersion of adsorbed polymer layers, the additional energy term, V_S, called the steric stabilization, is included in Equation (4.73):

$$V_T = V_R + V_A + V_S \qquad (4.80)$$

Schematic potential energy diagrams for two particles are depicted in Figure 4.34. As two particles approach, the presence of the adsorbed polymer molecules around the particles leads to a steric interaction in which the thickness of the adsorbed layer is greater than half the surface separation distance. Therefore, the particles do not get close to the primary minimum. The steric interaction V_S is influenced by two parameters:

1. The elastic or volume restriction based on the perturbation of the conformational freedom of the adsorbed molecules
2. The osmotic or mixing based on the release of the solvent into the normal bulk solvent

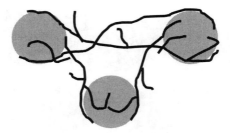

FIGURE 4.35 Bridging model for the flocculation of a colloidal particle by lyophilic polymers.

In general, the electrostatic repulsion is evident at a shorter distance than the steric interaction as long as the adsorbed molecules do not desorb from the particle surface. When three interactions (i.e., electrostatic, van der Waals, and steric) are combined, a primary maximum energy at a large distance results.

Addition of small amounts of anionic polyelectrolytes in the negatively charged particle dispersion destabilizes the dispersion (i.e., aggregation or flocculation). This case cannot be easily explained by a simple electrostatic theory. A *bridging* mechanism has been introduced to furnish a qualitative model for the destabilization. Upon contact with the colloidal particles, some segments of the polyelectrolyte and the lyophilic polymer chains are adsorbed at the particle surface and the rest extends into the dispersion medium. The important interactions between the particle surface and the polymer chains in the adsorption process are electrostatic interaction, hydrophobic bonding, hydrogen bonding, and ion binding. When these extended segments come into contact with other particles that have unoccupied sites, attachment to these sites results in flocculation (see Figure 4.35). The polymer chains serve as a bridge among the particles. Such destabilization normally occurs over a very narrow range of polymer concentrations. Restabilization is established when high concentrations are sufficient enough to cover the particle surface, thus creating a protective action through steric stabilization. Extended agitation may help restabilize a flocculated dispersion because the bridge can be broken and subsequently the free segment can be folded back to the particle surface.

4.3.3 SEDIMENTATION OF DILUTE SUSPENSIONS

Settling of a particle with radius a in a dilute suspension is hindered by the drag exerted in a dispersion medium. The resistance of the medium is proportional to the settling velocity of the particle. In a very short time, the particle reaches a constant velocity, known as the terminal velocity. The gravitational force on the particle balances the hydrodynamic resistance of the medium as given by:

$$\frac{4}{3} \pi \, a^3 (\rho_o - \rho) g = 6\pi \, \eta \, a \, V_o$$

or

$$V_o = \frac{2a^2 (\rho_o - \rho) g}{9\eta}$$

(4.81)

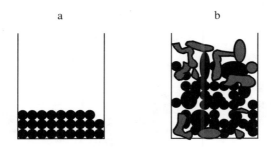

FIGURE 4.36 Sedimentation volumes for (a) cake and (b) flocculated sediments.

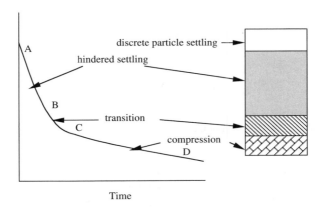

FIGURE 4.37 Settling of flocculated dispersions.

where ρ is the density of the medium, ρ_o is the density of the particles, η is the viscosity of the medium, V_o is the settling velocity, and g is the local gravity of acceleration. Equation (4.81) is called Stoke's law.

The positive density difference between the particles and the dispersing medium leads to the buildup of a sediment, provided that Brownian motion is not present. The pressure on the individual particles can lead to dense packing with small spaces between them. As a result, such dense sediment resists any exerting force and is difficult to redisperse. On the other hand, the aggregated or flocculated particles settle as flocs, and not as individual particles, to give a loose sediment of intra-aggregate water. The network structure of the flocs can extend through the entire system and further settle, leaving a clear supernatant (see Figure 4.36). It is easier to redisperse these flocculated particles. In an extreme case, the sedimentation volume of a flocculated suspension may be equal to the original volume of suspension, showing no clear supernatant liquid at the top. Such a suspension is a pharmaceutically favorable one.

The sedimentation velocity of the flocculated particles is determined by plotting the height of the sedimentation layer (H) as a function of time. Three types of plots exist, depending on the volume fraction of the flocs (φ), as shown in Figure 4.37:

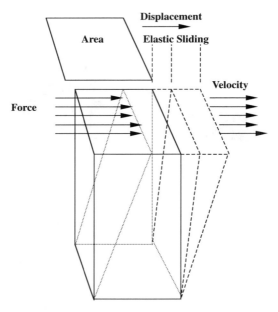

FIGURE 4.38 Laminar flow of a liquid.

For very dilute suspensions (φ <0.01), H decreases linearly to a constant level. The flocs individually settle rather than as networked clusters. As the concentration of flocs increases, the sedimentation velocity rapidly reduces and the increase in mixing boosts the settling rate, indicating that larger aggregated flocs are produced.

For concentrated suspensions (φ >0.25), on the other hand, there is no free-fall sedimentation because the intra-aggregate water is forced out slowly as the settled flocs merge.

In the intermediate range of floc concentrations, the flocculated particles settle at a constant rate in region A–B, known as hindered settling. This is followed by a transitional change in the region B–C, where the settling rate decreases. Consolidation (or compression) of the settled flocs occurs in region C–D, in which the flocs are supported by the underlying flocculated particles.

The sedimentation of pharmaceutical dispersions in non-Newtonian polymer solutions is of some practical interest. These polymers are used not only to stabilize colloidal particles but also to slow down (or prevent) settling, thus preventing cake formation. *Newtonian fluids* are defined as simple fluids that show a linear relationship between the rate of flow or shear (G) and the applied (or shearing) stress (F) at a constant viscosity (η) as shown in Figure 4.38:

$$G = \frac{F}{\eta} \tag{4.82}$$

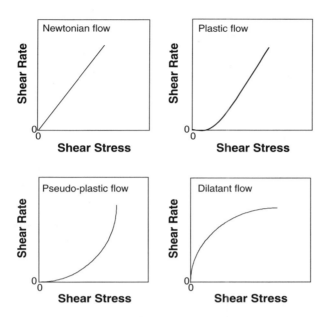

FIGURE 4.39 The behaviors of Newtonian and non-Newtonian fluids.

Fluids that deviate from this relationship are called *non-Newtonian* fluids. For many pure fluids and solutions (e.g., water, alcohol, and syrup), the viscosity is independent of G and F provided that the flow is laminar. For many pharmaceutical fluids, however, the viscosity varies with applied stress.

There are three types of non-Newtonian fluids: plastic, pseudoplastic, and dilatant. Figure 4.39 shows the rheological behaviors of Newtonian and non-Newtonian fluids. A *plastic fluid* does not move until the shear stress exceeds a certain minimum value, known as the yield value (f), and is expressed mathematically:

$$G = \frac{F - f}{\eta_P} \tag{4.83}$$

where η_P is the plastic viscosity. The main cause for this plasticity is the formation of a structural network throughout the solution, which must be broken before flow can be restored. Polymer melts, concentrated polymer solutions, and concentrated suspensions, particularly if the particles are flocculated, exhibit plastic flow. Even though the plastic fluids increase the viscosity of suspensions, which in turn slows down the settling rate of particles, there is a problem with pouring the pharmaceutical suspensions.

Unlike plastic flow, *pseudoplastic flow* is characterized as the flow that occurs as soon as a shear stress is applied and the apparent viscosity decreases with increasing shear stress (i.e., shear-thinning) without exhibiting a yield value, as illustrated in Figure 4.39. Empirically, the quantitative relationship is given by:

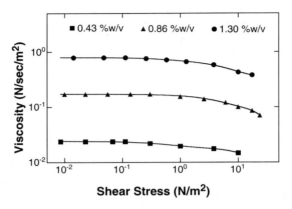

FIGURE 4.40 Viscosity vs. shear stress for aqueous solution of ethyl hydroxyethylcellulose. [Graph reconstructed from data by Buscall et al., *J. Colloid Interface Sci.,* 85, 78 (1982).]

$$G = \frac{F^n}{\eta'} \tag{4.84}$$

where η' is the apparent viscosity and n is the constant. As n becomes less than 1, the fluid behaves in a non-Newtonian fashion

As shear stress is applied to aqueous solutions of hydrocolloids such as polyethylene oxide, methylcellulose, or xanthan gum, the polymer molecules disentangle and align themselves in the same direction of flow. Consequently, the solvent immobilized by the polymers is released, thus lowering the apparent viscosity of the system. During standing, the pharmaceutical suspensions have a very high viscosity, which slows down the sedimentation of the particles. On shaking (or applying stress), the viscosity of the suspensions becomes less. Thus it is easy to pour them.

Figure 4.40 shows the shear-thinning behavior of an aqueous solution of ethyl hydroxyethylcellulose as a function of the concentration. The pseudoplastic behavior is observed at lower polymer concentrations as the molecular weight of the polymer increases. An aqueous solution of ethyl hydroxyethylcellulose becomes pseudoplastic at concentrations of less than 1%. Above the critical value of the shear stress the flow behavior is non-Newtonian, and viscosity decreases with the increasing shear stress. The critical stress is in the range of 0.1 N/m^2 for the solution.

A *dilatant flow* is characterized by the opposite type of pseudoplastic flow in which the apparent viscosity increases with the increase in shear stress (i.e., shear-thickening). The empirical equation described for the dilatant flow is similar to Equation (4.84) but the exponent n is greater than 1. This behavior is not common for all pharmaceutical solutions and dispersions but it is exhibited by pastes of small, deflocculated particles (solid content $\geq 50\%$). There is only a limited amount of fluid that can fill the interparticulate voids.

As the shear stress is increased, the limited fluid leaks out of the voids and clumps are produced so that the flow is greatly resisted and the viscosity increases. An extreme situation is one in which the flow may be stopped when the shear stress

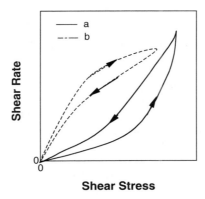

FIGURE 4.41 Thixotropic behaviors of silicate materials.

is overloaded. This problem may occur during wet granulation of pharmaceutical powders.

In the Newtonian and non-Newtonian fluids described above, replicate experiments would produce the same rate of shear (or viscosity) on the same shear stress. The determination of the viscosity is independent of the past history of the solution. In this case, the solutions respond and adapt immediately to a new shear environment. However, certain non-Newtonian fluids, containing particularly fine inorganic materials (e.g., silicates, clays, oxides), do not follow this mode. Such solutions are called *thixotropic,* meaning "to change by touch." Similarly, in a pseudoplastic flow, the apparent viscosity will decrease as the applied shear stress increases. However, the rate of shear and the viscosity will also decrease with time. This is in part due to the different time response of the system during structural breakdown at high shear stress and structure reformation at low shear stress. In other words, once the stress is removed, the broken structure does not return back to its original state immediately, even if it eventually regains back its original structure. Therefore, a hysteresis loop of the nonequilibrium downcurve and upcurve can be obtained (Figure 4.41). When unsheared, thixotropic materials form a three-dimensional gel-like structure in the medium due to the interactions (i.e., secondary bonds) between the inorganic materials. When the high rate of shear is imparted, these interactive three-dimensional network arrangements (e.g., intermolecular attractions and entanglements) are disrupted to a two-dimensional alignment and the viscosity falls (i.e., gel–sol transformation). When the stress is removed, the two-dimensional structure reforms the three-dimensional network but at a slower rate; meanwhile, Brownian motion restores the molecules back to their original state. The area within the hysteresis loop indicates the degree of breakdown. Thixotropy is particularly important for pharmaceutical suspensions, since it is desirable that on shaking (high shear stress), the suspension should pour (or flow) easily from its container and on standing, its viscosity rises to prevent (or slow down) settling. Sometimes shear stress leads to an irreversible structural breakdown between the elements of a material so that the original structural condition is never restored. Such behavior is known as "shear destruction." In some circumstances, an accelerated recovery of the original condition can be observed (Figure 4.41). For example, bentonite suspensions slowly recover back to their original state upon standing but they quickly return to the original state when the suspensions are gently disturbed.

4.3.4 PREVENTION OF CAKE FORMATION

As shown in Equation (4.81), suspended particles eventually settle and form dilatant (cake) sediments, which are difficult to redisperse. Several methods to control sedimentation and cake formation will be described here.

As seen clearly from Equation (4.81), the settling rate will be zero when the density difference between the particles and the dispersing medium is zero (i.e., $\rho_o - \rho = 0$). This method can only be applied to systems with smaller density differences because of the limitation to increase the density of the continuous medium by dissolving some inert simple molecules (e.g., sugar and water-miscible solvents) in Newtonian fluids. In addition, even if the matched density is obtained at one temperature, it cannot be maintained at other temperatures.

Equation (4.81) also clearly shows that an increase in the viscosity of the dispersion medium decreases the sedimentation rate. Natural or synthetic polymers (e.g., tragacanth, xanthan gum, hydroxyethylcellulose, and polyethylene oxide) that have the characteristics of pseudoplastic flow can be used. As mentioned before, the apparent viscosity of the polymer solutions is dependent on the applied shear stress. The amount of polymer required to reduce the rate of sedimentation is significantly less with increasing molecular weight of the polymer. At relatively high concentrations, the polymer chains will interact with each other to possibly lead to flocculation of the suspension. In addition, the polymer solution becomes viscoelastic when the polymer coils overlap with each other. The elastic component of the polymer solution reduces the settling rate and prevents cake formation. At a concentration of xanthan gum ($MW > 10^6$) of <0.1%, the solution becomes viscoelastic due to the polymer chain interactions. However, careful evaluation should be made of the characteristics of the interactions of the polymer coils with the polymer coils and the polymer coils with the suspended particles. Aging of polymer solutions, particularly those from natural origins, should be carefully considered because there is the possibility of chemical or microbial degradation, which reduces the viscosity of the dispersion medium. This would lead to sedimentation and cake formation on prolonged storage. If the rheological property changes greatly with temperature (i.e., refrigeration or thermal gelation), the suspension may form a cake at either low or high temperatures.

When fine inorganic materials (e.g., bentonite, oxides) are added to water containing suspended particles, the dispersion becomes thixotropic and the inorganic materials form a three-dimensional network (i.e., gel) structure in the medium. The gel network has sufficient elastic properties. It entraps the particles and prevents settling and cake formation. The network structure is broken down upon shaking, thus facilitating pouring. However, the gel structure is influenced by pH and electrolyte concentration.

The use of mixtures of hydrocolloids and fine inorganic materials can overcome some of the problems encountered for each of them alone. In the mixtures, the

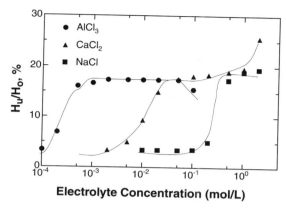

FIGURE 4.42 Height of sedimentation volume of griseofulvin as a function of electrolyte concentrations in pH 3. [Graph reconstructed from data by Mathews and Rhodes, *J. Pharm. Sci.*, 59, 521 (1970).]

amounts of polymers and inorganic materials can be lowered and the dispersion is then less dependent on the temperature and degradation. In addition, the influence of the pH and electrolyte can be significantly reduced. For example, mixtures of carboxymethylcellulose and bentonite (50:50 ratio) and methylcellulose and Veegum (magnesium aluminum silicate), assuming well-balanced suspensions, yield a "three-dimensional network" of trapped particles, which slows settling and prevents cake formation. The network results from the bentonite alone and the adsorption of the polymers in the bentonite and/or suspended particle surfaces (i.e., bridging). The mechanism of network formation is a complicated one and depends on the suspended particles, inorganic materials, hydrocolloids, and conditions (e.g., pH, electrolyte, and temperature).

According to DLVO theory, the flocculated particles can be obtained by careful control of the electrolyte concentration in the medium (i.e., zeta potential). The Schulz–Hardy rule states that the higher the electrolyte valence needs, the lower the electrolyte concentration, as illustrated in Figure 4.42. Above the critical coagulation concentration, the height of the sediment volume increases, and redispersion can be easily achieved. Addition of a polyelectrolyte in the right concentration range leads to flocculation by "bridging," as mentioned in the previous section. There may not be any problems producing flocculated particles on a large scale. However, some problems might be expected when transferring the flocculated dispersion into smaller bottles, since flocs may quickly settle during transfer, and each final product may end up with different dose levels. Figure 4.43 shows the controlled flocculation of bismuth subnitrate by KH_2PO_4. When the concentration of KH_2PO_4 is in the range of 6 to 60 mmol/L, the zeta potential approaches zero, and a high sedimentation height results.

A close look at Equation (4.81) indicates that a variable that makes a great impact on the settling rate is the particle size. For example, the reduction of a particle radius from 10 to 1 μm leads to a reduction in the settling rate of 10^2 times. Pharmaceutical suspensions should be manufactured from the smallest particles

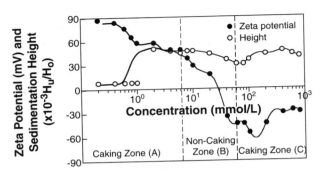

FIGURE 4.43 Controlled flocculation of bismuth subnitrate as a function of KH_2PO_4 concentration. [Graph reconstructed from data by Haines and Martin, *J. Pharm. Sci.,* 50, 753 (1961).]

possible and dispersed in dispersion medium containing both hydrocolloids and finely divided inorganic materials. One example of such a commercial product is Pepto-Bismol®, which uses methylcellulose and magnesium aluminum silicate as suspending agents.

SUGGESTED READINGS

1. M. E. Aulton (Ed.), *Pharmaceutics: The Science of Dosage Form Design,* Churchill and Livingstone, London, 1988, Chapters 2, 4, 6, 15, and 16.
2. J. T. Davies and E. K. Rideal, *Interfacial Phenomena,* Academic Press, New York, 1961, Chapter 8.
3. P. H. Elworthy, A. T. Florence, and C. B. Macfarlane, *Solubilization by Surface-Active Agents,* Chapman and Hall, London, 1968.
4. A. T. Florence and D. Attwood, *Physicochemical Principles of Pharmacy,* 2nd Ed., Chapman and Hall, New York, 1988, Chapters 2, 6, and 7.
5. W. C. Griffin, *J. Soc. Cosmet. Chem.,* 5, 1 (1954).
6. P. C. Hiemenz, *Principles of Colloid and Surface Chemistry,* 2nd Ed., Marcel Dekker, New York, 1986.
7. K. J. Laidler and J. H. Meiser, *Physical Chemistry,* Benjamin/Cummings, Menlo Park, CA, 1982, Chapter 17.
8. H. A. Lieberman, M. M. Rieger, and G. S. Banker, *Pharmaceutical Dosage Forms: Disperse Systems,* Vols. 1 and 2, Marcel Dekker, New York, 1988 and 1989.
9. A. Martin, *Physical Pharmacy,* 4th Ed., Lea and Febiger, Philadelphia, 1993, Chapters 14, 15, 17, and 18.
10. H. Schott, Comments on Hydrophile–Lipophile Balance Systems, *J. Pharm. Sci.,* 79, 87 (1990).
11. D. J. Shaw, *Introduction to Colloid and Surface Chemistry,* 4th Ed., Butterworth and Heinemann, Oxford, England, 1992.
12. T. F. Tadros (Ed.), *Solid/Liquid Dispersions,* Academic Press, New York, 1987.
13. W. J. Weber, Jr., *Physicochemical Processes for Water Quality Control,* Wiley Interscience, New York, 1972, Chapters 2, 3, and 5.
14. V. R. Williams, W. L. Mattice, and H. B. Williams, *Basic Physical Chemistry for the Life Sciences,* 3rd Ed., W. H. Freeman and Co., San Francisco, 1978, Chapter 9.

PROBLEMS

1. Varying amounts of activated carbon were added to 500 mL of a drug solution (MIK 6836X) with an initial concentration of 95 mg/L. The solutions were allowed to reach equilibrium for 5 days. The filtrate of the solution was analyzed as:

Carbon added (g)	0.60	0.35	0.3	0.25	0.15	0.03
Filtrate concentration (mg/L)	6.0	11.2	18.1	31.3	45.1	83.8

Determine the parameters for the Langmuir and Freundlich isotherms.

2. Determine the amount of surfactants (Span 60, HLB = 4.7 and Tween 60, HLB = 14.9) required to obtain an O/W emulsion as:

Mineral oil (HLB = 12)	36%
Beeswax (HLB = 9)	2%
Wool fat (HLB = 10)	1%
Cetyl alcohol (HLB = 15)	1%
Emulsifiers	5%
Water, to make	100%

3. The following surface tensions vs. concentration were obtained for an aqueous solution of a surfactant at 25°C. Determine the critical micelle concentration and the area per molecule occupied by the surfactant.

c (10^{-4} mol/dm^3)	0.1	1.0	2.0	5.0	8.0	10.0	30.0
γ (mN m^{-1})	63.8	46.4	41.1	33.5	30.1	29.2	29.0

4. The following critical micelle concentration of a surfactant in an aqueous medium vs. temperature was measured as:

Temperature (°C)	15	20	25	30	40	50
c.m.c. (mmol/dm^3)	21.7	20.7	19.7	19.0	17.6	16.1

Calculate the enthalpy change of micellization.

5. Determine the thickness of the electrical diffuse double layer for a negatively charged solid particle in the following aqueous electrolyte solutions at 20°C: a) 0.1 mol/L NaCl, b) 0.001 mol/L CaCl$_2$, c) 0.0001 mol/L AlCl$_3$.

5 Kinetics

When developing final dosage forms, it is important to know whether the product is safe for its intended therapeutic use over a long period of storage time. Compounds used in the final product as well as active ingredients should be stable at normal environmental conditions. If the ingredients undergo chemical degradation, one should know the pathway of degradation, the byproducts, and their safety to the recipients. In addition, administered drugs undergo biotransformation in biological fluids and body organs. In this chapter, kinetic analysis of the degradation and biotransformation of chemical compounds will be emphasized.

5.1 PATHWAYS OF DRUG DEGRADATION

A number of drug substances and excipients employed in pharmaceutical products have a variety of chemical structures, which may be broken down under certain environmental conditions. Major degradation routes are hydrolysis, oxidation, and photolysis.

5.1.1 HYDROLYSIS

Drug substances having ester and amide labile groups in their molecular structure degrade via hydrolysis in the presence of water. The degradation process by hydrolysis accelerates in the presence of hydrogen or hydroxyl ions, and hydrolytic reactions involve nucleophilic attack of the labile groups. Hydrolysis is one of the most common degradation paths encountered with pharmaceuticals.

Common ester labile bonds are formed between an alcohol and a carboxylic acid. The ester bond is hydrolyzed by hydrogen and hydroxyl ions as shown:

The acyl oxygen in the ester group is protonated and the carboxyl group is further polarized. Nucleophilic attack at the acyl carbon is increased by water. A base, which is the powerful nucleophile, attacks on the acyl carbon and the carbon–oxygen bond is broken.

TABLE 5.1
Effects of Types of Substituents
of Benzoates on the Rate Constants

Y	R_2	Rate Constant, k_{OH} ($\times 10^{-4} M^{-1} sec^{-1}$)
H	CH_3	6.08
H	C_2H_5	1.98
H	$n\text{-}C_3H_7$	1.67
H	C_2H_4Cl	12.4
H	$C_2H_3Cl_{12}$	31.9
Cl	CH_3	19.1
NO_2	CH_3	276

Source: Taken from K. A. Connors, G. L. Amidon, and L. Kennon, *Chemical Stability of Pharmaceuticals: A Handbook for Pharmacists,* Wiley Interscience, New York, 1979.

The rate of degradation of an ester labile group is dependent on the characteristics of R_1 and R_2. For a given R_1, the rate of degradation decreases with the higher alkyl group of R_2OH, because the higher the alkyl, the fewer electrons are withdrawn whereas for a given R_2, the degradation rate increases with the increase in electron-withdrawing group (e.g., Cl, NO_2) of R_1COOH. Table 5.1 shows the effects of substitution types of benzoates on the rate constant. The rate of degradation by hydrolysis increases by replacing methyl to ethyl and propyl. The higher alkyl groups possessing the greater electron-donating characteristics increase the electron density at the acyl carbon, and thus the attack of OH^- is inhibited. On the contrary, electron-attracting groups such as chlorine and NO_2 increase the rate of degradation. There are other mechanisms of ester hydrolysis: steric factors, leaving groups, and neighboring charges (see Ref. 4).

Another chemical structure in pharmaceuticals is an amide group, which is formed between a carboxylic acid and an amine and is less susceptible than ester groups to hydrolysis. This is due to the lesser electrophilicity of the carbon–nitrogen bond. The amide group is hydrolyzed as:

The rate of degradation of the amide group by hydrolysis is dependent on the characteristics of the substituents R_1, R_2, and R_3. Antibiotics possessing the β-lactam structure, which is a cyclic amide, are hydrolyzed rapidly by ring opening of the β-lactam group. The ring opening of the β-lactam is much faster than that of other amide groups because a four-membered ring is joined to a five- or six-membered ring and a weaker bond exists between carbon and nitrogen of β-lactam. Penicillins and cephalosporins belong to this category.

5.1.2 OXIDATION

Oxygen is one of the abundant elements in the environment. Upon exposure to oxygen, pharmaceuticals that are not in their most oxidized state may decompose. Oxidation/reduction reactions involve the transfer of electrons or the transfer of oxygen or hydrogen from a substance. There should be the drug molecules to be oxidized (i.e., reducing agents) and other substances to be reduced (i.e., oxidizing agents) in a same system. Oxidation of inorganic and organic compounds is easily explained by a loss of electrons and the loss of a molecule of hydrogen, respectively, as:

Inorganic compounds: $SO_3^{-2} + 2OH^- \rightleftharpoons SO_4^{-2} + H_2O + 2e^-$

Organic compounds: loss of hydrogen

The rate of oxidation of organic compounds may be dependent on the concentration of H^+ or pH. At low pH, the rate of degradation of many compounds decreases.

When an oxidation reaction involves molecular oxygen, the reaction occurs spontaneously under mild conditions. It is known as *autooxidation.* In an autooxidation process, free radicals, formed by thermal or photolytic cleavage of chemical bonds (e.g., peroxide, ROOH) or redox processes with metal ions present in raw material impurities, are involved

$$Fe^{+2} + ROOH \longrightarrow Fe^{+3} + OH^- + RO*$$

The free radical formed, RO^*, reacts with oxygen to produce a peroxide radical, and the reaction propagates as:

$$RO* + O_2 \longrightarrow ROOO*$$

$$ROOO* + RH \longrightarrow ROOOH + RO*$$

The free radical reaction continues until all the free radicals are consumed or destroyed.

5.1.3 PHOTOLYSIS

Light energy, similar to heat, provides the activation necessary for oxidation to take place. After a drug substance has absorbed radiant light energy (hυ, where h is

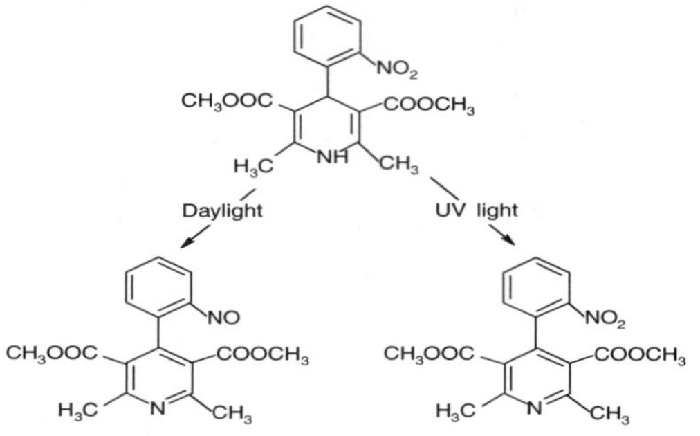

FIGURE 5.1 Pathways of photolysis of nifedipine.

Planck's constant and υ is the frequency of the light), it becomes an unstable, excited species. The activated species either emits radiant light of a different wavelength (no decomposition occurs) or decomposes. Oxidation very often accompanies photodegradation in the presence of oxygen and light. The photolysis of a drug substance may cause discoloration of the product and packaging materials in addition to chemical degradation. The pathways of photolysis are generally very complex and depend on drug molecules (e.g., see Figure 5.1).

The rest of this chapter will deal with kinetic interpretation of chemical degradation.

5.2 SINGLE AND MULTIPLE REACTIONS, ELEMENTARY REACTIONS, MOLECULARITY, AND ORDER OF REACTIONS

In a reaction, reactants yield products. One should consider whether a reaction takes place via a single stoichiometric equation that has a single rate expression (i.e., *single reaction*) or whether more than one stoichiometric equation must be used to express the rate of reaction of all the reaction constituents (i.e., *multiple reactions*).

Consider the following reaction with stoichiometric equation:

$$A + B \longrightarrow P \tag{5.1}$$

The rate of the reaction (rate of disappearance of reactants A and B or rate of production of product P) is proportional to the concentration of the reactants in the mixture. The rate equation for this stoichiometric reaction is:

$$\text{Rate} = k\,[A][B] \tag{5.2}$$

where k is the rate constant and the square brackets in Equation (5.2) indicate the concentrations of each reactant. The above reaction is called an *elementary reaction.*

When the rate equation does not correspond stoichiometrically, the reaction is called a *nonelementary reaction.* Consider the thermal decomposition of nitrous oxide to nitrogen and oxygen as follows:

$$N_2O \longrightarrow N_2 + \frac{1}{2}O_2 \qquad (5.3)$$

which has a rate equation:

$$Rate = \frac{k_1[N_2O]^2}{1 + k_2[N_2O]} \qquad (5.4)$$

Nonelementary reactions, such as Equation (5.4), are expressed as a single reaction [i.e., Equation (5.3)] because the overall reaction is the result of sequential elementary reactions and the intermediates are very small, unnoticeable, and difficult to isolate. Therefore, some of these intermediates do not appear in the stochiometric equation of the reaction. In this chapter (and generally in pharmaceutical sciences), nonelementary reactions will be ignored.

The *molecularity* of a single elementary reaction is the number of molecules engaged in the reaction. A simple elementary reaction is referred to as uni-, bi-, or termolecular if one, two, or three chemical species are involved in the chemical reaction, respectively:

$$Unimolecular: \quad A \longrightarrow B + C$$

$$Bimolecular: \quad A + B \longrightarrow C + D$$

$$Termolecular: \quad A + 2B \longrightarrow C + D$$

For a general single elementary reaction,

$$\alpha A + \beta B + \gamma C + \cdots \longrightarrow \omega X + \sigma Y + \tau Z + \cdots \qquad (5.5)$$

The rate of the reaction, r, is given by:

$$r = -\frac{1}{\alpha}\frac{d[A]}{dt} = -\frac{1}{\beta}\frac{d[B]}{dt} = -\frac{1}{\gamma}\frac{d[C]}{dt} \cdots = \frac{1}{\omega}\frac{d[X]}{dt} = \frac{1}{\sigma}\frac{d[Y]}{dt} = \frac{1}{\tau}\frac{d[Z]}{dt} \cdots \qquad (5.6)$$

Often the rate of the reaction is expressed as:

$$r = k[A]^a[B]^b[C]^c \cdots \qquad a + b + c \cdots = n \qquad (5.7)$$

where the exponents a, b, c, $\cdots$ do not necessarily correspond to the stoichiometric coefficients α, β, γ $\cdots$. The exponents are determined experimentally and not necessarily by an integer. The reaction is of the ath order with respect to reactant A, b^{th} order with respect to reactant B and so on. The total order of the reaction is to the nth in Equation (5.7).

Regardless of the order of the reactions, the rate of reaction has the units of concentration/time (i.e., mole/L sec). The units of the rate constant are dependent on the overall order of the reaction:

$$k = (\text{concentration})^{1-n}(\text{time})^{-1} \qquad (5.8)$$

5.3 IRREVERSIBLE REACTIONS

5.3.1 ZERO-ORDER REACTIONS

In a zero-order reaction [i.e., $n = 0$ in Equation (5.7)], the rate of an elementary unimolecular reaction is expressed as:

$$r = -\frac{d[A]}{dt} = k_o \qquad (5.9)$$

where k_o is the zero-order rate constant and t is the time. The rate of reaction is independent of the concentration of the reactants and constant. Integrating Equation (5.9) yields:

$$\int_{[A]_o}^{[A]} d[A] = -k_o \int_0^t dt \quad \text{or} \quad [A] = [A]_o - k_o t \qquad (5.10)$$

where the subscript o denotes the initial concentration. A plot of the remaining drug concentration, [A], vs. t gives a straight line with a slope of $-k_o$, which has the same units as the rate of reaction [i.e., (concentration)(time)$^{-1}$].

The *half-life* ($t_{0.5}$) and *shelf-life* ($t_{0.9}$) are defined as the times required for the concentration of the drug to decrease by 50 and 10%, respectively. For zero-order reactions,

$$t_{0.5} = \frac{0.5[A]_o}{k_o} \qquad (5.11a)$$

$$t_{0.9} = \frac{0.1[A]_o}{k_o} \qquad (5.11b)$$

The half-life of a zero-order reaction is directly proportional to $[A]_o$. Unlike other reaction kinetics, it is possible to determine the time required for 100% of the drug in a formulation to completely decompose. It takes two half-lives for complete degradation for zero-order reactions.

It is hard to find many examples in the pharmaceutical field that follow zero-order reaction kinetics. Figure 5.2 shows the degradation of vitamin A acetate to anhydrovitamin A.

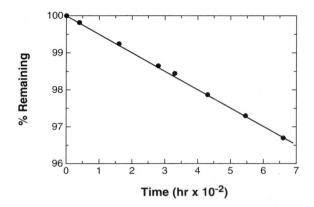

FIGURE 5.2 Degradation of vitamin A acetate in ethanol/water (95%/5%). [Graph reconstructed from data by Higuchi and Rheinstein, *J. Am. Pharm. Assoc., Sci. Ed.*, 48, 155 (1959).]

Example 5.1

The degradation of a colorant in a solid dosage form was found to follow a zero-order reaction with a rate constant of 3.1×10^{-4} absorbance units per hour at 37°C. What is the half-life of the preparation with an initial absorbance of 0.56 at 486 nm? This dosage form should be discarded when the absorbance is below 0.34. Calculate the predicted life of the dosage form at 37°C.

Solution

$$t_{0.5} = \frac{0.5[A]_o}{k_o} = \frac{0.5 \times 0.56 \text{ absorbance}}{3.1 \times 10^{-4} \text{ absorbance / hr}} = 903.2 \text{ hr} = 37.6 \text{ days}$$

$$[A] = [A]_o - k_o t$$

$$t = \frac{[A]_o - [A]}{k_o} = \frac{(0.56 - 0.34) \text{ absorbance}}{3.1 \times 10^{-4} \text{ absorbance / hr}} = 709.7 \text{ hr} = 29.6 \text{ days}$$

5.3.2 FIRST-ORDER REACTIONS

The rate of the first-order degradation kinetics ($A \longrightarrow B$) is written as:

$$r = -\frac{d[A]}{dt} = k_1[A] \tag{5.12}$$

where k_1 is the first-order rate constant. Integrating Equation (5.12) yields:

$$\int_{[A]_o}^{[A]} \frac{d[A]}{[A]} = -k_1 \int_0^t dt \quad \text{or} \quad \ln\left(\frac{[A]}{[A]_o}\right) = -k_1 t \tag{5.13}$$

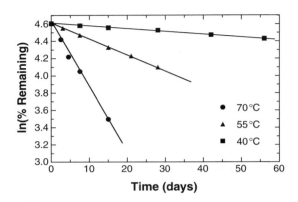

FIGURE 5.3 Degradation of gemcitabine HCl at pH 3.2 at different temperatures. [Graph reconstructed from data by Jansen et al., *J. Pharm. Sci.,* 89, 885 (2000).]

A plot of the logarithm of the fraction remaining (as ordinate) as a function of time (as abscissa) gives a straight line with a slope of $-k_1$, as shown in Figure 5.3. The first-order rate constant, k_1, has the units of time^{-1}. The half-life and shelf-life for first-order reactions are given by:

$$\ln\left(\frac{0.5[A]_o}{[A]_o}\right) = -k_1 t_{0.5} \quad \text{or} \quad t_{0.5} = \frac{-\ln 0.5}{k_1} = \frac{0.693}{k_1} \tag{5.14a}$$

$$\ln\left(\frac{0.9[A]_o}{[A]_o}\right) = -k_1 t_{0.9} \quad \text{or} \quad t_{0.9} = \frac{-\ln 0.9}{k_1} = \frac{0.105}{k_1} \tag{5.14b}$$

As shown in Equation (5.14a) and Equation (5.14b), the half-life and the shelf-life are constant and independent of the drug concentration, $[A]_o$. For example, if the half-life of a first-order reaction is 124 days, it takes 124 days for a drug to decompose to $0.5\,[A]_o$. Also it takes another 124 days for 50% of the remaining 50% of the drug to decompose. In Equation (5.13), the time required for 100% degradation cannot be calculated because $\ln([A]/[A]_o)$ is an indefinite number.

For a very stable dosage form, the decrease of $[A]$ with time is very small and within the allowed experimental error. However, the change of $[B]$ (product) is noticeable and can be plotted as the appearance of the product with respect to time:

$$[B] = [A]_o\left(1 - e^{-k_1 t}\right) \tag{5.15}$$

where $[A]_o = [A] + [B]$.

Example 5.2

A drug product is known to be ineffective after it has decomposed by 23%. The initial concentration of the product was 11.5 mg/mL. After 1 year, the drug concentration in the product was found to be 7.4 mg/mL. Assuming that the drug degradation is first-order, what should the expiration date be and what is the half–life of the product?

Solution

$$[A]_o = 11.5 \text{ mg / mL}$$

$$\text{after t = 12 months,} \quad [A] = 7.4 \text{ mg / mL}$$

$$\ln\left(\frac{7.4 \text{ mg / mL}}{11.5 \text{ mg / mL}}\right) = -k_1(12 \text{ mon}) \qquad k_1 = \frac{-\ln(7.4 / 11.5)}{12 \text{ mon}} = 0.037 \text{ mon}^{-1}$$

The expiration date and half-life can be determined as:

$$\ln(0.77) = -(0.037 \text{ mon}^{-1}) \text{ t} \quad \text{or} \quad t = \frac{-\ln 0.77}{0.037 \text{ mon}^{-1}} = 7.1 \text{ mon}$$

$$t_{0.5} = \frac{0.693}{k_1} = 18.7 \text{ mon}$$

5.3.3 APPARENT ZERO-ORDER REACTIONS

As mentioned before, not many zero-order degradation reactions exist in pharmaceutics. However, some drugs in certain common dosage forms, such as suspensions, follow zero-order kinetics. Looking at the phase where the degradation takes place, first-order degradation kinetics is observed. But the overall degradation kinetics in the entire dosage form is a zero-order rate. Drug degradation kinetics in an aqueous phase of a suspension dosage form is expressed as:

$$\frac{d[A]}{dt} = -k_1[A] \tag{5.12}$$

In suspension formulations, the concentration of the drug in the aqueous phase remains constant (i.e., saturated) until the suspended drug particles are completely exhausted:

$$k_1[A] = k_1[A]_s = k_o \tag{5.16}$$

where $[A]_s$ is the solubility of a drug. Substituting Equation (5.16) into Equation (5.12) yields:

$$\frac{d[A]}{dt} = -k_o \tag{5.9}$$

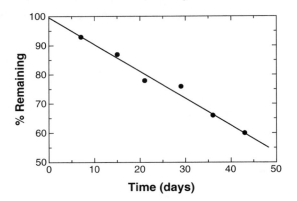

FIGURE 5.4 Hydrolysis of aspirin in an aqueous suspension at 34°C. [Graph reconstructed from data by K. C. James, *J. Pharm. Pharmacol.*, 2, 363 (1958).]

Example 5.3

The degradation of aspirin by hydrolysis in an aqueous suspension was carried out and is represented in Figure 5.4. What is the apparent rate constant for the hydrolysis of the aqueous aspirin suspension? What is the hydrolysis rate constant in an aqueous phase? Assume the initial concentration is 0.21 mole/L. The solubility of aspirin is 0.0183 mole/L.

Solution

$$[A]_o = 0.21\ M \quad [A] = 0.13\ M \quad \text{at } t = 43 \text{ days}$$

$$k_o = \frac{[A]_o - [A]}{t} = \frac{(0.21 - 0.13)\ \text{moles}}{43\ \text{days}} = 1.86 \times 10^{-3}\ M\,/\,\text{day}$$

$$k_1[A]_s = k_1 \times (0.0183\ M) = 1.86 \times 10^{-3}\ M\,/\,\text{day}$$

The hydrolysis rate constant in the aqueous phase is given by $k_1 = 0.10\,/\,\text{day}$.

Example 5.4

The hydrolysis of aspirin in aqueous suspension is zero-order. Aspirin was suspended in an aqueous solution, which was maintained at pH 2.5. The amount of aspirin suspended initially was 70 g/L. After 2 weeks, a 5 ml aliquot of the suspension was withdrawn and found by analysis to contain 0.3375 g aspirin. (a) What is the rate constant for the hydrolysis of aspirin in suspension, expressed in g/L/day? (b) How long will it take for 10% of the aspirin suspended initially to hydrolyze? (c) After 50% of the aspirin suspended initially is hydrolyzed, how much additional time is required for 50% of the remaining aspirin to hydrolyze?

Solution

(a)   Final concentration after 2 weeks (14 days):

$$[A] = \frac{0.3375g}{5mL} \times \frac{1000mL}{L} = 67.5g / L$$

$$[A]_o - [A] = k_o t, \qquad (70 - 67.5)g / L = k_o (14 \text{ days})$$

$$k_o = \frac{2.5g / L}{14 \text{ days}} = 0.1785g / L / day$$

(b) $t_{0.9} = \dfrac{0.1[A]_o}{k_o} = \dfrac{0.1 \times 70g / L}{0.1785g / L / day} = 39.2 \text{ days}$

(c) $t_{05} = 5 \times t_{0.9} = 196 \text{ days}$

After 196 days, 50% of the aspirin (35 g/L) has been destroyed. Therefore, 35 g/L (70 g/L – 35 g/L) remains. The time required for 50% of the remaining aspirin to be hydrolyzed:

$$t_{0.5} = \frac{0.5 \times [A]_o}{k_o} = \frac{0.5 \times 35g / L}{0.1785g / L / day} = 98 \text{ days}$$

5.3.4 SECOND-ORDER REACTIONS

There are two types of second-order reactions:

$$\text{Type I:} \quad A + A \longrightarrow P$$

$$\text{Type II:} \quad A + B \longrightarrow P$$

For type I second–order reactions, the rate of reaction is given by:

$$\frac{d[A]}{dt} = -k_2 [A]^2 \tag{5.17}$$

where k_2 is the second-order rate constant. Integration of Equation (5.17) yields:

$$\int_{[A]_o}^{[A]} \frac{d[A]}{[A]^2} = -k_2 \int_0^t dt \quad \text{or} \quad \frac{1}{[A]} - \frac{1}{[A]_o} = -k_2 t \tag{5.18}$$

The half-life of a second-order reaction is given by:

$$\frac{1}{0.5[A]_o} - \frac{1}{[A]_o} = -k_2 t_{0.5} \quad \text{or} \quad t_{0.5} = \frac{1}{k_2[A]_o} \tag{5.19}$$

The half-life of a second-order reaction is inversely proportional to $[A]_o$.
For type II second-order reactions, the rate can be expressed as:

$$\frac{d[A]}{dt} = -k_2[A][B] \tag{5.20}$$

At time t, the amounts of A and B reacted are equal (i.e., stoichiometrically 1:1 ratio and $[A]_o X_A = [B]_o X_B$, where X_A and X_B are the fractional conversions of A and B, respectively). Equation (5.20) can then be written in terms of X_A as:

$$[A]_o \frac{dX_A}{dt} = k_2[A]_o^2(1-X_A)(M-X_A) \tag{5.21}$$

where $M = [B]_o / [A]_o$. Integrating Equation (5.21):

$$\int_0^{X_A} \frac{dX_A}{(1-X_A)(M-X_A)} = k_2[A]_o \int_0^t dt \tag{5.22a}$$

or
$$\ln \frac{[B][A]_o}{[A][B]_o} = k_2([B]_o - [A]_o)t \tag{5.22b}$$

If the initial concentrations of A and B are the same, Equation (5.20) is the same as Equation (5.18) for type I. For type I, the plot of 1/[A] vs. t gives a straight line with a slope of k_2, as shown in Figure 5.5b. An example of a second-order reaction can be obtained by comparing the excessive amount of B over A. As concentration [B] remains constant, Equation (5.20) becomes a first-order reaction. Figure 5.6 shows the linear plot of the concentration, ln([B]/[A]) vs. time t, for second-order reactions.

Example 5.5
Some experimental data for the hydrolysis of ethyl acetate ($[A]_o = 0.01211$ gmol / L) with NaOH ($[B]_o = 0.02578$ gmol / L) at 15.8°C are given in Table 5.2. Calculate the rate constant of the second-order reaction.

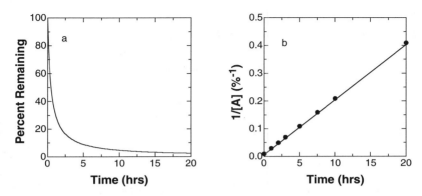

FIGURE 5.5 Linear plot of kinetic data for a second-order reaction.

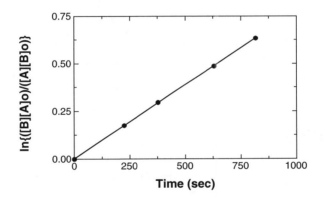

FIGURE 5.6 Alkaline hydrolysis of ethyl acetate at 15.8°C.

TABLE 5.2
Hydrolysis of Ethyl Acetate at 15.8°C

Time (sec)	[A] (g mole/L)	[B] (g mole/L)
224	0.00889	0.02256
377	0.00734	0.02101
629	0.00554	0.01921
816	0.00454	0.01821

Solution

Data given in Table 5.2 are rearranged according to Equation (5.22b):

Time (sec)	$\frac{[B][A]_o}{[A][B]_o}$
224	1.192
377	1.345
629	1.629
816	1.884

The plot of $\ln\left([B]/[A]\times[A]_o/[B]_o\right)$ against t gives a straight line with a slope of 0.000775, as shown in Figure 5.6, which is equal to $k_2([B]_o-[A]_o)$. Therefore,

$$k_2 = \frac{slope}{[B]_o-[A]_o} = \frac{0.000775}{0.01367} = 0.0566 \text{ (L / mole / sec)}$$

Example 5.6

A drug compound degrades by a second-order kinetics, and 14% of the compound is decomposed in 10 minutes. How long would it take to decompose by 35%?

Solution

At t = 10 min, $[A] = 0.86[A]_o$

From Equation (4.18),

$$\frac{1}{0.86[A]_o} - \frac{1}{[A]_o} = k_2 \times 10 \text{ min, } \quad \text{or} \quad k_2 = \frac{0.0163}{[A]_o}$$

For 35% degradation,

$$\frac{1}{0.65[A]_o} - \frac{1}{[A]_o} = \frac{0.0163}{[A]_o} \times t, \quad t = 33 \text{ min.}$$

5.4 DETERMINATION OF THE ORDER OF REACTION AND ITS RATE CONSTANT

The methods used to determine the order of the reaction and its rate constant may be divided into two groups: (1) differentiation method and (2) integration method.

5.4.1 DIFFERENTIATION METHOD

In the differentiation method, the rate of degradation with respect to time is calculated from the experimental data for concentration vs. time. Two techniques

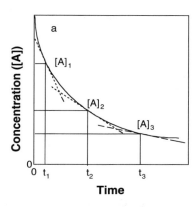
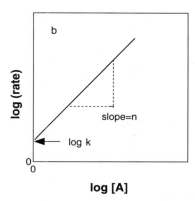

FIGURE 5.7 Procedures for determining the order of reaction and its rate constant: (a) concentration vs. time and (b) log (rate) vs. log (concentration).

of the differentiation method are the complete experimental run and the initial rate run. The analysis of the single experimental run plots the concentration vs. time followed by smoothing of the data (probably via regression analysis). From the regressed curve, one determines the slope at suitable time values, which gives the rate (i.e., $-d[A]/dt$). For a single reaction, the general form of the rate expression is given by:

$$-\frac{d[A]}{dt} = k[A]^n \tag{5.23a}$$

Taking the logarithm on both sides results in:

$$\log\left(-\frac{d[A]}{dt}\right) = \log k + n \log[A] \tag{5.23b}$$

The rate constant k and the order of reaction can be determined from the plot of log $(-d[A]/dt)$ vs. log [A]. Figure 5.7 illustrates these procedures. First, the rate is determined from the concentration vs. time curve (Figure 5.7a). Second, the rate vs. concentration is plotted in a log–log plot (Figure 5.7b). The slope and the y-intercept furnish the order of reaction and the rate constant, respectively.

If the reaction is expressed by multimolecular reactions:

$$-\frac{d[A]}{dt} = k[A]^a[B]^b[C]^c\dots\dots \tag{5.24}$$

Taking the logarithm of Equation (5.24) yields:

$$\log\left(-\frac{d[A]}{dt}\right) = \log k + a \log[A] + b \log[B] + c \log[C] + \cdots \tag{5.25}$$

TABLE 5.3
Data Workup for Example 5.7

Time (h)	% Remaining	Rate ($\Delta\%/\Delta t$)	Mean % Remaining
60	77	0.30	71
100	65	0.23	58
160	51	0.20	45
220	39	0.14	33.5
300	28	0.11	24

Equation (5.25) can be solved using a nonlinear regression method with the logarithmic values of each reactant against the rate. The y-intercept gives the rate constant whereas the coefficients represent the exponents of each reactant. The overall order of the reaction is the summation of each coefficient.

Example 5.7
Experimental data for the degradation of clindamycin in 0.1 *M* HCl at 59°C are shown in Table 5.3. Determine the order of reaction and its rate constant.

Solution
The rate ($-d[A]/dt$) in Equation (5.23a) can be obtained in two different ways: (1) the concentration vs. time is plotted and the slope at various times is calculated; or (2) the simple numerical differentiation between two adjacent points is determined (the third column in Table 5.3). The mean concentration between two points (the fourth column in Table 5.3) is determined from the corresponding values of the rates.

The log–log plot of rate vs. mean concentration [Equation (5.23b)] is presented in Figure 5.8. The slope of this plot is 0.92, which is rounded off to 1.0 (first-order). The intercept of the plot is −2.23, which gives $k = 5.9 \times 10^{-3}$ / hr.

Another technique of the differentiation method is the initial rate measurement. A series of experiments are carried out for different initial concentrations over a short time period (5 to 10% or less conversion). This approach is different from the experimental run discussed in Figure 5.7. Each rate measurement requires a new experiment with a different initial concentration. The initial rate of the reaction is determined from the curve of the concentration vs. time, as shown Figure 5.9a. The log of the initial rate is then plotted against the log of the initial concentration (Figure 5.9b). If the order of the reaction calculated from the concentration–time curve is different from the one determined by initial rate experiments, interference by the reaction products is expected, leading to complex reaction kinetics.

5.4.2 INTEGRATION METHOD

The integration method is based on comparisons between the observed experimental data (concentration vs. time) and the calculated values of the analytical equations. The equations are obtained from the integration of the mathematical expressions of the rate of the reaction. There are two techniques in the integration method: the

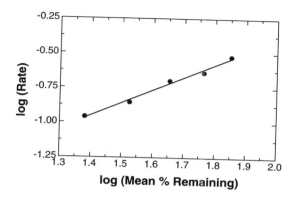

FIGURE 5.8 Log–log plot of rate vs. mean concentration.

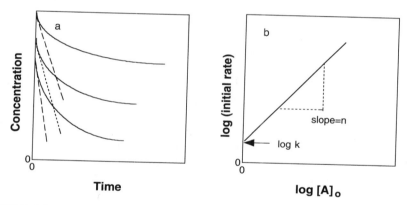

FIGURE 5.9 Method of initial rate measurement for determining the order of reaction.

general integration method and the fractional life method (i.e., half-life). The general integration method will be discussed first.

Example 5.8

The decomposition of an active drug in an aqueous solution is investigated over a period of time at a constant temperature. The resulting data of the concentration vs. time are shown in Table 5.4. What is the approximate order of the degradation kinetics and its rate constant?

Solution

First assume that either first-order or second-order reactions are applicable to the experimental data. Use Equation (5.13) and Equation (5.18) for the first-order and second-order reactions, respectively.

TABLE 5.4
Kinetic Data for Drug Degradation

T (day)	Concentration (mg/L)	k_1 (day^{-1})	k_2 (L/mg/day)
0	10.0		
5	6.5	8.62×10^{-2}	1.08×10^{-2}
10	4.8	6.06	1.09
20	3.2	4.05	1.04
30	2.4	2.88	1.04
40	1.9	2.34	1.10
50	1.6	1.72	0.99
60	1.34	1.77	1.21
70	1.17	1.36	1.08
80	1.04	1.18	1.07

$$\ln\left(\frac{[A]}{[A]_o}\right) = -k_1 t \qquad (5.13)$$

$$\frac{1}{[A]} - \frac{1}{[A]_o} = k_2 t \qquad (5.18)$$

If Equation (5.13) or Equation (5.18) fits the experimental data, the calculated values of the rate constant at various time intervals should all be the same or have small variations without any definite trend. The calculations of k_1 and k_2 based on the first point are shown below, and subsequent calculations are shown in Table 5.4.

$$k_1 = -\frac{1}{t}\ln\left(\frac{[A]}{[A]_o}\right) = -\frac{1}{5}\ln\frac{6.5}{10} = 8.62 \times 10^{-2}\,\text{day}^{-1}$$

$$k_2 = \frac{1}{t}\left(\frac{1}{[A]} - \frac{1}{[A]_o}\right) = \frac{1}{5}\left(\frac{1}{6.5} - \frac{1}{10}\right) = 1.08 \times 10^{-2}\,\text{L}/\text{mg}/\text{day}$$

In Table 5.4 the k_1 values show a definite trend with time; while the k_2 values show small variations with no definite trend. Therefore, the first-order reaction mechanism does not adequately describe the experimental kinetic data.

The next step is to plot the experimental data according to Equation (5.13) and Equation (5.18), as ln [A] vs. t and 1/[A] vs. t, respectively. Figure 5.10 shows that Equation (5.18) fits the experimental data well. The slope of this straight line gives the value of k_2:

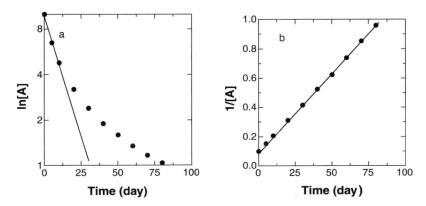

FIGURE 5.10 Comparative results of general integration method for first-order and second-order reactions: (a) first-order plot and (b) second-order plot.

$$\text{slope} = k_2 = \frac{0.15 - 0.96}{5 - 80} = 1.08 \text{ L / mg / day}$$

The *half-life* method (in general, the fractional-life method) is very useful in preliminary estimates of the order of the reaction. A series of experimental runs is carried out with different initial concentrations. If an irreversible reaction is considered:

$$\alpha A + \beta B + \gamma C + \cdots \longrightarrow \text{products}$$

The rate of reaction is given by the following equation:

$$-\frac{d[A]}{dt} = k[A]^a[B]^b[C]^c \cdots \tag{5.24}$$

If the stoichiometric ratios among the reactants are constant, Equation (5.24) can be rearranged to:

$$-\frac{d[A]}{dt} = k[A]^a\left(\frac{\beta}{\alpha}[A]\right)^b\left(\frac{\gamma}{\alpha}[A]\right)^c \cdots = k\left(\frac{\beta}{\alpha}\right)^b\left(\frac{\gamma}{\alpha}\right)^c \cdots [A]^{a+b+c\cdots} \tag{5.25}$$

or

$$-\frac{d[A]}{dt} = k'[A]^n \tag{5.26}$$

where

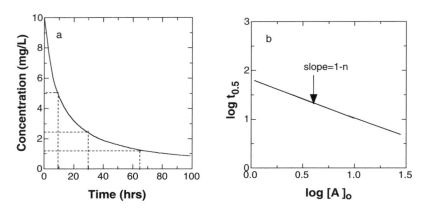

FIGURE 5.11 Concentration vs. time for the half-life method.

$$k' = k\left(\frac{\beta}{\alpha}\right)^b \left(\frac{\gamma}{\alpha}\right)^c$$

and n is $a + b + c + \ldots$.

Assume $n \neq 1$. Integrating Equation (5.26) and solving for the half-life yields

$$t_{0.5} = \frac{2^{n-1} - 1}{k'(n-1)} [A]_o^{1-n} \tag{5.27}$$

Taking the logarithms of Equation (5.27) gives:

$$\log t_{0.5} = \log\left(\frac{2^{n-1} - 1}{k'(n-1)}\right) + (1-n) \log [A]_o \tag{5.28}$$

Plotting $\log t_{0.5}$ against $\log [A]_o$ results in a straight line with a slope of $(1-n)$ as shown in Figure 5.11. If $n = 1$ (i.e., first-order reaction), Equation (5.14a) should be used instead. The order of the reaction should be rounded off to the integer closest to n, especially in pharmaceutical applications. An exact integrated equation is then used to determine the reaction rate constant.

Example 5.9

The degradation of a drug A with a reagent B was carried out using equal initial concentrations of the reactants. The following degradation data were obtained:

Time (sec)	0	50	100	150	200	250
$[A] \times 10^3$ mol/L	5.00	3.28	2.44	1.94	1.61	1.38

Determine the order of the degradation reaction using the half-life method.

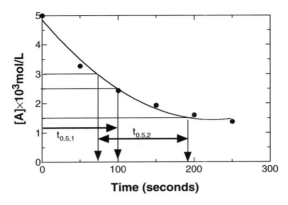

FIGURE 5.12 Graphical presentation for Example 5.9.

Solution

First construct a graph of the experimental data as shown in Figure 5.12. Second, obtain a regression analysis (t vs. [A]):

$$t = 487.8 - 2.133 \times 10^5 [A] + 2.326 \times 10^7 [A]^2$$

Half-life with $[A]_o = 5.0 \times 10^{-3} \, mol/L$, $t_{0.5} = 99.93$ sec

Half-life with $[A]_o = 3.0 \times 10^{-3} \, mol/L$, $t_{0.5} = (220.19 - 57.24)$ sec $= 162.95$ sec

Equation (5.28) can be rearranged to:

$$\frac{t_{0.5,1}}{t_{0.5,2}} = \left(\frac{[A]_{o,2}}{[A]_{o,1}} \right)^{n-1} \quad \text{or} \quad n = \frac{\log(t_{0.5,1/t_{0.5,2}})}{\log([A]_{o,2}/[A]_{o,1})} + 1 \quad (5.29)$$

Therefore,
$$n = \frac{\log(99.93/162.95)}{\log(3.0 \times 10^{-3}/5 \times 10^{-3})} + 1 = 1.93 \approx 2$$

5.5 OTHER IRREVERSIBLE REACTIONS

5.5.1 Autocatalytic Reactions

When the product is involved in a chemical reaction with the reactant, this is known as an autocatalytic reaction. The equation for this reaction is:

$$A + P \longrightarrow P + P$$

The rate of the reaction is given by:

$$-\frac{d[A]}{dt} = k_a[A][P] \tag{5.30a}$$

$$\frac{d[P]}{dt} = k_a[P]([A]_o + [P]_o - [P]) \tag{5.30b}$$

where k_a is the autocatalytic reaction rate constant. The total number of moles of the reactant (A) and the product (P) do not change throughout the reaction at any time:

$$[T] = [A] + [P] = [A]_o + [P]_o = \text{constant} \tag{5.31}$$

where [T] is the total concentration.

Equation (5.30b) becomes:

$$-\frac{d[P]}{[P]([T]-[P])} = k_a dt \tag{5.32}$$

Integrating and rearranging Equation (5.32) yields:

$$-\int_{[P]_o}^{[P]} \frac{d[P]}{[P]([T]-[P])} = -\frac{1}{[T]}\left(\int_{[P]_o}^{[P]} \frac{d[P]}{[P]} + \int_{[P]_o}^{[P]} \frac{d[P]}{[T]-[P]}\right) = k_a \int_0^t dt \tag{5.33a}$$

or $\quad \ln\left(\frac{[P][A]_o}{[P]_o([A]_o + [P]_o - [P])}\right) = \ln\left(\frac{[P][A]_o}{[A][P]_o}\right) = [T]k_a t = ([A]_o + [P]_o)k_a t \tag{5.33b}$

Equation (5.33b) yields:

$$[P] = \frac{[A]_o + [P]_o}{1 + ([A]_o/[P]_o)e^{-([A]_o+[P]_o)k_a t}} \tag{5.34}$$

Substituting Equation (5.34) into Equation (5.30a) and solving [A] yields:

$$[A] = \frac{[A]_o + [P]_o}{1 + ([P]_o/[A]_o)e^{([A]_o+[P]_o)kt_a}} \tag{5.35}$$

In an autocatalytic reaction, the rate of the reaction increases as the product forms and reaches a maximum at $[A] = [P]$. Then, the rate becomes zero as the reactant completely disappears, as shown in Figure 5.13. It is presumed that some

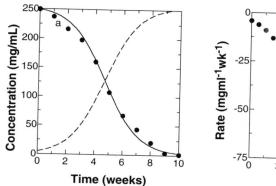
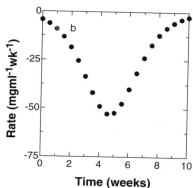

FIGURE 5.13 Autocatalytic reaction of obidoxime chloride with $k = 3.27 \times 10^{-3} mL(mg \cdot wk)^{-1}$: (a) concentration vs. time and (b) rate vs. time. [Graph reconstructed from data by Rubnov et al., *J. Pharm. Pharmcol.*, 51, 9 (1999).]

of product P must be present at t = 0 in order to proceed with the autocatalytic reaction. To test for an autocatalytic reaction, plot the time and concentration terms of Equation (5.33b) to see the straight line passing through the origin.

Example 5.10

As shown in Figure 5.13, obidoxime HCl underwent an autocatalytic reaction. Assume $[A]_o = 250$ mg / L and $[P]_o = 2.5$ mg / L. Calculate the rate constant.

Solution

Numerical data were extracted from Figure 5.13 as:

Time (weeks)	[A]	[P]	$\dfrac{[P][A]_o}{[A][P]_o}$
0	250.0	2.5	
1	237.5	15.0	6.3
2	216.2	36.3	16.8
3	197.5	55.0	27.9
4	160.0	92.5	57.8
5	107.5	145.0	134.9
6	67.5	185.0	274.1
7	43.8	208.7	476.5
8	21.3	231.2	1085.4
9	3.8	248.7	6544.7
10	1.3	251.2	19323.1

The plot of the final column against time gives a slope of 0.958/week (Figure 5.14), which is equal to $k_a([A]_o + [P]_o)$. Therefore,

$$k_a = \frac{0.958 / wk}{252.5 mg / mL} = 3.8 \times 10^{-3} \ mL / mg / wk$$

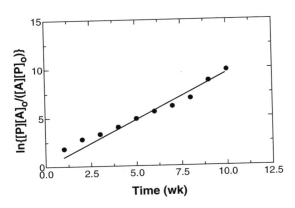

FIGURE 5.14 Determination of the rate constant of an autocatalytic reaction.

5.5.2 PARALLEL REACTIONS

Let us consider that a compound A decomposes by several paths as follows:

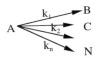

The reaction rate expression for compound A is written as:

$$-\frac{d[A]}{dt} = (k_1 + k_2 + \cdots + k_n)[A] = [A]\sum_{i=1}^{n} k_i \qquad (5.36)$$

Integrating Equation (5.36) gives:

$$\ln\left(\frac{[A]}{[A]_o}\right) = -\sum_{i=1}^{n} k_i t \qquad (5.37)$$

The rate expression for the other species (e.g., B) is given by:

$$-\frac{d[B]}{dt} = k_1[A] \qquad (5.38)$$

Substituting Equation (5.37) into Equation (5.38) and integrating the resulting equation yields:

$$[B] = [B]_o + \frac{k_1[A]_o}{\sum\limits_{i=1}^{n} k_i}\left[1 - \exp\left(-\sum_{n=1}^{n} k_i t\right)\right] = [B]_o + \frac{k_1}{\sum\limits_{i=1}^{n} k_i}([A]_o - [A]) \qquad (5.39)$$

Similar equations can be derived for other species. From the stoichiometry, the total concentrations of all the products remain unchanged at any given time (i.e., $[A]+[B]+\cdots+[N]=[A]_o$). Thus, the following expressions can be obtained:

$$\frac{[B]-[B]_o}{[C]-[C]_o}=\frac{k_1}{k_2}, \quad \frac{[B]-[B]_o}{[D]-[D]_o}=\frac{k_1}{k_3} \quad \text{etc.} \tag{5.40}$$

If the initial concentration of the products is zero, then the amount of each product present in the reaction mixture is in the ratio of:

$$[B]:[C]:[D]:\cdots:[N]=k_1:k_2:k_3:\cdots:k_n \tag{5.41}$$

When the reaction is complete or has gone for an infinite time, the mole fraction of each product can be expressed as:

$$\frac{[B]_\infty}{[B]_\infty+[C]_\infty+\cdots+[N]_\infty}=\frac{[B]_\infty}{[A]_o}=\frac{k_1}{\sum\limits_{i=1}^{n}k_i} \tag{5.42}$$

Similar expressions can be obtained for other species. From Equation (5.37), the slope is:

$$\text{slope}=-\sum_{n=1}^{n}k_i=-k_T \tag{5.43}$$

The rate constants for each product ($k_1, k_2,\cdots$) are then determined from Equation (5.42) and Equation (5.43).

Figure 5.15 shows the parallel degradation of cadralazine to triazolone, pyridazinone, and pyridazine at pH 7.4 and 80°C.

Example 5.11

The degradation rate constant of the cadralazine degradation reaction has been determined based on the data given in Figure 5.15 as $k_T=0.024/\text{hr}$. It was found that the fractional concentration of all species (A, B, C, and D) with respect to the initial concentration of [A] was 0.46, 0.31, 0.18, and 0.05, respectively, at t = 6 hr. Calculate the individual rate constants.

Solution

$[B]_o=[C]_o=[D]_o=0$. Then, Equation (5.39) can be transformed to:

$$\frac{[B]/[A]_o}{(1-[A]/[A]_o)}=\frac{0.31}{(1-0.46)}=0.574=\frac{k_1}{k_T}=\frac{k_1}{0.024/\text{hr}}, \quad k_1=0.014/\text{hr}$$

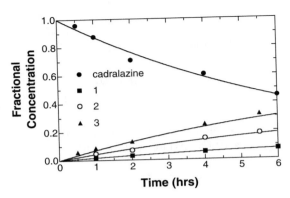

FIGURE 5.15 Parallel degradation of cadralazine to triazolone (1), pyridazinone (2), and pyridazine (3). [Graph reconstructed from data by Visconti et al., *J. Pharm. Sci.*, 73, 1812 (1984).]

Likewise,

$$k_2 = 0.33 \times 0.024 \,/\, hr = 0.008 \,/\, hr \quad \text{and} \quad k_3 = 0.096 \times 0.024 \,/\, hr = 0.002 \,/\, hr.$$

5.5.3 CONSECUTIVE REACTIONS

The first product of a chemical degradation reaction successively undergoes another degradation reaction to give a second intermediate or a final product. Consecutive unimolecular first-order reactions are represented as:

$$A \xrightarrow{k_1} B \xrightarrow{k_2} C \tag{5.44}$$

The rate equations for the three compounds are :

$$\frac{d[A]}{dt} = -k_1[A] \tag{5.45}$$

$$\frac{d[B]}{dt} = k_1[A] - k_2[B] \tag{5.46}$$

$$\frac{d[C]}{dt} = k_2[B] \tag{5.47}$$

Integrating equation (5.45) yields:

$$[A] = [A]_o \, e^{-k_1 t} \tag{5.48}$$

Substituting Equation (5.48) into Equation (5.46) gives:

$$\frac{d[B]}{dt} + k_2[B] = k_1[A]_o e^{-k_1 t} \tag{5.49}$$

which is an ordinary first-order differential equation and can be solved as:

$$[B]e^{\int k_2 dt} = \int k_1[A]_o e^{-k_1 t} e^{\int k_2 dt} dt + \text{constant} \tag{5.50}$$

Solving Equation (5.50), under the condition of $[B]_o = 0$ at $t = 0$, yields:

$$[B] = k_1[A]_o \left(\frac{e^{-k_1 t}}{k_2 - k_1} + \frac{e^{-k_2 t}}{k_1 - k_2} \right) \tag{5.51}$$

Notice that the total number of moles present during the reaction has remained constant. Then, the concentration of C can be determined:

$$[C] = [A]_o - [A] - [B] = [A]_o \left(1 + \frac{k_2}{k_1 - k_2} e^{-k_1 t} + \frac{k_1}{k_2 - k_1} e^{-k_2 t} \right) \tag{5.52}$$

Equation (5.51) can also be used for the concentration–time profile of a drug in plasma after the drug has been orally administered (one-compartment model):

$$\boxed{\text{Drug in GI}} \xrightarrow{\text{absorption}, k_1} \boxed{\text{Drug in Plasma}} \xrightarrow{\text{elimination}, k_2}$$

The values of the rate constants (k_1 and k_2) dictate the maximum concentration of B and its location. The time (t_{max}) needed to reach the maximum concentration of B (i.e., $[B]_{max}$) can be obtained by differentiating Equation (5.51) with respect to time and setting $d[B]/dt = 0$.

$$\frac{d[B]}{dt} = [A]_o k_1 \left(\frac{-k_1 e^{-k_1 t}}{k_2 - k_1} - \frac{k_2 e^{-k_2 t}}{k_1 - k_2} \right) = 0 \tag{5.53}$$

$$t_{max} = \frac{\ln(k_2 / k_1)}{k_2 - k_1} \tag{5.54}$$

Substituting Equation (5.54) into Equation (5.51) gives:

$$[B]_{max} = [A]_o \frac{k_1}{k_2 - k_1} \left\{ e^{-\frac{k_1}{k_2 - k_1}\ln\left(\frac{k_2}{k_1}\right)} - e^{-\frac{k_2}{k_2 - k_1}\ln\left(\frac{k_2}{k_1}\right)} \right\} = [A]_o \left(\frac{k_1}{k_2} \right)^{k_2/(k_2 - k_1)} \tag{5.55}$$

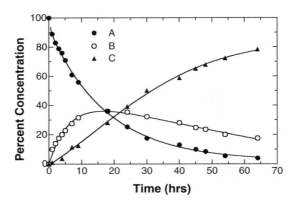

FIGURE 5.16 Time–concentration curves for irreversible consecutive reactions of a hydro-cortisone hemiester (A), a hydrocortisone alcohol (B), and the degradation products (C) at 70°C and pH 6.9. [Graph reconstructed from data by Mauger et al., *J. Pharm. Sci.,* 58, 574 (1969).]

Figure 5.16 shows the time–concentration curves for the three species. The concentration of A decreases exponentially. The concentration of B gradually increases up to a maximum and then goes down. The concentration of C increases sigmoidally, with the highest rate of increase at t_{max}.

Example 5.12

For the reaction in series ($A \rightarrow B \rightarrow C$), calculate the maximum concentration of B and its time if $k_1 = k_2$.

Solution

If $k_1 = k_2$, substituting Equation (5.54) into Equation (5.55) yields an indefinite value for $[B]_{max}$. Then, take Equation (5.45), Equation (5.46), and Equation (5.47) and derive the solution once again because Equation (5.54) and Equation (5.55) are only obtained when $k_1 \neq k_2$. Equation (5.46) can then be written as:

$$\frac{d[B]}{dt} = k_1[A] - k_1[B] \qquad (5.56)$$

Substituting Equation (5.48) into Equation (5.56) gives:

$$\frac{d[B]}{dt} + k_1[B] = k_1[A]_0 e^{-k_1 t} \qquad (5.57)$$

which is a first-order linear differential equation. Equation (5.57) is solved as:

$$[B]e^{\int k_1 dt} = \int k[A]_0 e^{-k_1 t} e^{\int k_1 dt} dt + \text{constant} \qquad (5.58)$$

Integrating Equation (5.58) with $[B]_o = 0$ at $t = 0$ yields:

$$[B] = k_1[A]_o\, t e^{-k_1 t} \tag{5.59}$$

Differentiating Equation (5.59) and setting $d[B]/dt = 0$ gives:

$$t_{max} = \frac{1}{k_1} \tag{5.60}$$

Substituting Equation (5.60) into Equation (5.59) yields:

$$[B]_{max} = \frac{[A]_o}{e} = 0.37[A]_o \tag{5.61}$$

Equation (5.61) implies that the yield of the product B cannot exceed 37% in this process.

Example 5.13
From Figure 5.16, calculate the rate constants and t_{max}.

Solution
The first-order rate constant of 0.062/hr for the reactant A (hydrocortisone hemiester) was determined by a simple least-square method of Equation (5.48). It was also determined from the graph that $[B]_{max} = 0.355\,[A]_o$.

$$\frac{[B]_{max}}{[A]_o} = \left(\frac{k_1}{k_2}\right)^{k_2/(k_2-k)_1} = 0.355$$

Taking logarithms on both sides gives:

$$\frac{k_2}{k_2-k_1}\log\left(\frac{k_1}{k_2}\right) = \frac{k_2}{k_2-0.062}\log\left(\frac{0.062}{k_2}\right) = -0.450$$

By trial and error, $k_2 = 0.066 / hr$ is determined. Then, $t_{max} = \ln(k_2/k_1)/(k_2-k_1) = 15.6$ hr.

5.6 REVERSIBLE REACTIONS

5.6.1 Reversible First-Order Reactions

Let us consider reactions for which reactants and products coexist at equilibrium with no complete conversion. The simplest case of these reactions is that the forward unimolecular reaction is opposed by the reverse unimolecular reaction as:

$$A \rightleftharpoons B \tag{5.62}$$

The rate expression is given as:

$$-\frac{d[A]}{dt} = k_f[A] - k_r[B] \tag{5.63}$$

where k_f and k_r are the forward and reverse reaction rate constants, respectively. Equation (5.63) can be rewritten in terms of the extent of reaction as:

$$\frac{[A]_o \, dx}{dt} = k_f([A]_o - [A]_o x) - k_r([A]_o M - [A]_o x) \tag{5.64}$$

where $M = [B]_o / [A]_o$ and x is the extent of reaction.

At equilibrium, the rate of the forward reaction is equal to that of the reverse reaction:

$$k_f[A]_\infty = k_r[B]_\infty \quad \text{or} \quad K = \frac{k_f}{k_r} = \frac{[B]_\infty}{[A]_\infty} = \frac{M + x_e}{1 - x_e} \tag{5.65}$$

where x_e is the equilibrium extent of reaction. Substituting Equation (5.65) into Equation (5.64) yields:

$$\frac{dx}{dt} = \frac{k_f(M+1)}{M + x_e}(x_e - x) \tag{5.66}$$

Integrating Equation (5.66) gives:

$$\ln\left(\frac{x_e - x}{x_e}\right) = \ln\left(\frac{[A] - [A]_\infty}{[A]_o - [A]_\infty}\right) = -\frac{M+1}{M + x_e} k_f t = -(k_f + k_r)t \tag{5.67}$$

A plot of $\ln[(x_e - x)x_e]$ vs. t or $\ln[([A] - [A]_\infty)/([A]_o - [A]_\infty)]$ versus t gives a straight line.

Figure 5.17 shows the interconversion of the lactone form of a semisynthetic analogue of camptothecin to its ring-opened carboxylate form. The lactone form predominates in low pH whereas the ring-opened carboxylate form prevails at neutral and alkaline pH, as illustrated in Figure 5.18.

Example 5.14

The lactone form of an analogue of camptothecin converts to its ring-opened carboxylate form. Both forms are in equilibrium. The following degradation data of the lactone form were collected:

Time (hr)	2	4	6	8	10	12	24	42	60
Conc. (%)	63	42	33	27	24	23	20	18	17

Calculate the forward and backward rate constants.

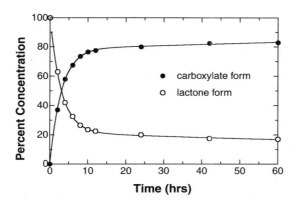

FIGURE 5.17 Hydrolytic degradation of an analogue of camptothecin at pH 7.11, I = 0.4 *M*, and 25°C. [Graph reconstructed from data by Kim et al., AAPS National Meeting, Paper No. 7916, Indianapolis, IN, Oct. 29, 2000.]

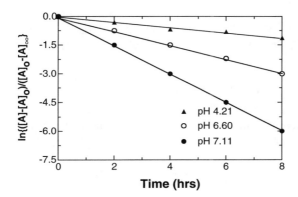

FIGURE 5.18 Determination of the rate constant of a reversible reaction.

Solution

First, one should extend the data to t = ∞ to obtain $[A]_\infty$ (= 16%). This leads to $[B]_\infty$ = 84%. The equilibrium constant becomes:

$$K = \frac{k_f}{k_r} = \frac{[B]_\infty}{[A]_\infty} = \frac{84}{16} = 5.25$$

According to Equation (5.67), the data are transformed to:

Time (hr)	2	4	6	8
$\ln\left[([A]-[A]_\infty)/([A]_0-[A]_\infty)\right]$	−1.50	−3.00	−4.50	−6.00

A plot of the second row vs. t will be a straight line with a slope of −0.75, which is equal to − ($k_f + k_r$). Then, the rate constants become:

$$k_f = 0.63 \, / \, hr \quad \text{and} \quad k_r = 0.12 \, / \, hr$$

5.6.2 Reversible Second-Order Reactions

Molecules may undergo more complex reactions than described by the first-order reversible steps. For example, two molecules react to produce one or two molecules, which in turn are in equilibrium with the two reactants. Consider the following chemical reaction:

$$A + B \rightleftarrows C + D \tag{5.68}$$

The rate is given in terms of the extent of reaction (x) (i.e., the decrease in the concentration of A with time) as:

$$\frac{dx}{dt} = k_f([A]_o - x)([B]_o - x) - k_r([C]_o + x)([D]_o + x) \tag{5.69}$$

If only A and B are presented initially (i.e., $[C]_o = [D]_o = 0$), then Equation (5.69) becomes:

$$\frac{dx}{dt} = k_f([A]_o - x)([B]_o - x) - k_r x^2 \tag{5.70}$$

When the equilibrium concentration is introduced, Equation (5.70) is further simplified. At $dx/dt = 0$, Equation (5.69) gives:

$$k_r = k_f \frac{([A]_o - x_e)([B]_o - x_e)}{x_e^2} \tag{5.71}$$

Substituting Equation (5.71) into Equation (5.70) yields:

$$\frac{dx}{dt} = k_f([A]_o - x)([B]_o - x) - k_f \frac{([A]_o - x_e)([B]_o - x_e)}{x_e^2} x^2 \tag{5.72}$$

Integration of Equation (5.72) by the partial fraction technique yields:

$$\ln\left(\frac{x[[A]_o[B]_o - ([A]_o + [B]_o)x_e] + [A]_o[B]_o x_e}{[A]_o[B]_o(x_e - x)} \right)$$
$$= k_f \frac{2[A]_o[B]_o - ([A]_o + [B]_o)x_e}{x_e} t \tag{5.73}$$

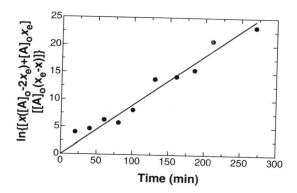

FIGURE 5.19 Degradation of 0.1 mg/L 5-aminolevulinic acid (ALA) followed by a reversible second-order reaction at pH 7.4 (200 mM NaHPO4). [Graph reconstructed from data by Bunke et al., *J. Pharm. Sci.*, 89, 1335 (2000).]

If $[A]_o = [B]_o$ or the reaction is $2A \rightleftharpoons C + D$, Equation (5.73) becomes:

$$\ln\left[\frac{x([A]_e - 2x_e) + [A]_o x_e}{[A]_o(x_e - x)}\right] = k_f \frac{2[A]_o([A]_o - x_e)}{x_e} t \qquad (5.74)$$

5-Aminolevulinic acid undergoes dimerization to 2,5-dicarboxyethyl-3,6-dihydropyrazine by a reversible second-order reaction. Figure 5.19 shows the plot of the left-hand side term of Equation (5.74) vs. time, which gives a straight line. Since this is second-order kinetics, the experimental data should demonstrate that the dimerization depends upon the initial concentration, with higher concentration leading to higher reaction rate.

A first-order reaction is often opposed by a second-order reaction and vice versa:

$$A \rightleftharpoons B + C \qquad (5.75a)$$

$$A + B \rightleftharpoons C \qquad (5.75b)$$

Equation (5.75a) is solved in exactly the same manner as Equation (5.68). The rate in terms of the extent of the reaction is then given by:

$$\frac{dx}{dt} = k_f([A]_o - x) - k_r x^2 \qquad (5.76)$$

Applying the equilibrium extent of the reaction to Equation (5.76) gives:

$$\frac{dx}{dt} = k_f([A]_o - x) - k_f \frac{([A]_o - x)}{x_e^2} x^2 \qquad (5.77)$$

Integration of Equation (5.77) by the partial fractions method yields:

$$\ln\left[\frac{[A]_o x_e + x([A]_o - x_e)}{[A]_o(x_e - x)}\right] = k_f \frac{2[A]_o - x_e}{x_e} t \qquad (5.78)$$

Likewise, the solution for Equation (5.75b) is given by:

$$\ln\left[\frac{x_e([A]_o^2 - x_e x)}{[A]_o^2(x_e - x)}\right] = k_r \frac{[A]_o^2 - x_e^2}{x_e} t \qquad (5.79)$$

5.7 REVERSIBLE AND SERIES REACTIONS (EIGENVALUE METHOD)

Many degradation and biotransformation reactions follow reversible and/or consecutive series pathways. Consider, for example, two reversible and consecutive first-order reactions:

$$X_1 \underset{k_{21}}{\overset{k_{12}}{\rightleftarrows}} X_2 \underset{k_{32}}{\overset{k_{23}}{\rightleftarrows}} X_3$$

The rate expressions for each compound are given by:

$$\frac{d[X_1]}{dt} = -k_{12}[X_1] + k_{21}[X_2] \qquad (5.80)$$

$$\frac{d[X_2]}{dt} = k_{12}[X_1] - (k_{21} + k_{23})[X_2] + k_{32}[X_3] \qquad (5.81)$$

$$\frac{d[X_3]}{dt} = k_{23}[X_2] - k_{32}[X_3] \qquad (5.82)$$

or, in a matrix form:

$$\frac{d}{dt}\begin{bmatrix} X_1 \\ X_2 \\ X_3 \end{bmatrix} = \begin{bmatrix} -k_{12} & k_{21} & 0 \\ k_{12} & -(k_{21} + k_{23}) & k_{32} \\ 0 & k_{23} & -k_{32} \end{bmatrix}\begin{bmatrix} X_1 \\ X_2 \\ X_3 \end{bmatrix} \qquad (5.83)$$

Simply,

$$\frac{dX}{dt} = KX \qquad (5.84)$$

where boldface symbols denote matrices.

Equation (5.80), Equation (5.81), and Equation (5.82) may be solved by analytical methods similar to those described in the previous sections and by the Laplace transform method, which will be dealt with in Section 5.8. In this section, the eigenvalue method is discussed. Equation (5.84) is a first-order equation, the solution of which is similar to that of the corresponding scalar equation, Equation (5.12):

$$X(t) = Ye^{Kt} \qquad (5.85)$$

A particular solution for each compound can be then written as:

$$[A] = Y_1 e^{-\chi t}, \quad [B] = Y_2 e^{-\chi t}, \quad [C] = Y_3 e^{-\chi t} \qquad (5.86)$$

Substituting Equation (5.86) into Equation (5.80), Equation (5.81), and Equation (5.82) yields:

$$(k_{12} - \chi)Y_1 \qquad\qquad - k_{21}Y_2 \qquad\qquad\qquad = 0$$

$$- k_{12}Y_1 + (k_{21} + k_{23} - \chi)Y_2 \qquad - k_{32}Y_3 \quad = 0 \qquad (5.87)$$

$$- k_{23}Y_2 + (k_{32} - \chi)Y_3 \quad = 0$$

where the Y_i terms are constants and χ is the parameter to be determined. Equation (5.87) is a set of simultaneous homogeneous linear equations. In a nontrivial solution, the determinant of the coefficients is zero:

$$\begin{vmatrix} k_{12} - \chi & - k_{21} & 0 \\ -k_{12} & k_{21} + k_{23} - \chi & - k_{32} \\ 0 & - k_{23} & k_{32} - \chi \end{vmatrix} = 0 \qquad (5.88)$$

or

$$\chi^3 - (k_{12} + k_{21} + k_{23} + k_{32})\chi^2 + (k_{12}k_{23} + k_{21}k_{32} + k_{12}k_{32})\chi = 0 \qquad (5.89)$$

where χ is the eigenvalue of this determinant. The three roots of χ are given by:

$$\chi_1 = 0, \quad \chi_2 = (\alpha + \beta)/2, \quad \chi_3 = (\alpha - \beta)/2 \tag{5.90}$$

where $\alpha = k_{12} + k_{21} + k_{23} + k_{32}$ and $\beta = \sqrt{\alpha^2 - 4(k_{12}k_{23} + k_{21}k_{32} + k_{12}k_{32})}$.
Substituting Equation (5.90) into Equation (5.86) then yields:

$$[X_1] = Y_{11}e^{-\chi_1 t} + Y_{12}e^{-\chi_2 t} + Y_{13}e^{-\chi_3 t} \tag{5.91a}$$

$$[X_2] = Y_{21}e^{-\chi_1 t} + Y_{22}e^{-\chi_2 t} + Y_{23}e^{-\chi_3 t} \tag{5.91b}$$

$$[X_3] = Y_{31}e^{-\chi_1 t} + Y_{32}e^{-\chi_2 t} + Y_{33}e^{-\chi_3 t} \tag{5.91c}$$

Of the three equations — Equation (5.80), Equation (5.81), and Equation (5.82) — only two are independent, while the remaining equation is dependent. Substituting Equation (5.91a) and Equation (5.91c) into Equation (5.80) and Equation (5.82), respectively, yields:

$$\frac{d[X_1]}{dt} = (-k_{12}Y_{11} + k_{21}Y_{21})e^{-\chi_1 t} + (-k_{12}Y_{12} + k_{21}Y_{22})e^{-\chi_2 t}$$
$$+ (-k_{12}Y_{f3} + k_{21}Y_{23})e^{-\chi_3 t} \tag{5.92a}$$

$$\frac{d[X_3]}{dt} = (k_{23}Y_{21} - k_{32}Y_{31})e^{-\chi_1 t} + (k_{23}Y_{22} - k_{32}Y_{32})e^{-\chi_2 t}$$
$$+ (k_{23}Y_{23} - k_{32}Y_{33})e^{-\chi_3 t} \tag{5.92b}$$

Taking the derivatives of Equation (5.91a) and Equation (5.91c) gives:

$$\frac{d[X_1]}{dt} = -\chi_1 Y_{11}e^{-\chi_1 t} - \chi_2 Y_{12}e^{-\chi_2 t} - \chi_3 Y_{13}e^{-\chi_3 t} \tag{5.93a}$$

$$\frac{d[X_3]}{dt} = -\chi_1 Y_{31}e^{-\chi_1 t} - \chi_2 Y_{32}e^{-\chi_2 t} - \chi_3 Y_{33}e^{-\chi_3 t} \tag{5.93b}$$

Substitute Equation (5.92a) into Equation (5.93a) and Equation (5.92b) into Equation (5.93b), and χ is solved. For $\chi = \chi_1$

$$(k_{12} - \chi_1)Y_{11} - k_{21}Y_{21} = 0 \tag{5.94a}$$

$$k_{23}Y_{21} + (\chi_1 - k_{32})Y_{31} = 0 \tag{5.94b}$$

$$Y_{21} = \frac{k_{12} - \chi_1}{k_{21}} Y_{11} = \frac{k_{12}}{k_{21}} Y_{11}, \qquad Y_{31} = \frac{k_{23}}{k_{32} - \chi_1} Y_{21} = \frac{k_{23}k_{12}}{k_{32}k_{21}} Y_{11} \qquad (5.94c)$$

For $\chi = \chi_2$

$$(\chi_2 - k_{12})Y_{12} + k_{21}Y_{22} = 0 \qquad (5.95a)$$

$$(k_{32} - \chi_2)Y_{32} - k_{23}Y_{22} = 0 \qquad (5.95b)$$

$$Y_{22} = \frac{k_{12} - \chi_2}{k_{21}} Y_{12}, \quad Y_{32} = \frac{k_{23}}{k_{32} - \chi_2} Y_{22} = \frac{k_{23}(k_{12} - \chi_2)}{k_{21}(k_{32} - \chi_2)} Y_{12} \qquad (5.95c)$$

For $\chi = \chi_3$

$$Y_{23} = \frac{k_{12} - \chi_3}{k_{21}} Y_{13}, \quad Y_{33} = \frac{k_{23}}{k_{32} - \chi_3} Y_{23} = \frac{k_{23}(k_{12} - \chi_3)}{k_{21}(k_{32} - \chi_3)} Y_{13} \qquad (5.96)$$

Substituting Equation (5.94c), Equation (5.95c), and Equation (5.96) into Equation (5.91a), Equation (5.91b), and Equation (5.91c), respectively:

$$[X_1] = Y_{11}e^{-\chi_1 t} + Y_{12}e^{-\chi_2 t} + Y_{13}e^{-\chi_3 t} \qquad (5.97a)$$

$$[X_2] = \left(\frac{k_{12}}{k_{21}}\right)Y_{11}e^{-\chi_1 t} + \left(\frac{k_{12} - \chi_2}{k_{21}}\right)Y_{12}e^{-\chi_2 t} + \left(\frac{k_{12} - \chi_3}{k_{21}}\right)Y_{13}e^{-\chi_3 t} \qquad (5.97b)$$

$$[X_3] = \left(\frac{k_{23}k_{12}}{k_{32}k_{21}}\right)Y_{11}e^{-\chi_1 t} + \left(\frac{k_{23}(k_{12} - \chi_2)}{k_{21}(k_{32} - \chi_2)}\right)Y_{12}e^{-\chi_2 t} + \left(\frac{k_{23}(k_{12} - \chi_3)}{k_{21}(k_{32} - \chi_3)}\right)Y_{13}e^{-\chi_3 t} \qquad (5.97c)$$

If $[X_1] = [X_1]_o$ and $[X_2]_o = [X_3]_o = 0$ at time $t = 0$, then

$$[X_1]_o = Y_{11} + Y_{12} + Y_{13} \qquad (5.98a)$$

$$0 = \left(\frac{k_{12}}{k_{21}}\right)Y_{11} + \left(\frac{k_{12} - \chi_2}{k_{21}}\right)Y_{12} + \left(\frac{k_{12} - \chi_3}{k_{21}}\right)Y_{13} \qquad (5.98b)$$

$$0 = \left(\frac{k_{23}k_{12}}{k_{32}k_{21}}\right)Y_{11} + \left(\frac{k_{23}(k_{12} - \chi_2)}{k_{21}(k_{32} - \chi_2)}\right)Y_{12} + \left(\frac{k_{23}(k_{12} - \chi_3)}{k_{21}(k_{32} - \chi_3)}\right)Y_{13} \qquad (5.98c)$$

Solving for Y_{11}, Y_{12}, and Y_{13} yields:

$$Y_{11} = \left(\frac{k_{21}k_{32}}{\chi_2\chi_3} \right)[X_1]_o \qquad (5.99a)$$

$$Y_{12} = \left(\frac{k_{12}(\chi_2 - k_{23} - k_{32})}{\chi_2(\chi_2 - \chi_3)} \right)[X_1]_o \qquad (5.99b)$$

$$Y_{13} = \left(\frac{k_{12}(k_{23} + k_{32} - \chi_3)}{\chi_3(\chi_2 - \chi_3)} \right)[X_1]_o \qquad (5.99c)$$

Substituting Equation (5.99a), Equation (5.99b), and Equation (5.99c) into Equation (5.97a), Equation (5.97b), and Equation (5.97c) yields:

$$[X_1] = [X_1]_o \left(\frac{k_{21}k_{32}}{\chi_2\chi_3} + \frac{k_{12}(\chi_2 - k_{23} - k_{32})}{\chi_2(\chi_2 - \chi_3)} e^{-\chi_2 t} + \frac{k_{12}(k_{23} + k_{32} - \chi_3)}{\chi_3(\chi_2 - \chi_3)} e^{-\chi_3 t} \right) \qquad (5.100a)$$

$$[X_2] = [X_1]_o \left(\frac{k_{12}k_{32}}{\chi_2\chi_3} + \frac{k_{12}(k_{32} - \chi_2)}{\chi_2(\chi_2 - \chi_3)} e^{-\chi_2 t} + \frac{k_{12}(\chi_3 - k_{32})}{\chi_3(\chi_2 - \chi_3)} e^{-\chi_3 t} \right) \qquad (5.100b)$$

$$[X_3] = [X_1]_o \left(\frac{k_{12}k_{32}}{\chi_2\chi_3} + \frac{k_{12}k_{23}}{\chi_2(\chi_2 - \chi_3)} e^{-\chi_2 t} - \frac{k_{12}k_{23}}{\chi_3(\chi_2 - \chi_3)} e^{-\chi_3 t} \right) \qquad (5.100c)$$

where

$$\chi_2\chi_3 = (\alpha^2 - \beta^2)/4 = k_{12}k_{23} + k_{21}k_{32} + k_{12}k_{32} \qquad (5.101)$$

Let us apply these general first-order solutions to two specific reactions: irreversible consecutive and simple reversible reactions. Consecutive reactions (A → B → C) do not have reverse reactions. This leads to:

$$k_{21} = k_{32} = 0 \qquad (5.102a)$$

$$\alpha = k_{12} + k_{23}, \qquad \beta = k_{12} - k_{23} \qquad (5.102b)$$

$$\chi_2 = k_{12}, \qquad \chi_3 = k_{23} \qquad (5.102c)$$

Substituting Equation (5.102a), Equation (5.102b), and Equation (5.102c) into Equation (5.100a), Equation (5.100b), and Equation (5.100c) yields:

$$[X_1] = [X_1]_o e^{-k_{12}t} \tag{5.103a}$$

$$[X_2] = [X_1]_o k_{12} \left(\frac{e^{-k_{12}t}}{k_{23} - k_{12}} + \frac{e^{-k_{23}t}}{k_{12} - k_{23}} \right) \tag{5.103b}$$

$$[X_3] = [X_1]_o \left(1 + \frac{k_{21}}{k_{12} - k_{23}} e^{-k_{12}t} + \frac{k_{12}}{k_{23} - k_{12}} e^{-k_{23}t} \right) \tag{5.103c}$$

Equation (5.103a), Equation (5.103b), and Equation (5.103c) are identical to Equation (5.48), Equation (5.51), and Equation (5.52), respectively, when $k_{12} = k_1$ and $k_{23} = k_2$.

Next, consider a simple reversible reaction (A $\rightleftarrows$ B). In this case, the following conditions are given:

$$k_{23} = k_{32} = 0 \tag{5.104a}$$

$$\alpha = \beta = k_{12} + k_{21} \tag{5.104b}$$

$$\chi_2 = k_{12} + k_{21}, \quad \chi_3 = 0 \tag{5.104c}$$

Substituting Equation (5.104a), Equation (5.104b), and Equation (5.104c) into Equation (5.100a) and Equation (5.100b) along with the initial conditions (i.e., $[A] = [A]_o$ and $[B] = [B]_o$ at t = 0) yields:

$$[X_1]_o = Y_{11} + Y_{12} \tag{5.105a}$$

$$0 = \frac{k_{12}}{k_{21}} Y_{11} - Y_{12} \tag{5.105b}$$

The solutions for Equation (5.105a) and Equation (5.105b) are:

$$Y_{11} = \frac{[X_1]_o}{1 + K}, \quad Y_{12} = \frac{K[X_1]_o}{1 + K} \tag{5.106a}$$

$$K = k_{12} / k_{21} \tag{5.106b}$$

The concentration of X_1 and X_2 with respect to time is:

$$[X_1] = \frac{[X_1]_o}{1 + K} \left(1 + K e^{-(k_{12} + k_{21})t} \right) \tag{5.107a}$$

$$[X_2] = \frac{K[X_1]_o}{1 + K} \left(1 - e^{-(k_{12} + k_{21})t} \right) \tag{5.107b}$$

At $t = \infty$, equilibrium is reached, and the equilibrium concentrations of X_1 and X_2 are given by:

$$[X_1]_\infty = \frac{[X_1]_o}{K+1}, \quad [X_2]_\infty = \frac{K[X_1]_o}{K+1} \tag{5.108}$$

Substituting Equation (5.108) into Equation (5.107a) and rearranging the resulting equation yields:

$$-\ln\left(\frac{[A]-[A]_\infty}{[A]_o-[A]_\infty}\right) = (k_{12} + k_{21})t \tag{5.109}$$

Equation (5.109) is identical to Equation (5.67) derived analytically.

5.8 USE OF LAPLACE TRANSFORM FOR DIFFERENTIAL RATE EQUATIONS

5.8.1 Definitions and Properties

Many drugs undergo complex *in vitro* drug degradations and biotransformations in the body (i.e., pharmacokinetics). The approaches to solve the rate equations described so far (i.e., analytical method) cannot handle complex rate processes without some difficulty. The Laplace transform method is a simple method for solving ordinary linear differential equations. Although the Laplace transform method has been used for more complex applications in physics, engineering, and other research areas, here it will be applied to ordinary differential equations of first-order rate processes.

The Laplace transformation of a function $f(t)$, $L[f(t)]$, is defined as:

$$L[f(t)] = \int_0^\infty e^{-st} f(t)dt \tag{5.110}$$

Two examples [$f(t) = t$ and $f(t) = e^{-at}$] are illustrated below:

$$L[t] = \int_0^\infty e^{-st}tdt = \left[-\frac{te^{-st}}{s} - \frac{e^{-st}}{s^2}\right]_0^\infty = \frac{1}{s^2} \tag{5.111}$$

$$L[e^{-at}] = \int_0^\infty e^{-st}e^{-at}dt = \left[\frac{-e^{-(s-a)t}}{s-a}\right]_0^\infty = \frac{1}{s-a} \tag{5.112}$$

If the derivative expression, $df(t)/dt$, is transformed, in Equation (5.110):

$$L[\frac{df(t)}{dt}] = \int\limits_0^\infty e^{-st} \frac{df(t)}{dt} dt = \left[e^{-st} f(t)\right]_0^\infty + s\int\limits_0^\infty e^{-st} f(t)dt \qquad (5.113)$$

If $f(t)$ is a continuous function at $t \geq 0$, Equation (5.113) becomes:

$$L[\frac{df(t)}{dt}] = sL[f(t)] - f(0) \qquad (5.114)$$

where $f(0)$ is the value of the function at $t = 0$.

Two important properties of Laplace transforms are their scaling and linearity as:

$$L[cf(t)] = cL[f(t)] \qquad (5.115)$$

$$L[f(t) + g(t)] = L[f(t)] + L[g(t)] \qquad (5.116)$$

Table 5.5 shows the Laplace transforms of many functions encountered in many drug degradation and biotransformation reactions. Once the rate equations are transformed into the s-domain, the inverse Laplace transformations of this s-domain expression are carried out to obtain the time domain solution for the rate equations.

5.8.2 APPLICATIONS OF LAPLACE TRANSFORMS FOR DRUG DEGRADATION AND BIOTRANSFORMATION

Consider, for example, a drug degradation or biotransformation reaction via hepatic metabolism undergoing the following pathways:

$$A \xrightarrow{k_1} B \xrightarrow{k_2} C \xrightarrow{k_3} D$$

The rate expressions for the four compounds are written as:

$$\frac{d[A]}{dt} = -k_1[A] \qquad (5.117a)$$

$$\frac{d[B]}{dt} = k_1[A] - k_2[B] \qquad (5.117b)$$

$$\frac{d[C]}{dt} = k_2[B] - k_3[C] \qquad (5.117c)$$

$$\frac{d[D]}{dt} = k_3[C] \qquad (5.117d)$$

The initial conditions are $[A] = [A]_o$ and $[B]_o = [C]_o = [D]_o = 0$ at $t = 0$. Taking the Laplace transforms of Equation (5.117a), Equation (5.117b), Equation (5.117c), and Equation (5.117d) yields:

TABLE 5.5
Laplace Transforms

$f(t)$	$L[f(t)]$
1	$1/s$
A	A/s
t	$1/s^2$
t^m	$\dfrac{m!}{s^{m+1}}$
Ae^{-at}	$\dfrac{A}{s+a}$
Ate^{-at}	$A/(s+a)^2$
$\dfrac{A}{a}(1-e^{-at})$	$\dfrac{A}{s(s+a)}$
$\dfrac{A}{a}e^{-(b/a)t}$	$\dfrac{A}{as+b}$
$\dfrac{(B-Aa_{})e^{-at}-(B-Ab)e^{-bt}}{b-a}\,(b\neq a)$	$\dfrac{As+B}{(s+a)(s+b)}$
$\dfrac{A}{b-a}(e^{-at}-e^{-bt})$	$\dfrac{A}{(s+a)(s+b)}$
$e^{-at}(A+(B-Aa)t)$	$\dfrac{As+B}{(s+a)^2}$
$-\dfrac{1}{PQR}\begin{bmatrix}P(Aa^2-Ba+C)e^{-at}\\ +Q(Ab^2-Bb+C)e^{-bt}\\ +R(Ac^2-Bc+C)e^{-ct}\end{bmatrix}$ $(p=b-c,\ Q=c-a,\ R=a-b)$	$\dfrac{As^2+Bs+C}{(s+a)(s+b)(s+c)}$
$A\left[\dfrac{1}{ab}+\dfrac{1}{a(a-b)}e^{-at}-\dfrac{1}{b(a-b)}e^{-bt}\right]$	$\dfrac{A}{s(s+a)(s+b)}$
$A\begin{bmatrix}\dfrac{1}{abc}-\dfrac{1}{a(a-b)(a-c)}e^{-at}-\dfrac{1}{b(b-c)(b-a)}e^{-b}\\ -\dfrac{1}{c(c-a)(c-b)}e^{-ct}\end{bmatrix}$	$\dfrac{A}{s(s+a)(s+b)(s+c)}$
$\dfrac{A}{a}t-\dfrac{A}{a^2}(1-e^{-at})$	$\dfrac{A}{s^2(s+a)}$
$\dfrac{B}{ab}-\dfrac{Aa-B}{a(a-b)}e^{-at}+\dfrac{Ab-B}{b(a-b)}e^{-bt}$	$\dfrac{As+B}{s(s+a)(s+b)}$
$\dfrac{B}{ab}-\dfrac{a^2-Aa+B}{a(b-a)}e^{-at}+\dfrac{b^2-Ab+B}{b(b-a)}e^{-bt}$	$\dfrac{s^2+As+B}{s(s+a)(s+b)}$

Source: Taken from Gibaldi and Perrier, *Pharmacokinetics,* Marcel Dekker, New York, 1975, p. 270.

$$sL[[A]] - [A]_o = -k_1 L[[A]], \quad L[[A]] = \frac{[A]_o}{s + k_1} \tag{5.118a}$$

$$sL[[B]] = k_1 L[[A]] - k_2 L[[B]] = \frac{k_1 [A]_o}{s + k_1} - k_2 L[[B]],$$

$$L[[B]] = \frac{k_1 [A]_o}{(s + k_1)(s + k_2)} \tag{5.118b}$$

$$sL[[C]] = k_2 L[[B]] - k_3 L[[C]] = \frac{k_1 k_2 [A]_o}{(s + k_1)(s + k_2)} - k_3 L[[C]],$$

$$L[[C]] = \frac{k_1 k_2 [A]_o}{(s + k_1)(s + k_2)(s + k_3)} \tag{5.118c}$$

$$sL[[D]] = k_3 L[[C]] = \frac{k_1 k_2 k_3 [A]_o}{(s + k_1)(s + k_2)(s + k_3)}$$

$$L[[D]] = \frac{k_1 k_2 k_3 [A]_o}{s(s + k_1)(s + k_2)(s + k_3)} \tag{5.118d}$$

Taking the inverse Laplace transforms of the Equation (5.118a), Equation (5.118b), Equation (5.118c), and Equation (5.118d) with the aid of Table 5.5 gives:

$$[A] = [A]_o e^{-k_1 t} \tag{5.119a}$$

$$[B] = \frac{k_1 [A]_o}{k_2 - k_1} \left(e^{-k_1 t} - e^{-k_2 t} \right) \tag{5.119b}$$

$$[C] = k_1 k_2 [A]_o \left(\frac{(k_2 - k_3)e^{-k_1 t} + (k_3 - k_1)e^{-k_2 t} + (k_1 - k_2)e^{-k_3 t}}{(k_2 - k_1)(k_1 - k_3)(k_3 - k_2)} \right) \tag{5.119c}$$

$$[D] = [A]_o - [A] - [B] - [C] = [A]_o \left(1 + \frac{k_2 k_3 e^{-k_1 t}}{(k_2 - k_1)(k_1 - k_3)} + \frac{k_1 k_3 e^{-k_2 t}}{(k_2 - k_1)(k_3 - k_2)} + \frac{k_1 k_2 e^{-k_3 t}}{(k_1 - k_3)(k_3 - k_2)} \right) \tag{5.119d}$$

Figure 5.20 shows concentration–time profiles for the decomposition of hydrocortisone butyrate at 60°C in a buffered aqueous propylene glycol (50 w/w%, pH 7.6). Consecutive, irreversible, first-order kinetic models [i.e., Equation (5.119a), Equation (5.119b), and Equation (5.119c)] fit reasonably well with the experimental

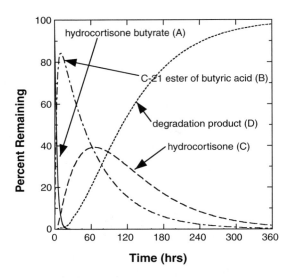

FIGURE 5.20 Concentration profiles of hydrocortisone C-17 butyrate, hydrocortisone C-12, and hydrocortisone at 60°C in a buffered aqueous propylene glycol solution (50 w/w%, pH 7.6). [Graph reconstructed from data by Yip et al., *J. Pharm. Sci.*, 72, 776 (1983).]

data. Because many kinetic parameters are involved in the degradation pathways, other kinetic models must be considered such as

$$A \rightleftharpoons B \longrightarrow C \longrightarrow D \quad \text{and} \quad A \longrightarrow B \longrightarrow C \longrightarrow D$$

In these cases, analysis of model discrimination should be carried out.

In chemical degradation kinetics and pharmacokinetics, the methods of eigen-value and Laplace transform have been employed for complex systems, and a choice between two methods is up to the individual and dependent upon the algebraic steps required to obtain the final solution. The eigenvalue method and the Laplace transform method derive the general solution from various possible cases, and then the specific case is applied to the general solution. When the specific problem is complicated, the Laplace transform method is easy to use. The reversible and consecutive series reactions described in Section 5.6 can be easily solved by the Laplace transform method:

$$A \underset{k_{21}}{\overset{k_{12}}{\rightleftharpoons}} B \underset{k_{32}}{\overset{k_{23}}{\rightleftharpoons}} C$$

The rate expressions for three compounds were given by Equation (5.80), Equation (5.81), and Equation (5.82). If only A is present initially, $[B]_o = [C]_o = 0$ and $[A]_o = [A] + [B] + [C]$, which is subsequently substituted into Equation (5.81) for $[C]$. Then, the Laplace transforms of Equation (5.80) and Equation (5.81) are given as:

$$sL[[A]] - [A]_o = -k_{12}L[[A]] + k_{21}L[[B]] \tag{5.120a}$$

or

$$L[[A]] = \frac{k_{21}L[[B]] + [A]_o}{s + k_{12}} \tag{5.120b}$$

$$sL[[B]] = (k_{12} - k_{32})L[[A]] - (k_{21} + k_{23} + k_{32})L[[B]] + \frac{k_{32}[A]_o}{s} \tag{5.121a}$$

Substituting Equation (5.120b) into Equation (5.121a) yields:

$$L[[B]] = \frac{k_{12}[A]_o(s + k_{32})}{s[s^2 + (k_{12} + k_{21} + k_{23} + k_{32})s + (k_{12}k_{23} + k_{12}k_{32} + k_{21}k_{32})]} \tag{5.121b}$$

Equation (5.121b) can be written as:

$$L[[B]] = \frac{k_{12}[A]_o(s + k_{32})}{s(s + \alpha)(s + \beta)} \tag{5.121c}$$

where

$$\alpha + \beta = k_{12} + k_{21} + k_{23} + k_{32} \tag{5.122a}$$

$$\alpha\beta = k_{12}k_{23} + k_{12}k_{32} + k_{21}k_{32} \tag{5.122b}$$

The partial fraction method is applied to Equation (5.121c), and then the inverse transform functions given in Table 5.5 are employed:

$$[B] = k_{12}[A]_o\left(\frac{k_{32}}{\alpha\beta} + \frac{k_{32} - \alpha}{\alpha(\alpha - \beta)}e^{-\alpha t} - \frac{k_{32} - \beta}{\beta(\alpha - \beta)}e^{-\beta t}\right) \tag{5.123}$$

Equation (5.123) is substituted into Equation (5.120b):

$$L[[A]] = [A]_o\left(\frac{s^2 + (k_{21} + k_{23} + k_{32})s + k_{21}k_{32}}{s(s + \alpha)(s + \beta)}\right) \tag{5.124}$$

From Table 5.5, the inverse transform equation for Equation (5.124) is given as:

$$[A] = [A]_o\left(\frac{k_{21}k_{32}}{\alpha\beta} + \frac{k_{12}(\alpha - k_{23} - k_{32})}{\alpha(\alpha - \beta)}e^{-\alpha t} - \frac{k_{12}(\beta - k_{23} - k_{32})}{\beta(\alpha - \beta)}e^{-\beta t}\right) \tag{5.125}$$

$$[C] = [A]_o - [A] - [B] = k_{12}k_{23}[A]_o \left(\frac{1}{\alpha\beta} + \frac{1}{\alpha(\alpha - \beta)} e^{-\alpha t} + \frac{1}{\beta(\beta - \alpha)} e^{-\beta t} \right) \quad (5.126)$$

Equation (5.123), Equation (5.125), and Equation (5.126) are identical to Equation (5.100a), Equation (5.100b), and Equation (5.100c), respectively, when $\alpha = \chi_1$ and $\beta = \chi_2$.

An anticancer drug, 5-fluorouracil, is metabolized by dihydropyrimidine dehydrogenase (DHPDH), dihydropyrinidase (DHP), and other enzymes (b-ureidopropionase and three aminotransferases). Patients who are deficient in these enzymes can suffer severe neurotoxicity if the drug is prescribed. The drug is biotransformed in four steps in humans as follows:

5,6-dihydro-5-fluorouracil   α-fluoro- β-
                              ureidopropionic acid   α-fluoro- β-alanine

Mathematical techniques described in Section 5.6 and Section 5.7 can be applied to the above complex pathways of the drug.

5.9 ENZYME–SUBSTRATE REACTIONS

5.9.1 ENZYME–SUBSTRATE REACTIONS WITHOUT INHIBITION

Enzymes are excellent catalysts in biological systems. They produce biologically active molecules by lowering the activation energy, thus causing the rate of biotransformation in the reaction to increase by several orders of magnitude. The general scheme for enzyme-catalyzed reactions is:

$$A \xrightarrow[\text{enzyme}]{} P$$

In the first step, the enzymes form an intermediate enzyme–substrate complex, $(A.E)^*$:

$$A + E \underset{k_2}{\overset{k_1}{\rightleftharpoons}} (A.E)^* \quad \text{fast} \quad (5.127)$$

where E is the enzyme. At high concentrations of substrate, all of the enzymes present are bound to the substrate, forming the enzyme–substrate complex.

In the second step, the enzyme–substrate complex is decomposed or hydrolyzed to the product and the enzyme:

$$(A.E)^* \xrightarrow[k_3]{} P + E \quad \text{slow} \tag{5.128}$$

The rates for the above reactions can be written as:

$$\frac{d[A]}{dt} = -k_1[A][P] + k_2[(A.E)^*] \tag{5.129}$$

$$\frac{d[(A.E)^*]}{dt} = k_1[A][P] - k_2[(A.E)^*] - k_3[(A.E)^*] \tag{5.130}$$

$$\frac{d[E]}{dt} = -\frac{d[(A.E)^*]}{dt} \tag{5.131}$$

$$\frac{d[P]}{dt} = k_3[(A.E)^*] \tag{5.132}$$

One may apply the analogous method described in Section 5.6 and Section 5.7 to solve for the above equations. Substituting $k_{32} = 0$ into Equation (5.81) and Equation (5.82) gives the exact solution as:

$$[A] = [A]_o \left(\frac{k_{12}(\chi_2 - k_{23})}{\chi_2(\chi_2 - \chi_3)} e^{-\chi_2 t} + \frac{k_{12}(k_{23} - \chi_3)}{\chi_3(\chi_2 - \chi_3)} e^{-\chi_3 t} \right) \tag{5.133a}$$

$$[B] = [A]_o \left(\frac{-k_{12}}{(\chi_2 - \chi_3)} e^{-\chi_2 t} + \frac{k_{12}}{(\chi_2 - \chi_3)} e^{-\chi_3 t} \right) \tag{5.133b}$$

$$[C] = [A]_o \left(\frac{k_{12}k_{23}}{\chi_2\chi_3} + \frac{k_{12}k_{23}}{\chi_2(\chi_2 - \chi_3)} e^{-\chi_2 t} - \frac{k_{12}k_{23}}{\chi_3(\chi_2 - \chi_3)} e^{-\chi_3 t} \right) \tag{5.133c}$$

where

$$\chi_2 = \tfrac{1}{2} \left[k_1 + k_2 + k_3 + \sqrt{(k_1 + k_2 + k_3)^2 - 4k_1 k_3} \right] \tag{5.134a}$$

$$\chi_2 = \tfrac{1}{2} \left[k_1 + k_2 + k_3 - \sqrt{(k_1 + k_2 + k_3)^2 - 4k_1 k_3} \right] \tag{5.134b}$$

However, a simpler approach may be employed to these enzyme reactions. First, assume that the concentration of the intermediate is not negligible and the total enzyme concentration ($[E]_o$) is the sum of the free ($[E]$) and bound enzyme $[(A.E)^*]$:

$$[E]_o = [E] + [(A.E)^*] \qquad (5.135)$$

The rate of formation of $(A.E)^*$ under steady-state approximation (which means that the concentration of $(A.E)^*$ is constant throughout the reaction and much smaller than those of $[E]$ and $[P]$) is:

$$\frac{d[(A.E)^*]}{dt} = k_1[A][E] - k_2[(A.E)^*] - k_3[(A.E)^*] = 0 \qquad (5.136)$$

from which

$$[(A.E)^*] = \frac{k_1[A][E]}{k_2 + k_3} \qquad (5.137)$$

Substituting Equation (5.135) into Equation (5.137) yields;

$$[(A.E)^*] = \frac{k_1[A][E]_o}{(k_2 + k_3) + k_1[A]} \qquad (5.138)$$

Substituting Equation (5.138) into Equation (5.134) results in:

$$\frac{d[P]}{dt} = \frac{k_3[A][E]_o}{K_m + [A]} \qquad (5.139)$$

where

$$K_m = \frac{k_2 + k_3}{k_1} \qquad (5.140)$$

From Equation (5.139), called the Michaelis–Menten equation, one sees that the rate of formation of P is proportional to the concentration of A at low concentrations (i.e., first-order) and independent of the concentration of A at high concentrations (i.e., zero-order). The general biphasic kinetic profile is shown in Figure 5.21. Usually, experimental runs are carried out in such a way that the concentration of A is very high compared to that of $[E]_o$. All of the enzyme is bound to the substrate and the reaction takes place at a maximum velocity. Then Equation (5.139) becomes:

$$V = V_m \frac{[A]}{K_m + [A]} \qquad (5.141)$$

where $V = d[P]/dt$ and $V_m = (d[P]/dt)_{max} = k_3[E]_o$. Rearranging equation (5.141) gives the Lineweaver–Burk plot (double recipocal form):

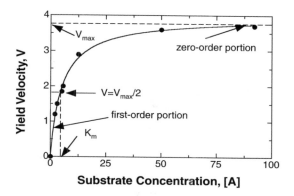

FIGURE 5.21 Yield–velocity vs. substrate concentration for an enzyme-catalyzed reaction.

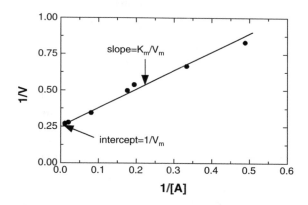

FIGURE 5.22 The Lineweaver–Burk plot for the data of Figure 5.21.

$$\frac{1}{V} = \frac{1}{V_m} + \frac{K_m}{V_m[A]} \qquad (5.142)$$

A plot of $1/V$ vs. $1/[A]$ gives a slope of K_m/V_m and an intercept of $1/V_m$, as shown in Figure 5.22.

Example 5.15.

Pyridoxal phosphate catalyzes the conversion of D-serine dehydratase to pyruvic acid:

$$CH_2OHCHNH_2COOH \longrightarrow CH_3COCOOH + NH_3$$

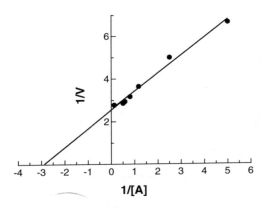

FIGURE 5.23 Lineweaver–Burk plot of 1/V vs. 1/[A] of Example 5.15.

The following experimental data were obtained based on the amount of pyruvic acid formed in 20 minutes. Calculate the apparent Michaelis–Menten constants.

Pyruvic acid, μM	0.1	0.2	0.275	0.315	0.340	0.350	0.360
Pyridoxal phosphate, M ($\times 10^5$)	0.20	0.40	0.85	1.25	1.70	2.00	8.00

Solution

The velocity of reaction can be measured by the formation of pyruvic acid. The reciprocals of the velocity of reaction and enzyme concentration are obtained:

1/V	6.66	5.00	3.64	3.17	2.94	2.86	2.78
1/[A] $\times 10^{-5}$	5.0	2.5	1.17	0.80	0.58	0.50	0.125

These values are plotted in Figure 5.23, resulting in a slope of 0.43 and y-intercept of 2.578 $(\mu M)^{-1}$, which enable the calculation of $V_m = 0.388\ \mu M$ and $K_m = 2.17 \times 10^{-5}\ \mu M$.

5.9.2 ENZYME–SUBSTRATE REACTION WITH INHIBITION

Enzyme activity may be inhibited by substances that inactivate the enzyme or occupy the active site of the enzyme before the substrate has a chance. As a result, the rate of transformation of the substrate to product is slowed. In *competitive inhibition,* similar substrates (or analogs) can bind to the same active site on the enzyme. Therefore, they compete with each other for the same active sites. This inhibition process is reversible and can be prevented or slowed by increasing the substrate concentration or by diluting the inhibitor in the solution. In this case, the enzyme already bound to the substrate is not inhibited. The effect of the competitive inhibitor (I) on the rate of enzyme reaction in Equation (5.129), Equation (5.130), Equation (5.131), and Equation (5.132) yields:

$$E + I \underset{k_5}{\overset{k_4}{\rightleftharpoons}} EI \qquad (5.143)$$

Three forms of enzyme are present: E, (A.E)*, and EI. The total enzyme concentration is given by:

$$[E]_o = [E] + [(A.E)^*] + [EI] \qquad (5.144)$$

Equation (5.143) gives the equilibrium constant as:

$$K_I = \frac{k_5}{k_4} = \frac{[I][E]}{[EI]} \qquad (5.145)$$

Substituting Equation (5.145) for [EI] into Equation (5.144) yields:

$$[E]_o = [(A.E)^*] + [E] + \frac{[I][E]}{K_I} = [(A.E)^*] + \left(1 + \frac{[I]}{K_I}\right)[E] \qquad (5.146)$$

Substituting Equation (5.137) into Equation (5.146) under steady-state approximations to the formation of (A.E)* yields:

$$[E]_o = [(A.E)^*] + \left(1 + \frac{[I]}{K_I}\right)\frac{K_m}{[A]}[(A.E)^*] \qquad (5.147)$$

Substituting Equation (5.147) into Equation (5.139) gives:

$$V = \frac{V_{max}[A]}{[A] + \left(1 + \dfrac{[I]}{K_I}\right)K_m} \qquad (5.148)$$

Rearranging Equation (5.148) to the form of a double reciprocal as Equation (5.142) gives:

$$\frac{1}{V} = \frac{1}{V_{max}} + \left(1 + \frac{[I]}{K_I}\right)\frac{K_m}{V_{max}}\frac{1}{[A]} \qquad (5.149)$$

If the inhibitor concentration is zero, Equation (5.149) becomes Equation (5.142).

Enzyme inhibition can occur by the reaction of an enzyme–substrate complex with an inhibitor and the reaction of a free enzyme with an inhibitor, which is called *noncompetitive inhibition*. These inhibitions are not reversible by increasing the concentration of the substrate in the enzyme solution. The reaction of the enzyme–substrate complex with an inhibitor can be expressed as:

$$(A.E)^* + I \underset{k_7}{\overset{k_6}{\rightleftarrows}} (AIE) \tag{5.150}$$

$$K_{II} = \frac{k_7}{k_6} = \frac{[I][(A.E)^*]}{[(AIE)]} \tag{5.151}$$

Four forms of enzyme are in the system: E, $(A.E)^*$, EI, and (AIE). Equation (5.144) becomes:

$$[E]_o = [E] + [(A.E)^*] + [EI] + [(AIE)] \tag{5.152}$$

Substituting Equation (5.145) and Equation (5.151) into Equation (5.152) gives:

$$[E]_o = [(A.E)^*] + \frac{[I][(A.E)^*]}{K_{II}} + [E] + \frac{[I][E]}{K_I} = [(A.E)^*]\left(1 + \frac{[I]}{K_{II}}\right) + \left(1 + \frac{[I]}{K_I}\right)[E] \tag{5.153}$$

Substitution of Equation (5.153) into Equation (5.139) and rearrangement to the double reciprocal form yields:

$$\frac{1}{V} = \left(1 + \frac{[I]}{K_I}\right)\frac{K_m}{V_{max}}\frac{1}{[A]} + \frac{1}{V_{max}}\left(1 + \frac{[I]}{K_{II}}\right) \tag{5.154}$$

If there is no reaction between the free enzyme and the inhibitor, and the inhibitor binds only to the $(A.E)^*$ complex, Equation (5.154) becomes the *uncompetitive inhibition* equation:

$$\frac{1}{V} = \frac{K_m}{V_{max}}\frac{1}{[A]} + \frac{1}{V_{max}}\left(1 + \frac{[I]}{K_{II}}\right) \tag{5.155}$$

The characteristics of the double reciprocal plots given by Equation (5.149), Equation (5.154), and Equation (5.155) determine what kind of enzyme inhibition may occur: competitive, noncompetitive, or uncompetitive. In a given concentration of enzyme and inhibitor, the substrate concentration is changed and the double reciprocal plot of 1/V against 1/[A] is drawn. Figure 5.24a illustrates the double

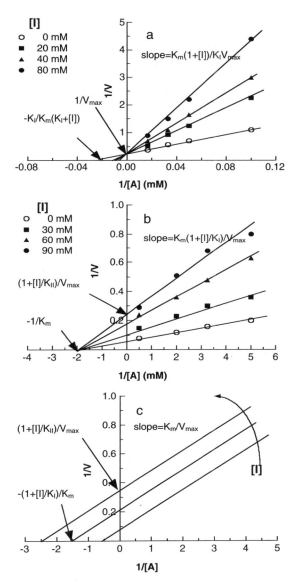

FIGURE 5.24 The double reciprocal plots of (a) competitive inhibition, (b) noncompetitive inhibition, and (c) uncompetitive inhibition. [Graph reconstructed from data by Nnane et al., *Br. J. Cancer*, 83, 74 (2000).]

reciprocal plot for competitive inhibition in the presence and absence of an inhibitor. With changing concentrations of the inhibitor, the common intercept is $1/V_{max}$, indicating that the maximum velocity does not change even in the presence of the inhibitor. At infinite substrate concentration (i.e., $1/[A] = 0$), excess substrate displaces the inhibitor from the active site of the enzyme, and V_{max} remains the same for the control and the inhibited systems.

In noncompetitive inhibition, a family of lines goes through the same intercept on the x-coordinate, which is $-1/K_m$. When K_I is equal to K_{II}, the inhibition is called a "simple linear noncompetitive inhibition" (Figure 5.24b). This indicates that V_{max} decreases as the inhibitor concentration increases and K_m for the substrate does not change. In an uncompetitive inhibition (Figure 5.24c), the family of lines is parallel to each other and has the same slope of K_m/V_{max}.

Example 5.16

It was reported that maltose inhibits the hydrolysis of starch by malt α-amylase. The following data were obtained:

Maltose Concentration (mg/mL)	α-Amylase Concentration (mg/mL)			
	11.52	5.76	2.8	1.44
	Relative Hydrolysis Velocity			
0.00	100	82	56	39
6.35	90	77	50	36
12.75	82	66	46	31
25.40	67	57	38	27

Calculate the values of K_m and K_I for the enzyme and inhibitor, respectively.

Solution

According to Equation (5.149), the data are transformed to:

Maltose Concentration [I]	α-Amylase Concentration (mg/mL)			
	11.52	5.76	2.88	1.44
	1/[A]0.087	0.174	0.348	0.695
mg/mL	1/V			
0.0	0.0100	0.0122	0.0178	0.0256
6.35	0.0111	0.0129	0.0200	0.0277
12.70	0.0122	0.0152	0.0217	0.0323
25.40	0.0149	0.0175	0.0263	0.0370

The plot of 1/V vs. 1/[A] for the hydrolysis reaction in the presence and absence of maltose is presented in Figure 5.25. From the x- and y-intercepts for the uninhibited hydrolysis, $K_m = 3.70$ mg/mL and $V_m = 135.1$ relative velocity units. The plot demonstrates that maltose is a noncompetitive inhibitor because of the same x-intercept. The value of K_I can be calculated from the slope:

$$slope = 0.0415 = \frac{K_m}{V_m}\left(1+\frac{[I]}{K_I}\right) = \frac{3.70}{135.1}\left(1+\frac{25.4}{K_I}\right), \quad K_I = 49.3 \text{ mg/mL}$$

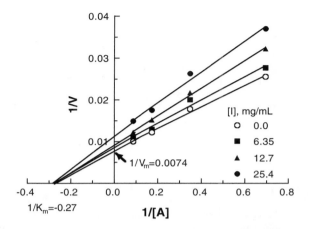

FIGURE 5.25 Lineweaver–Burk plot of the hydrolysis of starch by α-amylase in the presence of maltose.

5.10 ACID–BASE CATALYZED DEGRADATION KINETICS

5.10.1 Acid–Base Catalyzed Hydrolysis of Neutral Chemicals

In an aqueous environment, the decomposition of a number of drugs via hydrolysis occurs much more rapidly than in the solid state, especially in the presence of hydrogen or hydroxyl ions. When the rate of degradation is expressed in an equation containing the hydrogen or hydroxyl ion terms, this degradation reaction is called an acid–base catalyzed hydrolysis. In addition, drug compounds with labile bonds, such as esters, amides, and aromatic ethers, undergo accelerated degradation in the presence of hydrogen or hydroxyl ions. For example, when a drug compound decomposes by an acid–base catalysis, the schematic process is as follows:

$$A + H^+ \xrightarrow{k_+} P \quad \text{for specific acid catalysis} \tag{5.156a}$$

$$A + OH^- \xrightarrow{k_-} P \quad \text{for specific base catalysis} \tag{5.156b}$$

$$A + H_2O \xrightarrow{k_o} P \quad \text{for noncatalysis (solvent alone)} \tag{5.156c}$$

The overall rate expression is given as:

$$-\frac{d[A]}{dt} = k_+[H^+][A] + k_-[OH^-]A + k_o[A] = [A]\left(k_+[H^+] + k_-[OH^-] + k_o\right) \tag{5.157}$$

For a given pH, the rate equation is:

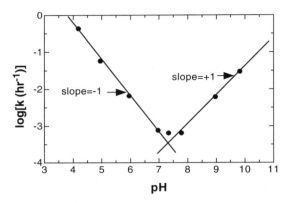

FIGURE 5.26 pH-rate constant profile for the specific acid–base catalyzed hydrolysis of a water-soluble diaziridinyl benzoquinone derivative. [Graph reconstructed from data by Jain et al., AAPS National Meeting, Paper No. 2268, Indianapolis, IN, Oct. 29, 2000.]

$$-\frac{d[A]}{dt} = k_{obs}[A] \tag{5.158a}$$

$$k_{obs} = k_{+}[H^{+}] + k_{-}[OH^{-}] + k_{o} \tag{5.158b}$$

where k_{obs} is the pseudo–first-order rate constant. Figure 5.26 illustrates the pH-rate profile for the specific acid–base catalyzed hydrolysis of a water-soluble diaziridinyl benzoquinone derivative (RH1). As the hydrogen concentration decreases, the pH increases from 1 to 7 and the rate of hydrolysis decreases. The term $k_{+}[H^{+}]$ is a dominating factor and is much larger than the sum of k_{o} and $k_{-}[OH^{-}]$. A further decrease in hydrogen ion concentration results in a linear increase in the rate of hydrolysis since the term $k_{-}[OH^{-}]$ then influences most of the hydrolysis. Near pH 7, the minimum rate of hydrolysis occurs. Either hydrogen or hydroxyl ions do not participate in the hydrolysis and the solvent (i.e., water) is the molecule responsible for the hydrolysis of RH1. These phenomena are predicted by Equation (5.158a). It is clear from Figure 5.26 that the degradation of the drug is catalyzed by both the acid and base which have slopes of −1 and +1, respectively. Possible forms of acid–base catalyzed hydrolysis of individual and combined effects are shown in Figure 5.27.

Solution dosage forms may contain a variety of other ingredients, including buffers used to maintain the pH. Buffer ingredients can catalyze the hydrolysis of active drugs; the process is called general acid–base catalyzed hydrolysis. For example, the active ingredient in a solution prepared with acetate buffer may undergo hydrolysis due to acetic acid and acetate species as well as the hydrogen and hydroxyl ions. The rate equation for this case is written:

$$-\frac{d[A]}{dt} = k_{+}[H^{+}][A] + k_{o}[A] + k_{-}[OH^{-}][A] + k_{HA}[HA][A] + k_{A}[Ac^{-}][A] \tag{5.159}$$

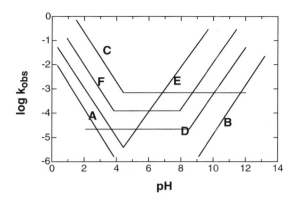

FIGURE 5.27 Possible forms of acid–base catalyzed hydrolysis.

where k_{HA} and k_A are the rate constants of the acetic acid, HA, and acetate, Ac⁻, respectively. The overall rate constant, k_{obs}, accounting for all the effects, can be written as:

$$k_{obs} = k_+[H^+] + k_o + k_-[OH^-] + k_{HA}[HA] + k_A[Ac^-] \qquad (5.160a)$$

or $$= k_o + \sum k_i[C_i]$$

where k_i is the hydrolysis rate constant due to species i and C_i is the concentration of species i. As a result of the effects of the buffer species on hydrolysis, the slopes may deviate from −1 and +1 at acidic and alkaline pHs, respectively, as shown in Figure 5.28.

Example 5.17

A drug is degraded by acid-catalyzed hydrolysis between pH 1.7 and 7.6. The specific rate constant of the hydrolysis of the drug at pH 4.7 is 0.47/month at 25°C. What pH should the drug solution be if the shelf-life is increased to 130 days?

Solution

The shelf-life of the drug at pH 4.7 is 0.1053/(0.47/month) = 6.72 days. Thus, 19.3 times the shelf-life is 130 days. The rate constant should be decreased by 19.3 times. This can be achieved by an increase in the pH of the solution by log 19.3 = 1.29 because the slope of the log k vs. pH relationship is −1. The pH of the solution should be 4.7 + 1.29 = 5.99 = 6.0.

Example 5.18

The following experimental data were obtained for the acid-catalyzed hydrolysis of a drug:

pH	1.30	1.40	1.50	1.70	2.00
k_{obs}, 10^{-3}/hr	5.16	8.30	12.0	14.6	17.8

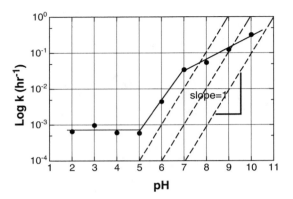

FIGURE 5.28 General acid–base catalyzed hydrolysis of dimethoxybiphenyl monocarbox-ylate HCl solutions in buffers of acetic acid/HCl (pH 2), acetate (pH 4 and 5), phosphate (pH 6 to 8), and borate (pH 9 and 10). [Graph reconstructed from data by Choi et al., *Arch. Pharm. Res.*, 24, 159 (2001).]

Calculate the rate constants for the solvent and acid.

Solution

Due to the very low pH, one can assume that the base-catalyzed hydrolysis is negligible in acidic conditions. Equation (5.158b) is applied to the above data with $[OH^-] \approx 0$ from which the regression is obtained:

$$k_{obs} = 2.0 \times 10^{-3} + 0.316[H^+]$$

from which

$$k_o = 2.0 \times 10^{-3} / hr \quad \text{and} \quad k_+ = 0.316 / hr$$

5.10.2 Acid–Base Catalyzed Hydrolysis of Polyprotic Weak Acids and Weak Bases

Ionic equilibrium will complicate the drug degradation process if the drug compound is a weak acid or weak base. A general approach for the acid–base catalyzed degradation of a weak acid or weak base is described as follows:

$$H_n A \rightleftharpoons H^+ + H_{n-1}A^- \tag{5.161}$$

$$K_i = \frac{[H^+][H_{n-i}A^{-i}]}{[H_{n-i+1}A^{1-i}]} \tag{5.162}$$

where K_i is the *i*th ionization constant of a polyprotic weak acid or weak base and $[H_{n-i}A^{-i}]$ is the *i*th deprotonated species.

The concentrations of the deprotonated species are determined as:

$$[H_{n-1}A^{-1}] = [H_nA]\frac{K_1}{[H^+]} \tag{5.163a}$$

$$[H_{n-2}A^{-2}] = [H_nA]\frac{K_1}{[H^+]}\frac{K_2}{[H^+]} \tag{5.163b}$$

The general expression for the concentration of the ith deprotonated compound is written as:

$$[H_{n-i}A^{-i}] = [H_nA]\frac{\prod\limits_{j=1}^{i}K_j}{[H^+]^i} \tag{5.163c}$$

When $K_0 = 1$, Equation (5.163c) can be further simplified to:

$$[H_{n-i}A^{-i}] = [H_nA]\frac{\prod\limits_{j=0}^{i}K_j}{[H^+]^i} \tag{5.163d}$$

Each compound (i.e., unprotonated and protonated species) in an aqueous solution undergoes acid–base catalyzed degradation (i.e., hydrolysis) as predicted in Equation (5.156a), Equation (5.156b), and Equation (5.156c). The pseudo–first-order degradation rate constant is:

$$k_{obs} = \frac{\sum\limits_{i=0}^{n}\dfrac{\prod\limits_{j=0}^{i}K_j}{[H^+]^i}\left(k_{i,+}[H^+] + k_{i,-}\dfrac{K_w}{[H^+]} + k_{i,o}\right)}{\sum\limits_{i=0}^{n}\dfrac{\prod\limits_{j=0}^{i}K_j}{[H^+]^i}} \tag{5.164}$$

where $k_{i,+}$, $k_{i,-}$, and $k_{i,o}$ are the rate constants of the acid catalysis, base catalysis, and noncatalysis reactions of the ith species, respectively, and K_w is the ionization constant of water.

Equation (5.164) can be rearranged for mono- and polyprotic weak acids (or weak bases) as follows:

For monoprotic weak acids, the pseudo–first-order rate constant is given by:

$$k_{obs} = \frac{k_{0,+}[H^+]^2 + [H^+](k_{0,o} + k_{1,+}K_1) + (k_{1,o}K_1 + k_{0,-}K_w) + \dfrac{k_{1,-}K_1K_w}{[H^+]}}{K_1 + [H^+]} \tag{5.165}$$

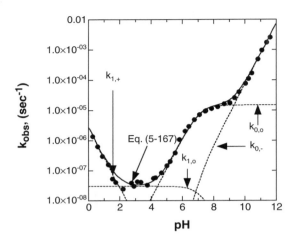

FIGURE 5.29 pH-rate constant profile for the degradation of L-phenylalanine methyl ester at 25°C. [Graph reconstructed from data by Skwierczynski and Connors, *Pharm. Res.*, 10, 1174 (1993).]

Equation (5.164) for monoprotic weak bases is written as:

$$k_{obs} = \frac{k_{1,+}[H^+]^2 + [H^+](k_{1,o} + k_{0,+}K_1) + (k_{0,o}K_1 + k_{1,-}K_w) + \dfrac{k_{0,-}K_1K_w}{[H^+]}}{K_1 + [H^+]} \qquad (5.166)$$

The second ($k_{1,o} + k_{0,+}K_1$) and third ($k_{0,o}K_1 + k_{1,-}K_w$) terms in the numerator of Equation (5.166) can be further simplified to $k_{1,o}$ and $k_{0,o}K_1$, respectively, when the hydrolysis of the undissociated species by H^+ and the protonated species by OH^- are assumed to be negligible. Equation (5.166) then becomes:

$$k_{obs} = \frac{k_{1,+}[H^+]^2 + k_{1,o}[H^+] + k_{0,o}K_1 + \dfrac{k_{0,-}K_1K_w}{[H^+]}}{K_1 + [H^+]} \qquad (5.167)$$

Figure 5.29 illustrates the pH-rate constant profile for the hydrolysis of L–phenylalanine methyl ester (weak base, $pK_a = 7.11$) at 25°C. When attempts are made to simulate the experimental data with Equation (5.167) over a wide range of pH values, the model seldom fits well, because the values of k_{obs} differ by several orders of magnitude and nonlinear regression analysis does not converge. Therefore, it is recommended that the kinetic values be within less than a few orders of magnitude. A localized and stepwise simulation process is recommended. At very low or high pH, Equation (5.167) simplifies to

$$k_{obs} = \frac{k_{1,+}[H^+]^2}{K_1 + [H^+]} \approx k_{1,+}[H^+] \quad \text{if} \quad [H^+] \gg K_1 \qquad (5.168a)$$

$$k_{obs} = \frac{k_{0,-}K_1K_w/[H^+]}{K_1+[H^+]} \approx \frac{k_{0,-}}{[H^+]} \quad \text{if} \quad [H^+] \ll K_1 \tag{5.168b}$$

When Equation (5.168a) and Equation (5.168b) are applied to the experimental data at low or high pH, $k_{1,+} = 2.5 \times 10^{-6} sec^{-1}M^{-1}$ and $k_{0,-} = 0.74 \ sec^{-1}M^{-1}$ are obtained. The second term in the numerator of Equation (5.167) is estimated from the plateau region (pH range of 2 to 4). Thus,

$$k_{obs} = \frac{k_{1,o}[H^+]}{K_1+[H^+]} \approx k_{1,o} \quad \text{if} \quad [H^+] \gg K_1 \tag{5.169}$$

$k_{1,o} \cong 3.5 \times 10^{-8} sec^{-1}M^{-1}$ is obtained.

The third term, $k_{0,o}$, is estimated from data at the pH range of 1 to 9 using the following equation:

$$k_{obs} = \frac{k_{1,+}[H^+]^2 + k_{1,o}[H^+] + k_{0,o}K_1}{K_1+[H^+]} \tag{5.170}$$

If only the protonated base is hydrolyzed, Equation (5.166) yields:

$$k_{obs} = \frac{k_{1,+}[H^+]^2 + k_{1,o}[H^+] + k_{1,-}K_w}{K_1+[H^+]} \tag{5.171}$$

Figure 5.30 shows the hydrolysis of chlordiazepoxide (weak base, $pK_a = 4.7$) at 79.5°C and I = 0.5 M. In this case, the rate constants are estimated by Equation (5.171). However, the rate constant of the protonated base by OH$^-$ (i.e., $k_{1,-}$) is easily calculated from the data at pH > 7.5:

$$k_{obs} = \frac{k_{1,-}K_w}{K_1+[H^+]} \approx \frac{k_{1,o}K_w}{K_1} \tag{5.172}$$

At very low pH (<1.5), the pseudo–first-order rate constant is expressed by Equation (5.168a).

It is interesting to take notice of the effect of an aromatic carboxylic acid group on hydrolysis. The effects of pH on the hydrolysis of aspirin and aspirin methyl ester have been investigated.

R = H   aspirin
R = CH$_3$ aspirin methyl ester

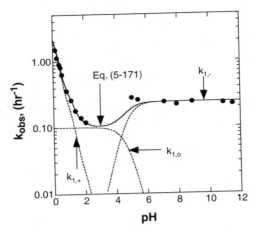

FIGURE 5.30 pH-rate constant profile of the hydrolysis of chlordiazepoxide ($pK_a = 4.7$) at 79.5°C and I = 0.5 M. [Graph reconstructed from data by Maulding et al., *J. Pharm. Sci.*, 64, 278 (1975).]

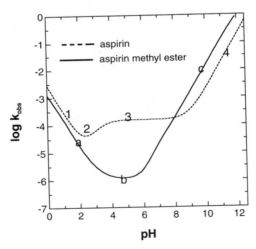

FIGURE 5.31 pH-rate constant profiles for the hydrolysis of aspirin (dotted line) and aspirin methyl ester (solid line). [Graph reconstructed from data by G. M. Loudon, *J. Chem. Ed.*, 68, 973 (1991).]

The pH-rate constant profiles of aspirin and aspirin methyl ester are shown in Figure 5.31. The profiles for aspirin methyl ester and aspirin are partitioned into three and four zones, respectively. Distinctively, the aspirin methyl ester profile is expressed by Equation (5.158b). The aspirin profile has similar hydrolysis rates in the zones of very low and very high pH to the aspirin methyl ester profile. However, in the range of pH 3 to 7, aspirin shows one upward bend at a pH close to 3.5, which is about the pK_a (=3.4) of aspirin. At pH 4 to 5, the hydrolysis rate of aspirin is

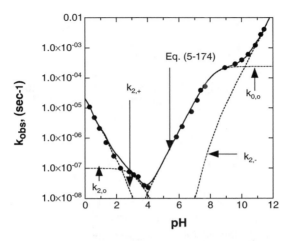

FIGURE 5.32 pH-rate constant profile of the hydrolysis of aspartame ($pK_{a1} = 3.19$ and $pK_{a2} = 8.14$) at 25°C in water. [Graph reconstructed from data by Skwierczynski and Connors, *Pharm. Res.,* 10, 1174 (1993).]

accelerated relative to aspirin methyl ester by about 150 times. This upward bend is observed at pH 5 for the hydrolysis of L-phenylalanine methyl ester (pK_a 4.7), as shown in Figure 5.29. Thus, this acceleration of hydrolysis is evidently related to the carboxylic acid group, presumably due to titration of aspirin. One may postulate that the aspirin anion undergoes much greater degradation than the analogous methyl ester. This leads to equating the dissociation constant (K_a) to the hydrolysis rate constant presented in Equation (5.167). The impact of K_a on the hydrolysis rate constant is negligible at zone 1.

For diprotic weak acids, Equation (5.164) becomes:

$$k_{obs} = \frac{\begin{aligned}&k_{0,+}[H^+]^3 + [H^+]^2(k_{0,o} + k_{1,+}K_1) \\ &+ [H^+](k_{2,+}K_1K_2 + k_{1,o}K_1 + k_{0,-}K_w) \\ &+ (k_{1,-}K_1K_w + k_{2,o}K_1K_2) + \dfrac{k_{2,-}K_1K_2K_w}{[H^+]}\end{aligned}}{[H^+]^2 + K_1[H^+] + K_1K_2} \tag{5.173}$$

Figure 5.32 shows the pH–pseudo–first-order rate constant profile of the degradation of aspartame (an ampholyte, $pK_{a1} = 3.19$ and $pK_{a2} = 8.14$). In the hydrolysis of aspartame, the protonated/undissociated form predominates at low pH (<3), while the deprotonated/dissociated form exists at high pH (>8). As demonstrated for monoprotic weak acids and weak bases, certain terms in the numerator of Equation (5.173) become negligible. For example, the hydrolysis of the protonated/undissociated form by OH⁻, of the protonated/dissociated form by H⁺ and OH⁻, and the deprotonated/dissociated form by H⁺ are not likely to occur. Then, Equation (5.173) for the ampholytic drug is written as:

$$k_{obs} = \frac{k_{2,+}[H^+]^3 + k_{2,o}[H^+]^2 + k_{1,o}K_1[H^+] + k_{0,o}K_1K_2 + \dfrac{k_{0,-}K_1K_2K_w}{[H^+]}}{[H^+]^2 + K_1[H^+] + K_1K_2}$$ (5.174)

At low pH (<1.5) and high pH (>11), the slopes, at the low and high pHs, of the plot of log k_{obs} vs. pH are −1.0 and +1.0, respectively. Thus, Equation (5.174) further simplifies to:

$$k_{obs} = k_{2,+}[H^+] \quad \text{and} \quad k_{obs} = \frac{k_{0,-}K_w}{[H^+]}$$

The values of $k_{2,+} = 2.05 \times 10^{-5} \sec^{-1} M^{-1}$ and $k_{0,-} = 1.50 \sec^{-1} M^{-1}$ are estimated. Substituting these values into Equation (5.174) followed by nonlinear regression analysis gives other k values. Intuitively from the profile of pH 2 to 4, one can assume $k_{1,o} = 0$. As demonstrated for monoprotic and diprotic weak acids and weak bases, the pH-rate constant profile is dependent on the kinetic pathway of the hydrolysis. It can be seen from Figure 5.32 that at pH 3 to 4 and pH 4 to 9, $k_{2,o}$ and $k_{0,o}$ are the predominant processes of the hydrolysis of aspartame, respectively.

For triprotic weak acids, Equation (5.164) becomes:

$$k_{obs} = \frac{M_1[H^+]^4 + M_2[H^+]^3 + M_3[H^+]^2 + M_4[H^+] + M_5 + \dfrac{M_6}{[H^+]}}{[H^+]^3 + K_1[H^+]^2 + K_1K_2[H^+] + K_1K_2K_3}$$ (5.175)

where

$$M_1 = k_{0,+}$$

$$M_2 = k_{0,o} + k_{1,+}K_1$$

$$M_3 = k_{2,+}K_1K_2 + k_{1,o}K_1 + k_{0,-}K_w$$

$$M_4 = k_{3,+}K_1K_2K_3 + k_{2,o}K_1K_2 + k_{1,-}K_1K_w$$ (5.176)

$$M_5 = k_{3,o}K_1K_2K_3 + k_{2,-}K_1K_2K_w$$

$$M_6 = k_{3,-}K_1K_2K_3K_w$$

The degradation kinetics of 7-N-(p-hydroxyphenyl)mitomycin C (M-83) ($pK_{a1} = 2.76$, $pK_{a2} = 9.41$, and $pK_{a3} = 10.9$) in aqueous solution are expressed by Equation (5.175). The drug exists as M-83$^+$, M-83°, M-83$^-$, and M-83^{-2}:

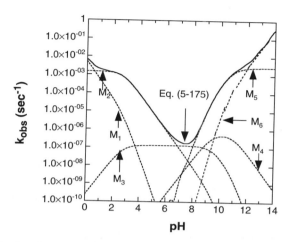

FIGURE 5.33 Simulated pH-rate constant profile for the hydrolysis of 7-*N*-(*p*-hydroxyphenyl) mitomycin C (M-83) ($pK_{a1} = 2.76$, $pK_{a2} = 9.41$, and $pK_{a3} = 10.9$). [Graph reconstructed from data by Beijnen et al., *Int. J. Pharm.*, 45, 189 (1988).]

$$H_3A^+ \underset{\longleftarrow}{\overset{K_1}{\rightleftharpoons}} H_2A \underset{\longleftarrow}{\overset{K_2}{\rightleftharpoons}} HA^- \underset{\longleftarrow}{\overset{K_3}{\rightleftharpoons}} A^{-2}$$

The individual rate constants incorporated in the single macro-reaction constants (Ms) are kinetically indistinguishable. As mentioned before, one term is often predominant over others in the macro-reaction constants. Unless the kinetic reaction pathways are distinctively singled out, the degradation process is assumed to have the following values for M: $M_1 = 5.3 \times 10^{-3}$ $M^{-4}\text{sec}^{-1}$, $M_2 = 1.5 \times 10^{-3}$ $M^{-3}\text{sec}^{-1}$, $M_3 = 2.3 \times 10^{-10}$ $M^{-2}\text{sec}^{-1}$, $M_4 = 4.3 \times 10^{-19}$ $M^{-1}\text{sec}^{-1}$, $M_5 = 2.2 \times 10^{-26}$ sec^{-1}, and $M_6 = 2.7 \times 10^{-38}$ $M\text{sec}^{-1}$. Figure 5.33 shows the contribution of the individual macro-reaction constants to the pseudo–first-order rate constant (k_{obs}). The solid line is the sum of the contributions of the macro-reaction constants. In the degradation of M-83, as seen in Figure 5.33, M_2 and M_5 are responsible for the pH-rate constant profile over a wide range of pH values. In addition, the acid-catalyzed hydrolysis of M-83+ and base-catalyzed hydrolysis of M-83^{-2} are the predominant processes at very low and very high pH values, respectively. M_3 and M_4 contribute to a lesser extent.

A few examples of pH-rate constant profiles have been demonstrated so far. The pH-rate constant profiles shown in Figure 5.29 through Figure 5.33 are segmental patterns of the generalized pH-rate constant profile polygon shown in Figure 5.34. Depending on the types of drugs (i.e., mono-, di-, triprotic weak acids or weak bases) and the degree of contribution of individual rate constants to the overall pseudo–first-order rate constant, many different configurations of the pH–k_{obs} relationship can be constructed. However, the connecting corners between the two lines are smooth curvatures in real cases.

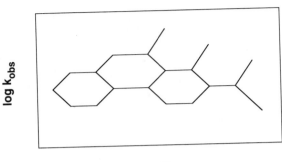

FIGURE 5.34 Generalized pH–k_{obs} polygon. [Graph reconstructed from J. T. Cartensen, *Drug Stability: Principles and Applications,* 2nd Ed., Marcel Dekker, New York, 1995. p 91.]

5.11 OXIDATION (FREE RADICAL REACTION)

Pharmaceutical compounds, containing phenolic hydroxyl, enolic hydroxyl, thiol, sulfide, ether, amine, unsaturated olefin, peroxide, or aldehyde groups undergo oxidative degradation in the presence of molecular oxygen. Most oxidation reactions are a series of slow chain reactions. First, organic compounds that yield free radicals (R*) by the catalytic action of light, heat, or trace metals initiate oxidation. Second, the free radicals react with oxygen to produce peroxide radicals (ROO*), which further react with the organic compounds to give rise to hydroperoxides and free radicals (R*). The reaction progresses until all the free radicals are consumed or destroyed. A series of simple free radical chain reactions is described by the following steps:

Initiation: organic compound (M_1) $\xrightarrow{k_1}$ R* + H*

Propagation: R* + O_2 $\xrightarrow{k_2}$ ROO*

ROO* + M_1 $\xrightarrow{k_3}$ ROOH + R*

Termination: 2ROO* $\xrightarrow{k_4}$ nonradical products

The overall rate of oxidation of the organic compound (M_1) is:

$$-\frac{d[M_1]}{dt} = k_1[M_1] + k_3[ROO*][M_1] \qquad (5.177)$$

The changes of free radical concentrations during the oxidation reaction are assumed to be the steady-state approximation:

$$\frac{d[R^*]}{dt} = 0 = k_1[M_1] - k_2[O_2][R^*] + k_3[M_1][ROO^*] \tag{5.178}$$

$$\frac{d[ROO^*]}{dt} = 0 = k_2[O_2][R^*] - k_3[M_1][ROO^*] - k_4[ROO^*]^2 \tag{5.179}$$

Adding Equation (5.178) into Equation (5.179) yields:

$$k_1[M_1] - k_4[ROO^*]^2 = 0 \quad \text{or} \quad [ROO^*] = \sqrt{\frac{k_1 M_1}{k_4}} \tag{5.180}$$

Substituting Equation (5.180) into Equation (5.177) gives:

$$-\frac{d[M_1]}{dt} = k_1[M_1] + k_3\sqrt{\frac{k_1 M_1}{k_4}}[M_1] \cong k_3\sqrt{\frac{k_1 M_1}{k_4}}[M_1] \tag{5.181}$$

The propagation reactions are faster than initiation and termination, and therefore the first term on the right-hand side of Equation (5.181) can be neglected.

To retard the rate of oxidation, antioxidants (AH) that do not completely inhibit the reaction are incorporated into drug products. The following reaction is added to the above chain reactions as follows:

$$ROO^* + AH \xrightarrow{k_5} ROOH + A^*$$

Equation (5.179) is then modified to:

$$\frac{d[ROO^*]}{dt} = 0 = k_2[O_2][R^*] - k_3[M_1][ROO^*]$$
$$- k_4[ROO^*]^2 - k_5[AH][ROO^*] \tag{5.182}$$

Adding Equation (5.178) into Equation (5.182) yields:

$$k_1[M_1] - k_5[AH][ROO^*] - k_4[ROO^*]^2 = 0 \tag{5.183}$$

The rate of termination is negligible compared to the rate of propagation, and Equation (5.183) then becomes:

$$k_1[M_1] - k_5[AH][ROO^*] = 0 \quad \text{or} \quad [ROO^*] = \frac{k_1[M_1]}{k_5[AH]} \tag{5.184}$$

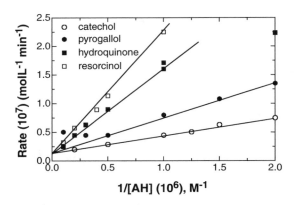

FIGURE 5.35 The retarded oxidation of benzaldehyde in the presence of antioxidants at 30°C. [Graph reconstructed from data by D. E. Moore, *J. Pharm. Sci.*, 65, 1447 (1976).]

Substituting Equation (5.184) into Equation (5.177) gives:

$$-\frac{d[M_1]}{dt} = k_1[M_1] + k_3 \frac{k_1[M_1]}{k_5[AH]}[M_1] = k_1[M_1]\left(1 + \frac{k_3[M_1]}{k_5[AH]}\right) \quad (5.185)$$

Figure 5.35 shows the retarded oxidation of benzaldehyde in the presence of antioxidants at 30°C. It is interesting to see a common intercept in the linear plots.

The initiation step normally does not involve molecular oxygen to yield free radicals. Certain compounds composing a structure of quinone and/or hydroquinone react readily with molecular oxygen to form a semiquinone or a free radical quinone. An example of this is the oxidation of morphine. This kind of oxidation process does not add oxygen to the compounds.

Metal ions very often catalyze oxidation. In this case, the metal ions are oxidized in the presence of oxygen at low pH. The oxidized metal ions react with organic compounds to yield free radical compounds. The free radical compounds couple to form dimers as follows:

$$2Mn^{+2} + 2H^+ + \tfrac{1}{2}O_2 \longrightarrow 2Mn^{+3} + H_2O$$

$$Mn^{+3} + RH \longrightarrow Mn^{+2} + H^+ + R*$$

$$2R* \longrightarrow R-R$$

A complete removal of oxygen in aqueous solution is not feasible and thus in practice, the metal ions are frequently complexed with chelating agents (EDTA, disodium edate, citric acid, etc.).

5.12 DEGRADATION KINETICS IN INCLUSION COMPLEXES, MICELLES, AND LIPOSOMES

The degradation of drug substances and excipients is influenced by many factors. In an effort to stabilize or minimize the degradation, complex formation between drugs and excipients and entrapment of drug substances in micelles and liposomes have been investigated. In this section, inclusion complex formation is discussed. The basic principles of inclusion complex formation have been presented in Chapter 3. Only the degradation of drugs in the 1:1 interaction complex system is considered. For 1:2 and 2:1 complexes, Chapter 3 should be consulted. Caffeine, aldehydes, and others have been used as ligands to form complexes but these are pharmacologically active. Recently, cyclodextrins and their derivatives have gained considerable attention because they may improve stability.

If drug A complexes with ligand L:

$$A + L \rightleftharpoons A - L$$
$$\mid \qquad\qquad \mid$$
$$k_f \qquad\qquad k_c$$

degradation products

The stability constant, K, is given by:

$$K = \frac{[A - L]}{[A]_f [L]_f} \qquad\qquad (5.186)$$

where $[A]_f$ and $[L]_f$ are the concentration of free drug and free ligand, respectively.

The overall degradation of drug in the presence of ligand is the sum of free drug A and complex A–L given by:

$$\frac{d[A]}{dt} = -(k_f [A]_f + k_c [A - L]) \qquad\qquad (5.187)$$

where k_f and k_c are the rate constant for the degradation of the drug in the absence of complex formation and in its complex form, respectively. Substituting Equation (5.186) into Equation (5.187) yields:

$$\frac{d[A]}{dt} = -(k_f + k_c K[L]_f)[A]_f [L]_f \qquad\qquad (5.188)$$

The apparent rate equation is given by:

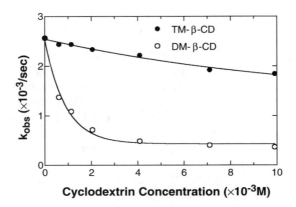

FIGURE 5.36 Stabilization of prostacyclin by the derivatives of cyclodextrin. [Graph reconstructed from data by Hirayama et al., *Int. J. Pharm.*, 35, 193 (1987).]

$$\frac{d[A]}{dt} = -k_{obs}[L]_f \left([A]_f + [A-L]\right) = k_{obs}[A]_f [L]_f (1 + K[L]_f) \qquad (5.189)$$

Substituting Equation (5.188) into Equation (5.189) and rearranging the resulting equation yields:

$$\frac{1}{k_{obs} - k_f} = \frac{1}{k_c - k_f} + \frac{1}{K(k_c - k_f)} \frac{1}{[L]_f} \qquad (5.190)$$

However, [L], the total concentration of ligand present in solution, can replace $[L]_f$, with the assumption that the ligand is present in excess of the drug or only small amounts of [L] form complexes.

The plot of the reciprocal of $k_{obs} - k_f$ against $1/[L]$ is linear, with a slope of $1/[K(k_c - k_f)]$ and an intercept of $1/(k_c - k_f)$. Figure 5.36 shows the stabilization of prostacyclin by the derivatives of β-cyclodextrin. However, not all inclusion complexes provide the stabilization of drugs. In many cases, drug degradation is enhanced via inclusion complex formation [e.g., prostaglandin E_1 and E_2/β-cyclodextrin (β-CD), aspirin/β-CD].

Example 5.19

Stabilization of prostacyclin in solution by β-cyclodextrin (βCD) was carried out with the following results:

βCD concentration, × $10^{-3}M$	0.0	0.6	1.1	2.0	4.1	7.1	9.9
k_{obs}, 10^{-3}/sec		2.60	2.12	1.90	1.54	1.32	1.11	1.09

Calculate the stability constant and the degradation rate constant of the complexed drug.

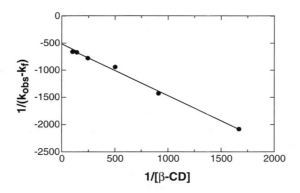

FIGURE 5.37 Determination of the stability constant and the degradation rate constant of Example 5.19.

Solution

Data are transformed according to Equation (5.190) as:

CD conc.	1/CD conc.	k_{obs}	$k_{obs} - k_f$	$1/(k_{obs} - k_f)$
$0.0 \times 10^{-3} M$		2.60×10^{-3}/sec		
0.6	1667	2.12	-0.48×10^{-3}/sec	-2083
1.1	909	1.90	-0.70	-1429
2.0	500	1.54	-1.06	-943
4.1	244	1.32	-1.28	-781
7.1	141	1.11	-1.49	-671
9.9	101	1.09	-1.51	-662

The plot of the fifth column against the second column is shown in Figure 5.37, and the slope and intercept are calculated.

$$\text{slope} = -0.9262 = \frac{1}{K(k_c - k_f)}, \quad \text{intercept} = -545 = \frac{1}{k_c - k_f}$$

$$K = \frac{\text{intercept}}{\text{slope}} = \frac{-545}{-0.9262} = 588\ M, \quad k_c = 2.6 \times 10^{-3} - \frac{1}{545} = 0.77 \times 10^{-3}\ /\ \text{sec}$$

Another way to stabilize drugs is to entrap them in micelles and liposomes. When surfactants, consisting of hydrophilic and lipophilic groups, in a solution reach up to a certain concentration (critical micelle concentration, c.m.c), they form micelles (see Chapter 4). If drugs (especially hydrophobic drugs) are entrapped inside micelles, which are hydrophobic in nature, the entrapped drugs are less vulnerable to degradation than unentrapped drugs due to the much smaller amount of water present within micelles. The degradation of a drug substance in a micellar system is dependent on the stability of entrapped drug and unentrapped drug and the quantity of micelles in the system.

The volume of micelles, V_m, in a solution is given by:

$$V_m = \frac{[S] - [S]_{cmc}}{\rho} \qquad (5.191)$$

where $[S]$ and $[S]_{cmc}$ are the concentration of surfactant and critical micelle concentration, respectively, and ρ is the density of the surfactant. The total amount of drug present in the system, A, is the sum of the amount of drug in the bulk phase, $[A]_b$, and in the micelles, $[A]_m$, as:

$$A = [A]_b (V - V_m) + [A]_m V_m = ([A]_m - K[A]_m)V_m + K[A]_m V \qquad (5.192)$$

where V and K are the total volume of the solution and the distribution coefficient $(= [A]_b / [A]_m)$, respectively.

Assuming that the degradation in the bulk phase and in micelles follows first-order kinetics, the total rate of degradation in mass is given by:

$$V_m \frac{d[A]_m}{dt} + (V - V_m) \frac{d[A]_b}{dt} = \frac{dA}{dt} = -k_m V_m [A]_m - k_b (V - V_m)[A]_b \qquad (5.193)$$

Equation (5.192) leads to:

$$[A]_m = \frac{A}{(1 - K)V_m + KV}, \qquad [A]_b = \frac{KA}{(1 - K)V_m + KV} \qquad (5.194)$$

Substituting Equation (5.194) into Equation (5.193) yields:

$$\frac{dA}{dt} = -\frac{k_m V_m A}{(1 - K)V_m + KV} - \frac{k_b K(V - V_m)A}{(1 - K)V_m + KV} = -k_{obs} A \qquad (5.195)$$

where

$$k_{obs} = \frac{k_m V_m + k_b K(V - V_m)}{(1 - K)V_m + KV} \qquad (5.196)$$

However, if a drug is dissolved in oil and emulsified with surfactants, the first term of the numerator in Equation (5.196) becomes negligible because the drugs in an oil droplet remain in the oil phase until coalescence occurs whereas micelles constantly change in a micellar system. Figure 5.38 shows the stabilization of indomethacin in the presence of cationic liposome at pH 9.37 (carbonic buffer) and 40°C.

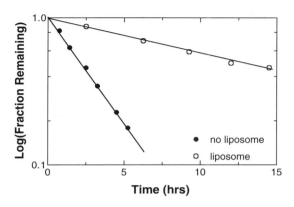

FIGURE 5.38 Stabilization of indomethacin in the presence of cationic liposome at pH 9.37 (carbonic buffer) and 40°C. [Graph reconstructed from data by D'Silva and Notari, *J. Pharm. Sci.*, 71, 1394 (1982).]

5.13 TEMPERATURE EFFECTS ON THE REACTION RATE CONSTANTS

The degradation of final dosage forms will occur over a long time at low temperature (i.e., 25°C). For example, it may take a year or more even for 5 to 10% of drugs to decompose. When one considers the errors in analytical assays, the degradation data may not be significant. To obtain degradation data within a reasonably short period of time, degradation experiments are carried out at higher temperatures. Then, the kinetic data at high temperatures are extrapolated to the corresponding kinetic data at 25°C. However, it is imperative to know the dependence of a degradation reaction on temperature. Two theories that describe the temperature dependence of the rate equation are: collision theory and transition-state theory.

The *collision theory*: In a gas, molecules A are moving and colliding together with molecules B. The total number of collisions of molecules A with molecules B, Z_{AB}, at a given time, Δt, is:

$$Z_{AB} = n_A n_B \sigma_{AB}^2 \sqrt{8\pi RT \frac{M_A + M_B}{M_A M_B}} \qquad (5.197)$$

where n_A and n_B are the numbers of moles of the molecules A and B in a unit volume, respectively, M_A and M_B are the molecular weights of the molecules A and B, respectively, and σ_{AB} is the mean collision diameter [$= \frac{1}{2}(\sigma_A + \sigma_B)$], where σ_A and σ_B are the diameters of molecules A and B, respectively. However, not every collision between molecules A and B leads to a reaction. Only a small fraction of the collisions leads to a reaction as a result of those molecules possessing energy in excess of the minimum energy, E. The collisions are then equal to the Boltzman factor ($e^{-E/RT}$), and the actual number of collisions for a given reaction is:

$$Z_{successful} = Z_{AB}e^{-E/RT} \qquad (5.198)$$

The rate for a bimolecular reaction is given as:

$$r_A = -k_{AB}[A][B] = (\text{collision rate}) \times (\text{fraction of effective collision})$$

$$= Z_{AB}e^{-E/RT}$$

$$= N_A\sigma_{AB}^2\sqrt{8\pi RT\frac{M_A + M_B}{M_A M_B}}e^{-E/RT}[A][B] \qquad (5.199)$$

Equation (5.199) shows that the rate constant is dependent on the temperature:

$$k_{AB} \propto \sqrt{T}e^{-E/RT} \qquad (5.200)$$

The *transition-state theory*: Molecules colliding or possessing sufficient energy can combine to form unstable intermediates, known as activated complexes. These activated complexes transiently exist and are spontaneously converted to products in a first-order rate process. They are also constantly in equilibrium with the reactants. Thus, reactions can be written:

$$A + B \underset{k_2}{\overset{k_1}{\rightleftarrows}} (AB)^* \xrightarrow{k_3} C \qquad (5.201)$$

where $(AB)^*$ is the transient activated complex.

The rate equations are:

$$K_{AB}^* = \frac{k_1}{k_2} = \frac{[(AB)^*]}{[A][B]} \qquad (5.202)$$

and
$$\frac{d[(AB)^*]}{dt} = k_3[(AB)^*] \qquad (5.203)$$

where K_{AB}^* is the equilibrium constant. The rate of spontaneous decomposition of the activated complex is an equation for the specific rate of any reaction and given as:

$$k_3 = \frac{kT}{h} \qquad (5.204)$$

where **h** is the Planck constant and k is the Boltzman constant. Substituting Equation (5.204) and Equation (5.202) into Equation (5.203) yields:

$$\frac{d[(AB)^*]}{dt} = \frac{kT}{h}[(AB)^*] = \frac{kT}{h}K_{AB}^*[A][B] \qquad (5.205)$$

The thermodynamic relationship between the standard free energy change and the equilibrium constant of the activated complex is given as:

$$\Delta G^* = -RT \ln K_{AB}^* = \Delta H^* - T\Delta S^* \qquad (5.206)$$

or
$$K_{AB}^* = \exp(-\Delta G^* / RT) = \exp(-\Delta H^* / RT)\exp(\Delta S^* / R) \qquad (5.207)$$

Substituting Equation (5.207) into Equation (5.205) gives:

$$\frac{d[(AB)^*]}{dt} = \frac{kT}{h}e^{-\Delta H^*/RT}e^{\Delta S^*/R}[A][B] \qquad (5.208)$$

The term $e^{\Delta S^*/R}$ in Equation (5.208) is less sensitive to the temperature effects than the terms kT/h and $e^{-\Delta H^*/RT}$. Thus, the rate constant k for equation (5.208) is:

$$k_1, k_2, \text{or } k_3 = \frac{kT}{h}e^{-\Delta H^*/RT}e^{\Delta S^*/R} \propto \frac{kT}{h}e^{-\Delta H^*/RT} \propto Te^{-\Delta H^*/RT} \qquad (5.209)$$

The enthalpy of activation is directly related to the Arrhenius activation energy.

$$E = \Delta H^* + RT \qquad (5.210)$$

The difference between E and ΔH^* is very small, and ΔH^* is replaced by E. Thus, Equation (5.209) approximates to:

$$k_1, k_2, \text{or } k_3 \propto Te^{-E/RT} \qquad (5.211)$$

Figure 5.39 shows the schematic diagram of the transition state for an exothermic reaction. The transition-state theory assumes that the rate of formation of a transition-state intermediate is very fast and the decomposition of the unstable intermediate is slow and is the rate-determining step. On the other hand, the collision theory states that the rate of the reaction is controlled by collisions among the reactants. The rate of formation of the intermediate is very slow and is followed by the rapid decomposition of the intermediates into products. Based on these two theories, the following expression can be derived to account for the temperature dependence of the rate constant:

$$k \propto T^m e^{-E/RT} = k_0^* T^m e^{-E/RT}, \qquad 0 \le m \le 1 \qquad (5.212)$$

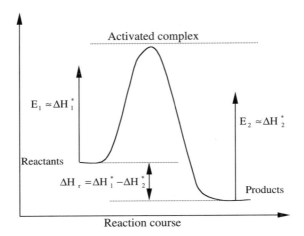

FIGURE 5.39 Schematic diagram of the transition state for an exothermic reaction.

where k_o^*, T, E, and R are the proportionality constant, the absolute temperature, the activation energy, and the gas constant, respectively.

Differentiating Equation (5.212) with respect to T and taking the logarithm yields:

$$\frac{d(\ln k)}{dT} = \frac{m}{T} + \frac{E}{RT^2} \tag{5.213}$$

For most chemical reactions, E >> mRT, and Equation (5.213) then becomes:

$$\frac{d(\ln k)}{dT} = \frac{E}{RT^2}, \quad \text{or} \quad k = Ae^{-E/RT} \tag{5.214}$$

where A is called the frequency factor. Equation (5.214) is known as Arrhenius' law. It was originally suggested by Arrhenius to fit chemical reaction experiments over a wide range of reaction temperatures.

A plot of ln k as a function of the reciprocal temperature gives a straight line with a slope of −E/R, from which E can be calculated. Another way to determine the activation energy is using two different values of k (k_1 and k_2) at two different temperatures (T_1 and T_2):

$$\ln k_1 = \ln A - \frac{E}{RT_1} \tag{5.215a}$$

$$\ln k_2 = \ln A - \frac{E}{RT_2} \tag{5.215b}$$

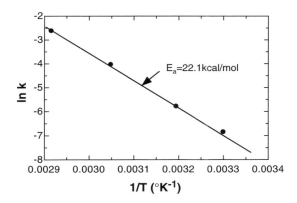

FIGURE 5.40 Arrhenius plot for the degradation of gemcitabine at pH 3.2. [Graph reconstructed from data by Jansen et al., *J. Pharm. Sci.,* 89, 885 (2000).]

Subtracting Equation (5.215b) from Equation (5.215a) yields:

$$\ln\left(\frac{k_1}{k_2}\right) = -\frac{E}{R}\left(\frac{1}{T_1} - \frac{1}{T_2}\right) = -\frac{E}{R}\left(\frac{T_2 - T_1}{T_1 T_2}\right) \tag{5.216}$$

Figure 5.40 shows the effect of the temperature (Arrhenius plot) on the degradation of gemcitabine at pH 3.2 (acetate buffer).

Example 5.20

What are the activation energy (kcal/mol) and the frequency factor A (hr^{-1}) for the decomposition of a drug if the rate constants at 120 and 140°C are 1.276 and 5.024/hr, respectively? Calculate the rate constant at 25°C.

Solution

Substituting all the information into Equation (5.216) gives:

$$\ln\left(\frac{1.276 / \text{hr}}{5.024 / \text{hr}}\right) = -\frac{E}{1.987}\left(\frac{413 - 393}{413 \times 393}\right)$$

$$E = 22{,}100 \text{ cal/mol} = 22.1 \text{ kcal/mol}$$

The rate constant at 25°C is calculated by:

$$\ln\left(\frac{k \, (\text{at } 25°\text{C})}{5.024 / \text{hr}}\right) = -\frac{22{,}100}{1.987}\left(\frac{413 - 298}{413 \times 298}\right)$$

$$k \, (\text{at } 25°\text{C}) = 1.54 \times 10^{-4}/\text{hr}$$

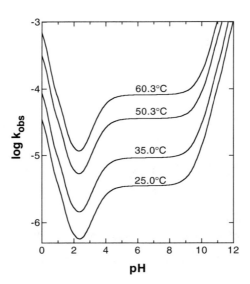

FIGURE 5.41 pH-rate constant profile for the hydrolysis of aspirin in 0.5% aqueous ethanol solution at four temperatures. [Graph simulated from data by E. R. Garret, *J. Am. Chem. Soc.,* 79, 3401 (1957).]

The frequency factor is calculated by:

$$\ln(1.276 \,/\, \mathrm{hr}) = \ln A - \frac{22,100}{1.987 \times 393} \qquad A = 2.5 \times 10^{12} \,/\, \mathrm{hr}$$

Example 5.21

Acetylsalicylic acid (aspirin) ($pK_a = 3.62$) undergoes acid–base catalyzed hydrolysis. The pseudo–first-order rate constants were determined at four different temperatures (25, 35, 50.3, and 60.3°C) as shown in Figure 5.41. The hydrolysis of aspirin follows Equation (5.167) with $k_{0,o} = 0$ and $k_{0,-} = 0$. Each rate constant is given by:

$$k_{0,+} = 10^{7.78}\, e^{-16,700/RT}, \qquad k_{1,+} = 10^{9.05}\, e^{-16,400/RT}$$

$$k_{1,o} = 10^{7.45}\, e^{-17,600/RT}, \qquad k_{1,-} = 10^{8.18}\, e^{-12,500/RT}$$

Calculate the pseudo–first-order rate constants at 45°C and at pH 6.

Solution

Each rate constant at 45°C is obtained as:

$$k_{0,+} = 10^{7.78} \exp\!\left(-\frac{16,700}{(1.987)(318.15)}\right) = 2.03 \times 10^{-4}\ \mathrm{Lmole^{-1}sec^{-1}}$$

$$k_{1,+} = 6.07 \times 10^{-3}, \quad k_{1,o} = 2.28 \times 10^{-5}, \quad k_{1,-} = 0.391$$

The pseudo–first-order rate constant at pH 6 is calculated as:

$$k_{obs} = \frac{k_{0,+}[H^+]^2 + k_{1,+}K_1[H^+] + k_{1,o}K_1 + \dfrac{k_{1,-}K_1K_w}{[H^+]}}{K_1 + [H^+]}$$

$$= \frac{2.03 \times 10^{-4} \times 10^{-12} + 6.07 \times 10^{-3} \times 10^{-3.62} \times 10^{-6} + 2.28 \times 10^{-5} \times 10^{-3.62} + 0.391 \times 10^{-3.62} \times 10^{-8}}{10^{-3.62} + 10^{-6}}$$

$$= 2.27 \times 10^{-5}/sec$$

SUGGESTED READINGS

1. J. T. Carstensen, *Drug Stability: Principles and Practices*, 2nd Ed., Marcel Dekker, New York, 1995.
2. R. Chang, *Physical Chemistry with Applications to Biological Systems*, 2nd Ed., Macmillan, New York, 1981, Chapter 12.
3. K. A. Connors, *Chemical Kinetics: The Study of Reaction Rates in Solution*, John Wiley and Sons, New York, 1990.
4. K. A. Connors, G. L. Amidon, and L. Kennon, *Chemical Stability of Pharmaceuticals: A Handbook for Pharmacists*, Wiley Interscience, New York, 1979.
5. S. Glastone and D. Lewis, *Elements of Physical Chemistry*, 2nd Ed., Van Nostrand Co., Mazuren Asian Ed., Tokyo, 1960, Chapter 16.
6. M. Gibaldi and D. Perrier, *Pharmacokinetics*, Marcel Dekker, New York, 1975.
7. O. A. G. J. van der Houwen et al., A General Approach to the Interpretation of pH Degradation Profiles, *Int. J. Pharm.*, 45, 181, (1988).
8. H. Kuhn and H.-D. Forsterling, *Principles of Physical Chemistry*, John Wiley and Sons, New York, 2000, Chapter 21.
9. O. Levenspiel, *Chemical Reaction Engineering*, 2nd Ed., John Wiley and Sons, New York, 1972, Chapters 2 and 3.
10. J. W. Moore and R. G. Pearson, *Kinetics and Mechanism*, Wiley Interscience, New York, 1981.
11. G. A. Russell, Fundamental Processes of Autooxidation, *J. Chem. Ed.*, 36, 111, (1959).
12. V. R. Williams, W. L. Mattice, and H. B. Williams, *Basic Physical Chemistry for the Life Sciences*, 3rd ed., W. H. Freeman and Co., San Francisco, 1978, Chapter 6.
13. S. Yoshioka and V. J. Stella, *Stability of Drugs and Dosage Forms*, Plenum Publishers, New York, 2000.

PROBLEMS

1. An initial assay of a solution product indicated a concentration of 5.5 mg/mL. Eighteen months later, however, an assay showed only 4.2 mg/mL. Assuming that both of the above assays were accurate, calculate the rate constant and shelf-life (10% degradation):
   a. If the degradation reaction follows zero-order kinetics with respect to the drug.
   b. If the degradation reaction is first-order with respect to the drug.

2. It was found that the degradation of a drug follows first-order kinetics. It took 36 days for 25% degradation of a drug formulation. How long does it take for 50% degradation of the remaining formulation?

3. A drug in a solution decomposes rapidly in an alkaline environment (pH 7 to 12) via base-catalyzed hydrolysis. A shelf-life of 23 days has been obtained at pH 9.4. What should the pH be if the shelf-life is increased to 2 years?

4. A drug is hydrolyzed via a first-order reaction in a solution. The solubility of the drug in water is 3.5 mg/100mL. A pharmacist made a suspension formulation of the drug containing 2.7 mg/mL. The shelf-life of the suspension was 15 days. Calculate the half-life of the solution.

5. Experimentally, it was found that the half-life for the hydrolytic degradation (first-order kinetics) of oxazepam in aqueous solution at pH 3.24 was 38.9 min at 80°C. However, 28% of the drug was hydrolyzed at 70°C after 25.4 min. Calculate the activation energy for the degradation, the degradation rate constant at 25°C, the shelf-life at 25°C, and what concentration of intact drug is left after 225 min. at 25°C, expressed as a percentage.

6. The following data were obtained for the hydrolysis of diazepam in a buffer solution at 80 and 90°C.

Time (min)	Concentration of Intact Diazepam (mol/L)	
	80°C	90°C
0	0.2000	0.2000
45	0.1334	0.0883
120	0.0679	0.0226

   a. What is the order of the degradation reaction?
   b. What are the values of the rate constants at 80°C and 90°C?
   c. What is the value of the activation energy for the degradation reaction?
   d. What is the value of the specific rate constant at 25°C?
   e. What is the shelf-life at 25°C?

7. One of the classical examples of a reversible reaction is the conversion of γ-hydroxybutyric acid into its lactone in an aqueous solution. In aqueous solution, the water concentration may be considered constant, so the reverse reaction follows pseudo–first-order kinetics. The following data were obtained. Determine the values of both first-order rate constants (forward and reverse). The initial acid concentration is 182.3 mol/L.

Time (ksec)	1.26	2.16	3.0	3.90	4.80	6.0	7.20	9.60	13.20
Lactone (mol/L)	24.1	37.3	49.9	61.0	70.8	81.1	90.0	103.5	115.5

8. In carrying out an enzyme assay it may be convenient to introduce an auxiliary enzyme to the system to affect the removal of a product produced by the first enzymatic reaction. The kinetics of these coupled enzyme assays can be expressed by:

$$A \xrightarrow{k_1} B \xrightarrow{k_2} C$$

If the first reaction is regarded as irreversible zero-order (i.e., the enzyme is saturated with substrate), and the second reaction is first-order in the product B, determine the time-dependent behavior of the concentration of intermediate B if no B is present initially. How long does it take to reach 98% of the steady-state value if $k_1 = 0.833$ mol/m^3/ksec and $k_2 = 0.767$/sec?

9. Many researchers studied the stability of a drug in the presence of β-cyclodextrin. The following data were obtained. Calculate the drug degradation rate constants of the drug inclusion complex.

Concentration β-CD	0	0.13	0.38	0.62	0.97	1.25
Pseudo–first-order rate constant (mol/L)	1.37	0.92	0.53	0.35	0.13	0.08

10. Derive the kinetic equation for the formation of HM via the following free-radical oxidation:

Initiation: organic compound $(M_2) \xrightarrow{k_1} 2R *$

Propagation: $R * + H_2 \xrightarrow{k_2} HM + H *$

$H * + M_2 \xrightarrow{k_3} HM + R *$

Inhibition: $H * + HM \xrightarrow{k_4} H_2 + R *$

Termination: $2R * \xrightarrow{k_5} M_2$

11. Sucrose is hydrolyzed by the catalytic action of sucrase. The following experimental data were obtained with $[A]_o = 1.0$ mmol/L and $[E]_o = 0.01$ mmol/L. Evaluate the Michaelis–Menten constants.

Time, hr	1	2	3	4	5	6	7	8	9	10	11
[A]	0.84	0.68	0.53	0.38	0.27	0.16	0.09	0.04	0.018	0.006	0.0025

12. The stability of penicillin G K (1 million units/L) in 5% dextrose at 24 hours at 25°C and various pH values is shown below. What is the expiration date of penicillin G K in 5% dextrose when the pH of the solution is (a) 4.5 and (b) 5.5?

13. From the result of an accelerated stability study, it was found that the first-order rate constants at 60 and 50°C were 0.08 and 0.06/day, respectively. What is the expiration date of the pharmaceutical product if it must be discarded when less than 88% of the labeled amount remains at 25°C?

14. If each reaction below is regarded as irreversible first-order and pure linoleic acid is the starting compound, derive the time–concentration equations of each species.

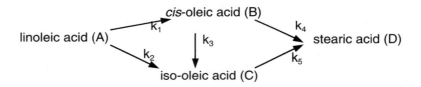

15. It was reported that the degradation of cefixime in an alkaline solution follows parallel and consecutive reactions as:

$$B \xleftarrow[k_2]{} A \xrightarrow{k_1} C \xrightarrow{k_3} D$$

Derive the time–concentrations of each species.

16. The hydrolysis of mitomycin follows the generalized acid–base catalyzed process in a phosphate buffer. It was found that dihydrogenphosphate ions are the only contributors to the hydrolysis along with hydrogen ions at low pH (3.5). At pH 3.5, the following data were obtained. Calculate the rate constants of the following expression:

$[H_2PO_4^-]$	0.01	0.05	0.1	0.2	0.3	0.4 mol/L
k_{obs}	1.30	1.32	1.34	1.40	1.45	1.56 ($\times 10^3$/sec)

$$k_{obs} = k_o + k_{H^+}[H^+] + k_{H_2PO_4^-}[H_2PO_4^-]$$

17. Derive the time–concentration expression of P in the following proposed reaction. At $t = 0$, $[A] = [A]_o$ and $[B] = [C] = [P] = 0$.

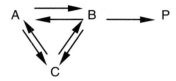

18. Degradation kinetics of methyl-*trans*-cinnamate in the presence of hydroxide ions follows second-order reaction kinetics. It was shown that the drug forms a complex with theophylline. The following kinetic data were obtained in the presence of theophylline and a great excess of hydroxide ion. Calculate the stability constant.

Theophylline (10^{-2} M)	9.46	6.43	4.93	3.42	2.65	2.08	0.0
k_{obs} (10^{-3}/sec)	2.54	2.93	3.24	3.54	3.76	4.01	4.99

6 Diffusion

When the conventional pharmaceutical dosage forms (i.e., tablets, capsules, or creams) are administered orally or topically, the active drug in the dosage form is rapidly released from the site of administration and absorbed into the systemic circulation. The release of the drug can occur within a short period of time (i.e., less than 30 min). As a result, the drug concentration in the blood quickly reaches a maximum level followed by an exponential decrease due to the elimination of the drug. Frequent administration of the medication or the use of controlled drug release dosage forms is necessary in order to maintain the therapeutic level of the drug concentration in the blood for an extended period of time. There are numerous ways to achieve this goal. One key method is for a drug to diffuse through polymers that slowly dissolve in water or are water insoluble. Either case allows a drug to find ways to get out of the interstices of the polymers. Here, we will discuss the diffusion processes of a drug through various systems.

6.1 DIFFUSION

6.1.1 TRANSPORT PROCESSES

The systems that have been considered in previous chapters are by and large at equilibrium and reversible. The movement of molecules from one position to another by processes such as diffusion, electrophoresis, and sedimentation is irreversible and at a distance from equilibrium. However, these transport processes have an interesting feature in that a system not in equilibrium proceeds to equilibrium. Moving toward equilibrium requires flow. Forces acting on the molecules drive the flow, and the forces result from the gradients (rate of change with distance) of potential energy (i.e., temperature/heat, pressure, mass/concentration, or external forces imposed on the system). When the gradients of potentials become uniform throughout the system, flow will stop. In other words, flow continues until these gradients disappear. The flow of mass is our focus here (e.g., the movement of smoke from chimney in air).

Where there exists only one kind of gradient of potential and one kind of flow, the flow (i.e., flux in mass, heat, momentum/area/time), J, at any point in the system, at any time, is directly proportional to the gradients of potentials in one direction as given by:

$$J = -L \frac{\partial U}{\partial x} \qquad (6.1)$$

where L is the proportionality constant and U is the potential. A negative sign is given in Equation (6.1) because the direction of flow is in the direction of decreasing

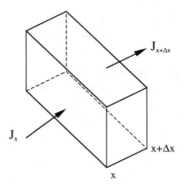

FIGURE 6.1 The change of mass in the plate within Δx.

potential. Equation (6.1) implies that the farther the system is removed away from a state of equilibrium, the faster it moves toward equilibrium. The flux is not readily measured, but the changes in potential with time in various positions are easily observed. Let us consider a thin plate in which the flow of mass occurs normal to the plate as shown in Figure 6.1. The net gain or loss of mass, Δm, through unit area of a plate, S, for a given time interval, Δt, is given by:

$$\Delta m = J_x S \,\Delta t - J_{x+\Delta x} S \,\Delta t \qquad (6.2)$$

The net change of concentration in the volume of the plate, $S \,\Delta x$, is given by:

$$\frac{\Delta m}{S \,\Delta x} = \Delta C = \frac{J_x - J_{x+\Delta x}}{\Delta x} \,\Delta t \qquad (6.3)$$

or
$$\frac{\Delta C}{\Delta t} = \frac{J_x - J_{x+\Delta x}}{\Delta x} \qquad (6.4)$$

When $\Delta t \to 0$ and $\Delta x \to 0$, Equation (6.4) becomes:

$$\frac{\partial C}{\partial t} = -\frac{\partial J}{\partial x} \qquad (6.5)$$

Equation (6.5) implies that the concentration will decrease in the volume of the plate if the rate of entering mass through the plate is slower than that of leaving mass.

Let us apply the above transport processes to the problem of interest, i.e., diffusion. The difference of chemical potential from one position to another drives the flow of mass to achieve uniform chemical potential throughout the system (i.e., equilibrium):

$$J_2 = -D_2 \frac{\partial C_2}{\partial x} \qquad (6.6)$$

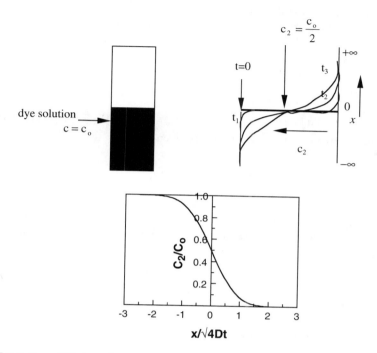

FIGURE 6.2 Free diffusion of a dye in liquid.

where subscript 2 denotes the solute and D_2 is called the diffusion coefficient of the solute. Equation (6.6) is referred to as Fick's first law of diffusion and says that the movement of mass will cease when no concentration gradient remains between two positions or that dC_2/dx approaches zero as diffusion occurs. Combining Equation (6.5) with Equation (6.6) yields:

$$\frac{\partial C_2}{\partial t} = D \frac{\partial^2 C_2}{\partial x^2} \tag{6.7}$$

Equation (6.7) is referred to as Fick's second law of diffusion and relates the temporal and spatial distribution of concentration of the system.

Let us consider two infinite length cylinders where one holding pure solvent is layered on top of the other holding a solution of dye as shown in Figure 6.2. The concentrations of each end ($x = +\infty$ and $x = -\infty$) remain zero and C_o, respectively. Initially, a sharp boundary is formed at $x = 0$. Under these initial and boundary conditions, Equation (6.7) is solved:

$$C_2 = \frac{C_o}{2} \left(1 - \frac{2}{\sqrt{\pi}} \int_0^{x/2\sqrt{Dt}} e^{-y^2} dy \right) \tag{6.8}$$

where the exponent y is a dummy variable of integration. Equation (6.8) gives a smooth S-shaped, time-dependent concentration curve as shown in Figure 6.2. The integral term is the error function erf ($x / \sqrt{4Dt}$). The complement error function erfc (z) = 1− erf(z). Then, Equation (6.8) can be rewritten as:

$$C_2 = \frac{C_o}{2} \, \text{erfc} \, (x / \sqrt{4Dt})$$

(6.9)

It is evident that C_2 equals $1/2C_o$ at $x = 0$ for all $t > 0$. The concentration difference at two positions (x_1 and x_2) is given by:

$$\Delta C_{2(x_1-x_2)} = \frac{C_o}{2}\left(\text{erfc}(x_1 / \sqrt{4Dt}) - \text{erfc}(x_2 / \sqrt{4Dt})\right)$$

(6.10)

The concentration difference rapidly reaches a maximum and slowly falls. Thus, at $t = t_{max}$ its derivative with respect to time, $\partial \Delta C_{2(x_1-x_2)} / \partial t$, becomes zero, resulting in:

$$x_1 e^{-\frac{x_1^2}{4Dt_{max}}} = x_2 e^{-\frac{x_2^2}{4Dt_{max}}}$$

(6.11)

Rearranging Equation (6.11) leads to:

$$D = \frac{x_2^2 - x_1^2}{4 \ln\left(x_2 / x_1\right)}$$

(6.12)

Another approach to determine the diffusion coefficient using Equation (6.8) is taking its derivative, which is the concentration gradient, and a shaped Gaussian "error" curve:

$$\frac{\partial C_2}{\partial x} = \frac{C_o}{2\sqrt{\pi Dt}} e^{-x^2/4Dt}$$

(6.13)

The area under the bell-shaped curve is obviously C_o:

$$C_o = \int_{-\infty}^{\infty}\left(\frac{\partial C_2}{\partial x}\right)dx = A$$

(6.14)

The concentration gradient at $x = 0$ is the height of the bell-shaped concentration curve given by:

$$\left(\frac{\partial C_2}{\partial x}\right)_{x=0} = \frac{C_o}{\sqrt{4\pi Dt}} = H$$

(6.15)

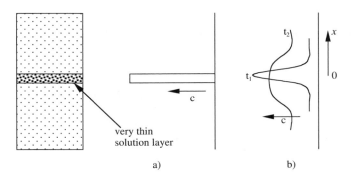

FIGURE 6.3 Diffusion of a dye from a very thin layer of solution: a) initial stage; b) concentration distributions after times t_1 and t_2.

Dividing Equation (6.14) by Equation (6.15) yields:

$$\frac{A}{H} = \sqrt{4\,\pi\,Dt} \qquad (6.16)$$

Plotting $(A/H)^2$ against t will give a straight line with the slope of $4\,\pi\,D$.

Another system can be postulated by placing a thin layer of a solution containing w grams of solute per unit cross-section sandwiched between layers of pure solvent, as shown in Figure 6.3. The concentration distribution at any position and time is given by:

$$C_2 = \frac{w}{\sqrt{4\pi\,Dt}}\,e^{-x^2/4DT} \qquad (6.17)$$

It is easy to see that Equation (6.17) is a solution of Equation (6.7) by taking its first derivative and second derivative with respect to t and x, respectively.

Diffusion is the random motion of molecules. The distance traveled between two positions is proportional to the square root of time. Einstein showed that the average of the square of the distance taken between the first position and the final position via many stops is related to the diffusion coefficient. The larger mean-square distance, the larger the diffusion coefficient expected. It can be seen that the mean-square displacement distance $<x^2>$ is related to the diffusion coefficient as given by:

$$<x^2> = \int_{-\infty}^{\infty} \frac{1}{\sqrt{4\pi\,Dt}} x^2 e^{-x^2/4Dt} = 2Dt \qquad (6.18)$$

Example 6.1

The diffusion coefficient of a bioactive protein has been determined to be 1.02×10^{-5} cm^2/min at 25°C in water. Calculate how long it takes the protein to diffuse a biological membrane whose thickness is 11.7 μm, assuming that there is no hindrance by the cell structure for diffusion.

Solution

The thickness of the membrane is the mean-square distance $<x^2>$. From Equation (6.18),

$$t = \frac{<x^2>}{2D} = \frac{(11.7 \times 10^{-4} \text{cm})^2}{2(1.02 \times 10^{-4} \text{cm}^2 / \text{min})} = 0.0067 \text{ min} = 0.40 \text{ sec}$$

For the Gaussian distribution shown in Equation (6.13) and Equation (6.17), the diffusion coefficient can be determined at half maximum as:

$$\frac{1}{2} = e^{-x^2/4Dt} \quad \text{or} \quad x = \pm\sqrt{4\pi \, Dt \, \ln 2} \tag{6.19}$$

The full width at half maximum becomes $4\sqrt{Dt \ln 2}$.

Example 6.2

A cylindrical syringe containing an agarose gel solution is layered on top of a solution of Rhodamine B ($C_o = 5 \times 10^{-4} M$). At 6 days, the following data were obtained. Calculate the diffusion coefficient of Rhodamine B in agarose gel.

Distance (mm)	1	3	5	7	9	11	13	15	17	19
C_i/C_o	0.96	0.89	0.81	0.74	0.67	0.59	0.53	0.47	0.43	0.37

Distance (mm)	21	23	25	27	29	33	37	41	45	49
C_i/C_o	0.32	0.26	0.23	0.19	0.16	0.12	0.08	0.05	0.03	0.01

Solution

Equation (6.13) can be modified:

$$\ln(\partial C_i / \partial x / C_o) = \ln(y_i / C_o) = -\frac{x_i^2}{4\pi Dt} - \ln(2\sqrt{\pi Dt})$$

$$\ln y_1 - \ln y_2 = -\frac{1}{4\pi Dt}(x_1^2 - x_2^2)$$

At $x = 14$ mm and $x = 16$ mm, $y_{14} / C_o = 0.02825$ and $y_{16} / C_o = 0.02585$

$$D = -\frac{(14\text{mm})^2 - (16\text{mm})^2}{4\pi \times 6\text{hr} \times (\ln 0.02825 - \ln 0.02585)} = 2.49 \times 10^{-5} \text{cm}^2 / \text{sec}$$

6.1.2 DIFFUSION COEFFICIENTS

As presented in the previous equations in this chapter, the diffusion coefficient is one of the important factors controlling the rate of diffusion and the spatial and temporal concentration distribution in the system. In problems of interest with regard to controlled release dosage forms, the kinetics of solute release from the dosage form is strongly dependent on the diffusion coefficient that is illustrated in the succeeding sections of this chapter. Only in rare situations do pharmaceutical scientists deal with diffusion in gases. Therefore, only the diffusion coefficients in liquids and polymers are presented in this section. Generally, two theories have been used to predict the diffusion coefficient: the hydrodynamic theory and the Eyring theory. In the Eyring theory, the solute molecules are assumed to form a cube lattice, and an equation for the diffusion coefficient is similar to the hydrodynamic theory described below, but it has been shown that the hydrodynamic theory fits the experimental data better than the Eyring theory. Therefore, the hydrodynamic theory is presented in the following section.

In the hydrodynamic theory, the diffusion coefficient of a solute molecule A or single particle through a stationary medium B, D_{AB}, is given by the Nernst–Einstein equation:

$$D_{AB} = kT \frac{u_A}{F_A} \qquad (6.20)$$

where k is the Boltzman constant, T is the absolute temperature, u_A is the steady state velocity, and F_A is the force. For very slow flow (i.e., the Reynolds number is less than 0.1), a relation between velocity and force for a solid sphere, under the possibility of "slip" between the solute or particle and the medium, is given by:

$$F_A = 6\pi \, \mu_B u_A r_A \left(\frac{2\mu_B + r_A \beta}{3\mu_B + r_A \beta} \right) \qquad (6.21)$$

where μ_B is the viscosity of the medium, r_A is the equivalent hydrodynamic radius of the solute, and β is the coefficient of the sliding friction.

For large spherical solute molecules or large spherical particles, the medium molecule has no tendency to slip at the surface of the solute molecule. Then, β becomes very large, resulting in:

$$F_A = 6\pi \, \mu_B u_A r_A \qquad (6.22)$$

which is Stokes' law. Substituting Equation (6.22) into Equation (6.20) yields:

$$D_{AB} = \frac{kT}{6\pi\mu_B \, r_A} \qquad (6.23)$$

which is called the Stokes–Einstein equation.

For smaller particles or smaller solute molecules, there is a great tendency for the medium to slip at the surface of the solute molecule and then $\beta = 0$. Thus, Equation (6.21) becomes:

$$F_A = 4\pi \mu_B u_A r_A \tag{6.24}$$

and Equation (6.20) reduces to:

$$D_{AB} = \frac{kT}{4\pi\mu_B r_A} \tag{6.25}$$

The radius of a solute molecule can be estimated, if the molecules are all alike and can be presumably packed in a cube lattice, by:

$$r_A \propto \left(\frac{N_A}{V_A}\right)^{1/3} \tag{6.26}$$

where N_A is Avogadro's number and V_A is the molar volume of the solute molecule as a liquid at its normal boiling point.

The theoretical approaches described in the foregoing equations have not been successful in predicting the diffusion coefficients. Thus, semiempirical relationships on the basis of the Stokes–Einstein equation have been developed. Wilke and Chang modified Equation (6.23), and their equation is good only for dilute concentrations of un-ionized solutes, as given by:

$$D_{AB} = 7.4 \times 10^{-8} \frac{(\varphi_B M_B)^{1/3} T}{\mu_B V_A^{0.6}} \tag{6.27}$$

where φ_B and M_B are the association parameters for the solvent and the molecular weight of the solvent, respectively. The values recommended for φ_B are 2.6 for water, 1.9 for methanol, 1.5 for ethanol, and 1.0 for other unassociated solvents.

The molar volume of the solute can be determined by Le Bas's approach, in which the constituent atoms and functional groups of a solute contribute additively to the property of the solute. Table 6.1 shows the additive-volume increment for the molar volume using Le Bas's approach. As shown in Figure 6.4, the experimental values of diffusion coefficients can be well predicted by the Wilke–Chang equation for the molar volume ranging from 50 to 1000 cm³/g mole. When the Stokes–Einstein equations [Equation (6.23) and Equation (6.25)] are applied, the predicted diffusion coefficients deviate greatly from the experimental ones. The error given by Equation (6.27) for dilute solutions of nondissociating molecules is within 10%. The solutes used for Figure 6.4 are both liquids and solids dissolved in water. The Wilke–Chang equation, originally developed for liquid solutes, can be used to predict the diffusion coefficients of solid solutes presumably because the molar volume is calculated at their boiling point.

Electrolyte solutes dissociate into cations and anions in water. They diffuse differently from undissociated solutes. However, cations should diffuse at the same rate as anions to balance the electroneutrality even though their sizes are different.

TABLE 6.1
Additive-Volume Increments for Atoms and Functional Groups Using Le Bas's Approach

	Increment (cm³/g mole)
Carbon	14.8
Hydrogen	3.7
Oxygen	7.4
In methyl esters and ethers	9.1
In ethyl esters and ethers	9.9
In higher esters and ethers	11.0
In acids	12.0
Joined to S, P, N	8.3
Nitrogen	
Double-bonded	15.6
In primary amine	10.5
In secondary amine	12.0
Bromine	27.0
Chlorine	24.6
Fluorine	8.7
Iodine	37.0
Sulfur	25.6
Ring, 3-membered	−6.0
4-membered	−8.5
5-membered	−11.5
6-membered	−15.0
Naphthalene	−30.0
Anthracene	−47.5

Source: Taken from R. Reid, J. M. Prausnitz, and B. E. Poling, *The Properties of Gases and Liquids*, 4th Ed., McGraw-Hill, New York (1987).

The diffusion coefficient of a single electrolyte at low concentrations is expressed by the Nernst–Haskell equation:

$$D = \frac{RT}{F_a^2}\left(\frac{1/z_+ + 1/z_-}{1/\lambda_+ + 1/\lambda_-}\right) \tag{6.28}$$

where λ_+ and λ_-, are the limiting ionic conductance (cm²/Ω/g equiv) and z_+ and z_- are the valences of cation and anion, respectively, and F_a is 96,500 Coulomb/g equiv.

From the viewpoint of pharmaceutical applications of diffusion, the diffusion of drugs through polymeric materials is more important than that in water or pure solvents (i.e., free diffusion) because various pharmaceutical dosage forms employ polymers to control or retard the diffusion of drugs. The characteristic of polymer

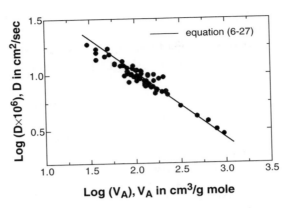

FIGURE 6.4 Plot of the predicted diffusion coefficients vs. the molar volumes of solutes along with the experimental data. [Graph reconstructed from data by Kuu et al. in *Treatise on Controlled Drug Delivery*, A. Kydonies (Ed.), Marcel Dekker, New York, 1992, p. 51.]

structure is one of the important parameters compared with the molecular size of diffusants. The hydrodynamic theory fails to describe the diffusion of solutes in polymers because there is no "continuum" in the polymer. Many semiempirical or empirical relationships have therefore been developed.

The characteristics of pore structure in polymers is a key parameter in the study of diffusion in polymers. Pore sizes ranging from 0.1 to 1.0 µm (macroporous) are much larger than the pore sizes of diffusing solute molecules, and thus the diffusant molecules do not face a significant hurdle to diffuse through polymers comprising the solvent-filled pores. Thus, a minor modification of the values determined by the hydrodynamic theory or its empirical equations can be made to take into account the fraction of void volume in polymers (i.e., porosity, ε), the crookedness of pores (i.e., tortuosity, τ), and the affinity of solutes to polymers (i.e., partition coefficient, K). The effective diffusion coefficient, D_e, in the solvent-filled polymer pores is expressed by:

$$D_e = D \frac{\varepsilon K}{\tau} \tag{6.29}$$

For pore sizes ranging from 50 to 200 Å, which are comparable to the sizes of the diffusing solute molecules and are called microporous, the diffusion of solutes may be substantially restricted by polymer materials. A diffusing molecule may be hindered from entering the pores and be chafed against the pores' walls. Equation (6.30) incorporates these factors into the effective diffusion coefficient as:

$$D_e = D(1-\gamma)^2(1-2.10\ 4\ \gamma + 2.09\ \gamma^3 - 0.95\ \gamma^5) \tag{6.30}$$

where γ is the ratio of the diameter of the diffusion solute to that of the pore. Equation (6.30) shows that the larger the values of γ, the smaller the diffusion coefficient will be. Equation (6.30) is useful up to $\gamma = 0.5$. Equation (6.30) can be applied to moderately swollen hydrophilic polymeric networks. However, the hydrodynamic theory has been successfully used to determine the diffusion coefficient for highly swollen gels such as 1% agarose gel.

Unlike linear polymers, cross-linked polymers do not have actual pores but there is a space between the polymer chains (mesh) ranging from 20 to 100 Å for diffusion of solutes. The mesh size is a key parameter for the diffusion of solutes through polymers in addition to the interaction between the diffusing solutes and the polymers. The diffusion of solutes in swollen cross-linked polymers is dependent on the degree of swelling, cross-linking density (i.e., mesh size), the molecular size of the solutes, and the molecular weight of the polymers. A typical equation used to calculate the effective diffusion coefficient is given by:

$$D_e = Df(\xi_p) \exp\left[\frac{-2\,\Delta E}{\overline{M}_n RT_f} (\overline{M}_n - \overline{M}_c) - \pi r_s^2 l_s \frac{v_s - v_p}{(Q_m - 1)v_s^2 + v_s v_p} \right] \quad (6.31)$$

where $f(\xi_p)$ is a function of the mesh size, ξ_p, ΔE is the penetration energy, $\overline{M}_n$ is the average molecular weight of the uncross-linked polymer, R is the gas constant, T_f is the temperature used to form the polymer, $\overline{M}_c$ is the number of average molecular weight between cross-links, r_s is the radius of the solute, l_s is the characteristic length of the solute, Q_m is the swelling ratio, v_s is the free volume of the solvent in the polymer network, and v_p is the free volume of the polymer. Equation (6.31) may be modified to simpler ones depending on the degrees of swelling and cross-linking density.

It should be pointed out that the characteristics of polymer structure (e.g., porosity, tortuosity, steric hindrance, mesh size, etc.) should be determined in order to calculate the diffusion coefficient of a specific molecule in a particular polymer. For cross-linked polymers, additional polymer properties should be characterized. Even though there are methods to determine these properties, a simple mathematical relationship between the diffusion coefficient of a solute and its molecular weight has been used due to the complexity of the experiment:

$$D_e \propto (M_w)^n \quad (6.32)$$

where n is a constant. Equation (6.32) can be used for the diffusion in liquids with the exponent of $-1/3$ since the molecular volume of a solute molecule is proportional to its molecular weight. Figure 6.5 shows the dependence of the diffusion coefficient on molecular weight.

6.2 DIFFUSION THROUGH A MEMBRANE

6.2.1 UNSTEADY-STATE DIFFUSION THROUGH A MEMBRANE

One of the ways to control drug release is to put a membrane barrier in the dosage form through encapsulation. The membrane barrier controls the transport of the drug

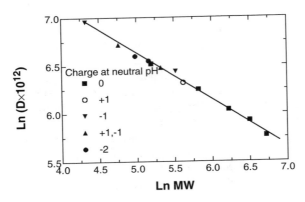

FIGURE 6.5 Dependence of diffusion coefficient on molecular weight for solutes in water and polymer. [Graph reconstructed from data by Haglund et al., *J. Chem. Ed.*, 73, 889 (1996)].

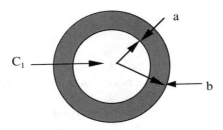

FIGURE 6.6 Schematic model for a membrane–reservoir sphere system.

or solvent (i.e., water). If the drug is encapsulated, it diffuses out of the membrane barrier, as shown in Figure 6.6. Fick's second law describes the diffusion process using a constant diffusion coefficient:

$$\frac{\partial C}{\partial t} = \frac{D}{r^2} \frac{\partial}{\partial r}\left(r^2 \frac{\partial C}{\partial r}\right)$$

(6.33)

with the initial and boundary conditions given as:

$$r = a \qquad C = C_1 \qquad t > 0 \qquad\qquad (6.34a)$$

$$r = b \qquad C = 0 \qquad t > 0 \qquad\qquad (6.34b)$$

$$a \leq r \leq b \qquad C = 0 \qquad t = 0 \qquad\qquad (6.34c)$$

Equation (6.33) has been solved for the concentration distribution in a spherical membrane as follows:

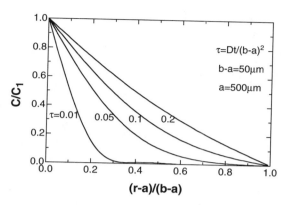

FIGURE 6.7 Drug concentration profiles with time in a membrane.

$$\frac{C}{C_1} = \frac{aK}{r} - \frac{aK(r-a)}{r(b-a)} + \frac{2aK}{r\pi} \sum_{n=1}^{\infty} \left(-\frac{1}{n}\right) \sin\left(\frac{n\pi(r-a)}{b-a}\right) \exp\left(-\frac{Dn^2\pi^2 t}{(b-a)^2}\right) \quad (6.35)$$

where K is the partition coefficient, which is the ratio of the drug concentrations in the membrane and in water. The concentration distribution in a membrane is shown in Figure 6.7. As $t \to \infty$, the concentration gradient in a spherical membrane barrier approaches a nonlinear steady-state pattern different from a sheet membrane barrier, which furnishes a linear gradient. The total amount diffused, M_t, through the membrane at the outer surface r = b, is obtained by integrating $-D\partial C / \partial r|_{r=b}$:

$$M_t = 4\pi ab(b-a)KC_1\left(\frac{Dt}{(b-a)^2} - \frac{1}{6}\right)$$

$$- \frac{8\pi ab(b-a)KC_1}{\pi^2} \sum_{n=1}^{\infty} \frac{(-1)^n}{n^2} \exp\left(-\frac{Dn^2\pi^2 t}{(b-a)^2}\right) \quad (6.36)$$

As time t approaches ∞, the last term in Equation (6.36) becomes zero and the total amount diffused through the membrane is:

$$M_t = 4\pi ab(b-a)KC_1\left(\frac{Dt}{(b-a)^2} - \frac{1}{6}\right) \quad (6.37)$$

Equation (6.37) is called the time-lag equation, with a lag time (t_{lag}) of:

$$t_{lag} = \frac{(b-a)^2}{6D} \quad (6.38)$$

When the membrane-encapsulated device has been stored before use, the drug migrates into the membrane and saturates it. The drug located near the surface of the membrane diffuses out first followed by diffusion of the drug from the core through the membrane-encapsulated device. The total amount of the drug released from the membrane is given by:

$$M_t = 4\pi ab(b-a)KC_1\left(\frac{Dt}{(b-a)^2} + \frac{b}{3a}\right)$$

$$-\frac{8\pi ab(b-a)KC_1}{\pi^2}\sum_{n=1}^{\infty}\frac{(-1)^n}{n^2}\exp\left(-\frac{Dn^2\pi^2t}{(b-a)^2}\right) \qquad (6.39)$$

As $t \rightarrow \infty$, Equation (6.39) becomes:

$$M_t = 4\pi ab(b-a)KC_1\left(\frac{Dt}{(b-a)^2} + \frac{b}{3a}\right) \qquad (6.40)$$

Equation (6.40) is called the burst-effect equation, with a burst-effect time (t_{burst}) of:

$$t_{burst} = -\frac{b(b-a)^2}{3aD} \qquad (6.41)$$

Figure 6.8 shows the plot of M_t vs. t for Equation (6.36). As time approaches infinite, the graph gives a straight line, which is a representation of Equation (6.37) for the time lag. The time intercept is calculated from Equation (6.38). This intercept and the slope [$= 4\pi ab(b-a)KC_1$], which is the steady-state release rate, are used to determine the diffusion and partition coefficients experimentally. Mathematical expressions, which include the amount of the drug diffused from freshly prepared and stored geometrical membranes (sheet and cylinder) at steady state are presented in Table 6.2.

Example 6.3
Paul and McSpadden studied the permeation of a red organic dye (Sudan III) in acetone through a silicone rubber membrane as shown in Figure 6.9. The partition coefficient of 0.148 has been independently determined for the dye in the membrane and in acetone by an extraction method. Calculate the diffusion coefficient and the solubility of the dye. Assume that the thickness and the diameter of the membrane are 0.15 cm and 8 mm, respectively.

Solution
From Figure 6.9,

TABLE 6.2
Cumulative Release from Membrane–Reservoir Systems

| **Time Lag** | **Burst Effect** |

Sheet: $\quad M_t = \dfrac{ADKC_1}{l}\left(t - \dfrac{l^2}{6D}\right)$ $\qquad\qquad M_t = \dfrac{ADKC_1}{l}\left(t + \dfrac{l^2}{3D}\right)$

Cylinder: $\displaystyle M_t = \frac{2\pi hDKC_1}{\ln(b/a)}\left(t - \frac{2\ln(b/a)}{D}\; \sum_{n=1}^{\infty}\frac{J_o(a\alpha_n)J_o(b\alpha_n)}{\alpha_n^2[J_o^2(b\alpha_n)-J_o^2(a\alpha_n)]}\right)$
$\displaystyle M_t = \frac{2\pi hDKC_1}{\ln(b/a)}\left(t + \frac{2\ln(b/a)}{D}\; \sum_{n=1}^{\infty}\frac{J_o^2(a\alpha_n)}{\alpha_n^2[J_o^2(a\alpha_n)-J_o^2(b\alpha_n)]}\right)$

Sphere: $\quad M_t = \dfrac{4\pi abDKC_1}{(b-a)}\left(t - \dfrac{(b-a)^2}{6D}\right)$ $\qquad M_t = \dfrac{4\pi abDKC_1}{(b-a)}\left(t + \dfrac{b(b-a)^2}{3aD}\right)$

Note: A = the surface area of a sheet; l = the thickness of a sheet membrane; h = the length of a cylinder; D = the diffusion coefficient; K = the partition coefficient; a and b = the inner and outer radii of a sphere or a cylinder, respectively; α_n = the positive roots of $J_o(a\alpha_n)Y_o(b\alpha_n) - J_o(b\alpha_n)Y_o(a\alpha_n) = 0$ where J_o, and Y_o = Bessel functions of the first and second kind of zero order, respectively.

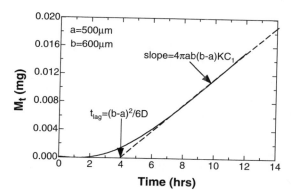

FIGURE 6.8 Cumulative drug release from a membrane–reservoir sphere (time lag).

$$\text{time lag} = 1.2\ \text{hr} = \frac{l^2}{6D},$$

$$D = (0.15\ \text{cm})^2\,/\,6\,/\,1.2\ \text{hr} = 3.125\times10^{-3}\ \text{cm}^2\,/\,\text{hr}$$

$$\text{slope} = \frac{DKC_1}{l} = 0.923 \qquad C_1 = \frac{0.923\times0.15}{0.148\times3.125\times10^{-3}} = 3.0\ \text{mg}\,/\,\text{cm}^3$$

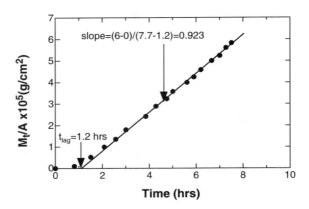

FIGURE 6.9 Permeation of a dye in a swollen silcone rubber membrane in acetone. [Graph reconstructed from data by Paul and McSpadden, *J. Membr. Sci.,* 1, 33 (1976).]

6.2.2 STEADY-STATE DIFFUSION THROUGH A MEMBRANE

6.2.2.1 Constant Activity Reservoir Systems

As shown in Figure 6.7, the concentration gradient in the membrane reaches a constant pattern over time (theoretically infinite time). A membrane-encapsulated sphere containing a saturated drug concentration (constant activity, C_s), has a constant rate of drug diffusion. In this case, Equation (6.33) becomes:

$$\frac{\partial}{\partial r}\left(r^2 \frac{\partial C}{\partial r}\right) = 0 \tag{6.42}$$

When the boundary conditions [Equation (6.34a) and Equation (6.34b)] are applied for a freshly coated membrane, the concentration distribution in the membrane is given by:

$$C = \frac{bKC_s(r-a)}{r(b-a)} \tag{6.43}$$

The amount of the drug diffused through the membrane at time t is given by:

$$M_t = \frac{4\pi abDKC_s}{(b-a)}t \tag{6.44}$$

The rate of drug diffusion through the membrane is determined by:

$$\frac{dM_t}{dt} = \frac{4\pi abDKC_s}{(b-a)} \tag{6.45}$$

6.2.2.2 Nonconstant Activity Reservoir Systems

A reservoir system is originally designed to have a constant activity. This activity diminishes after some time due to continuous drug depletion and influx of water. The rate of drug diffusion from a nonconstant activity reservoir is given by the mass balance as:

$$\frac{dM_t}{dt} = -\frac{4\pi a^3}{3}\frac{dC_1}{dt} \tag{6.46}$$

where C_1 is the time-dependent drug concentration in the reservoir. Under a pseudo–steady-state approximation, the rate of drug diffusion is given by Equation (6.45). Substituting Equation (6.46) into Equation (6.47) yields:

$$\frac{C_1}{C_{1o}} = \exp\left(-\frac{3bDK}{a^2(b-a)}t\right) \tag{6.47}$$

where C_{1o} is the initial drug concentration in the reservoir.

Differentiating Equation (6.47) and substituting the resulting equation into Equation (6.45) yields:

$$\frac{dM_t}{dt} = \left(\frac{4\pi abDKC_{1o}}{(b-a)}\right)\exp\left(-\frac{3bDK}{a^2(b-a)}t\right) \tag{6.48}$$

Integrating Equation (6.48) gives:

$$\frac{M_t}{M_\infty} = 1 - \exp\left(-\frac{3bDK}{a^2(b-a)}t\right) \tag{6.49}$$

where $M_\infty = 4\pi a^3 C_{1o}/3$ is the total amount of the drug in the reservoir.

The cumulative drug release and the drug release rate for constant activity and nonconstant activity reservoirs of other geometrical barriers are shown in Table 6.3.

Example 6.4

A drug diffusion experiment has been carried out over a long period of time to reach a steady-state condition. The data shown in Figure 6.10 have been collected. Calculate the partition coefficient and the drug solubility. The drug diffusion coefficient of 2×10^{-6} cm²/sec was independently determined by a time-lag experiment. The surface area, volume, and thickness of the membrane reservoir are 1.2 cm², 32.4 cm³, and 50 μm, respectively. The total amount of drug in the membrane reservoir is 25 mg.

Solution

From Figure 6.10,

TABLE 6.3

The Cumulative Drug Release and Release Rate for Constant Activity and Nonconstant Activity Reservoirs

	Drug Release	Release Rate
	Constant Activity	
Sheet	$\dfrac{M_t}{M_\infty} = \dfrac{ADKC_s}{l}t$	$\dfrac{dM_t}{dt} = \dfrac{ADKC_s}{l}$
Cylinder	$\dfrac{M_t}{M_\infty} = \dfrac{2\pi hDKC_s}{\ln(b/a)}t$	$\dfrac{dM_t}{dt} = \dfrac{2\pi hDKC_s}{\ln(b/a)}$
Sphere	$\dfrac{M_t}{M_\infty} = \dfrac{4\pi abDKC_s}{(b-a)}t$	$\dfrac{dM_t}{dt} = \dfrac{4\pi abDKC_s}{(b-a)}$
	Nonconstant Activity	
Sheet	$\dfrac{M_t}{M_\infty} = 1-\exp\left(-\dfrac{ADK}{V_1 l}t\right)$	$\dfrac{dM_t}{dt} = \dfrac{ADKC_{1o}}{V_1 l}\exp\left(-\dfrac{ADK}{V_1 l}t\right)$
Cylinder	$\dfrac{M_t}{M_\infty} = 1-\exp\left(-\dfrac{2DK}{a^2\ln(b/a)}t\right)$	$\dfrac{dM_t}{dt} = \dfrac{2\pi hDKC_{1o}}{a^2\ln(b/a)}\exp\left(-\dfrac{2DK}{a^2\ln(b/a)}t\right)$
Sphere	$\dfrac{M_t}{M_\infty} = 1-\exp\left(-\dfrac{3bDK}{a^2(b-a)}t\right)$	$\dfrac{dM_t}{dt} = \dfrac{4\pi abDKC_{1o}}{a^2(b-a)}\exp\left(-\dfrac{3bDK}{a^2(b-a)}t\right)$

Note: V_1: the volume of the reservoir; C_s: the solubility of drug; l: the thickness of the membrane.

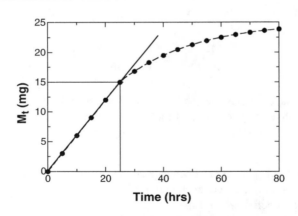

FIGURE 6.10 Steady-state diffusion of a drug through a sheet membrane.

$$\text{slope} = \frac{ADKC_s}{l} = \frac{15 \text{ mg}}{25 \text{ hr}} = 0.6 \text{ mg / hr}$$

$$KC_s = \frac{0.6 \times 0.005}{1.2 \times 2 \times 10^{-6} \times 3600} = 0.347 \text{ mg / cm}^3$$

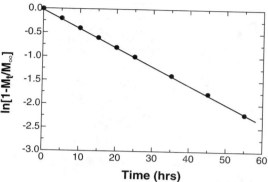

FIGURE 6.11 Plot of $\ln\left(1-\dfrac{M_t}{M_\infty}\right)$ vs. time.

Since 15 mg of the drug have been released under constant activity, the saturated concentration is 15 mg/32.4 cm³ = 0.463 mg/cm³ and K = 0.347/0.463 = 0.75. Under the nonconstant activity reservoir condition, the K value is equal to or close to 0.75; knowing this can predict the remaining portion of the release profile for the system.

At time = 25 hr, the drug reservoir becomes unsaturated. A new table is then formulated. The equation given in Table 6.3 for the nonconstant activity reservoir (sheet) is rearranged to:

t	new t	M_t	new M_t	$\ln\left(1-\dfrac{M_t}{M_\infty}\right)$
25	0	15.0 mg	0 mg	0.0
30	5	16.8	1.8	−0.198
35	10	18.3	3.3	−0.400
40	15	19.5	4.5	−0.598
45	20	20.5	5.5	−0.799
50	25	21.3	6.3	−0.994
60	35	22.5	7.5	−1.386
70	45	23.3	8.3	−1.772
80	55	23.9	8.9	−2.207

$$\ln\left(1-\frac{M_t}{M_\infty}\right)=-\frac{ADK}{V_1 l}t$$

From Figure 6.11,

$$\text{slope} = -\frac{ADK}{V_1 l} = -0.04,$$

$$K = \frac{0.04 \times 32.4 \times 0.005}{1.2 \times 2 \times 10^{-6} \times 3600} = 0.75$$

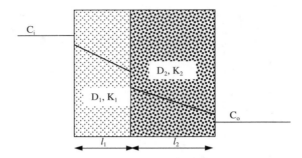

FIGURE 6.12 Drug diffusion through a laminated film with drug concentration C_i on the donor side and C_o on the receiver side.

6.2.3 MULTI-LAYER MEMBRANE DEVICES

A drug may diffuse through a series of barrier layers — drug diffusion through hydrophobic stratum corneum and hydrophilic-viable epidermis in series or multi-laminated films. Figure 6.12 shows the diffusion of a drug through two layers in a series of the thickness of l_1 and l_2. As shown in Table 6.3, the rate of drug diffusion per flat surface area (mass flux) is given by:

$$\frac{dM_t}{Adt} = \frac{D_1 K_1}{l_1}(C_i - C_1) = \frac{D_2 K_2}{l_2}(C_1 - C_o) \tag{6.50}$$

The drug concentration in the membrane layers is not easily determined, and Equation (6.50) is rearranged, using the known concentrations of C_i and C_o, to:

$$\frac{dM_t}{Adt} = \frac{C_i - C_o}{\dfrac{l_1}{D_1 K_1} + \dfrac{l_2}{D_2 K_2}} \tag{6.51}$$

The time-lag equation (t_{two}) for a two-layer film is:

$$t_{two} = \frac{\dfrac{l_1^2}{D_1}\left(\dfrac{l_1}{6D_1 K_1} + \dfrac{l_2}{2D_2 K_2}\right) + \dfrac{l_2^2}{D_2}\left(\dfrac{l_1}{2D_1 K_1} + \dfrac{l_2}{6D_2 K_2}\right)}{\dfrac{l_1}{D_1 K_1} + \dfrac{l_2}{D_2 K_2}} \tag{6.52}$$

Example 6.5

Tojo et al. studied the permeation across the skin, which consists of the lipophilic stratum corneum and hydrophilic viable epidermis. Drug concentration in the donor side is kept at a saturated level (i.e., C_i = drug solubility = 208 $\mu g \,/\, mL$) in 40% (v/v) aqueous PEG 400 solution. Two permeation experiments, as shown in Figure 6.13, were carried out under a sink condition using intact skin (two-layer)

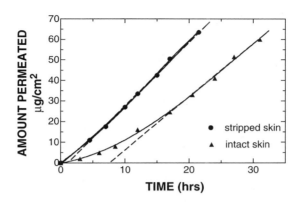

FIGURE 6.13 Permeation of progesterone across intact and stripped skins. [Graph reconstructed from data by Tojo et al., *J. Pharm. Sci.,* 76, 123 (1987).]

and stripped skin (viable skin) with thicknesses of 380 and 370 μm, respectively. Calculate the drug diffusivity and solubility in the stratum corneum.

Solution

$C_o = 0$ (sink condition),

Equation (6.51) is rearranged to the ratio of the flux across the two-layer skin to that across the single layer of skin (viable skin) [$\eta = \left(dM_t / (Adt) \right) / \left(dM_t / (Adt) \right)_1$] by:

$$\frac{dM_t}{Adt} = \frac{C_s}{\dfrac{l_2}{D_2 K_2}\left(\dfrac{1}{1-\eta}\right)} \tag{6.53}$$

The drug diffusivity across layer two (stratum corneum) is determined from:

$$D_2 = \left(\frac{1}{1-\eta}\right)\left(\frac{l_2}{K_2 C_s}\right)\left(\frac{dM_t}{Adt}\right) = \left(\frac{1}{1-\eta}\right)\left(\frac{l_2}{C_2}\right)\left(\frac{dM_t}{Adt}\right) \tag{6.54}$$

Substituting Equation (6.53) and Equation (6.54) into Equation (6.52) yields:

$$t_{two} = t_1(3-2\eta) + \frac{l_2}{6}\left(\frac{(1+2\eta)(1-\eta)C_2}{(dM_t / Adt)}\right) \tag{6.55a}$$

or $$C_2 = \frac{1-3(t_1/t_{two})+2\eta(t_1/t_{two})}{(1+2\eta)(1-\eta)}\left(\frac{6t_{two}}{l_2}\right)\left(\frac{dM_t}{Adt}\right) \tag{6.55b}$$

where

$$t_1 = \frac{l_1^2}{6D_1}$$

For the stripped skin (viable skin), the following equations are used to determine the drug diffusivity and solubility as:

$$D_1 = \frac{l_1}{C_1}\left(\frac{dM_t}{Adt}\right)_1, \quad C_1 = \frac{6t_1}{l_1}\left(\frac{dM_t}{Adt}\right)_1 \tag{6.56}$$

From Figure 6.13, the time-lag and the steady-state flux for the intact skin and stripped skin are:

$$t_1 = 1.2 \text{ hr}, \quad t_{two} = 7.6 \text{ hr}$$

$$\left(\frac{dM_t}{Adt}\right)_1 = \frac{60}{20-1.2} = 3.19 \ \mu g/cm^2/hr, \quad \left(\frac{dM_t}{Adt}\right) = \frac{60}{31-7.6} = 2.56 \ \mu g/cm^2/hr$$

$$\eta = \frac{2.56}{3.19} = 0.80$$

For the stripped skin,

$$C_1 = \frac{6 \times 1.2 \times 3.19}{0.037} = 621 \ \mu g/cm^3,$$

$$D_1 = \frac{0.037^2}{6 \times 1.2} = 1.9 \times 10^{-4} cm^2/hr$$

For the two-layer intact skin:

$$C_2 = \frac{1-3(1.2/7.6)+2(0.80)(1.2/7.6)}{(1+2\times0.80)(1-0.80)}\left(\frac{6\times7.6}{0.038}\right)(2.56) = 4602 \ \mu g/cm^3$$

$$D_2 = \left(\frac{1}{1-0.80}\right)\left(\frac{0.038}{4602}\right)(2.56) = 1.01 \times 10^{-4} cm^2/hr$$

6.3 DIFFUSION IN A MONOLITHIC MATRIX

6.3.1 Dissolved Drug in Polymeric Drug Carriers

Instead of diffusing through a membrane barrier, a drug is distributed within a polymer matrix or dissolved in a polymer. The drug concentration in the matrix is much less than the solubility of the drug in the polymer. When the matrix is in contact with a solvent (i.e., water), the drug starts diffusing out through the interstices of the polymer structure. If the distributed drug is a solid, then the solvent rapidly penetrates the polymer, dissolves the entire drug and forms an unsaturated drug solution. The mathematical expression for the drug diffusion through a matrix (slab geometry) is:

$$\frac{\partial C}{\partial t} = D \frac{\partial^2 C}{\partial x^2} \tag{6.57}$$

where x is the distance from the center of the slab. Equation (6.57) is then subjected to the following initial and boundary conditions:

$$C = C_o \qquad -l \le x \le l \qquad t = 0 \tag{6.58a}$$

$$C = 0 \qquad x = l, \quad x = -l \qquad t > 0 \tag{6.58b}$$

where l is the half thickness of the slab and C_o is the initial concentration of drug in the slab.

The concentration distribution in the matrix becomes:

$$\frac{C}{C_o} = \frac{4}{\pi} \sum_{n=0}^{\infty} \frac{(-1)^n}{2n+1} \exp\left(-\frac{D(2n+1)^2 \pi^2}{4l^2} t\right) \cos\left(\frac{(2n+1)\pi x}{2l}\right) \tag{6.59}$$

Equation (6.59) converges very slowly for the small values of time (or Dt/l^2). Thus, the corresponding equation used, for these small values of times, becomes:

$$\frac{C}{C_o} = 1 - \sum_{n=0}^{\infty} (-1)^n \operatorname{erfc} \frac{(2n+1)l - x}{2\sqrt{Dt}} - \sum_{n=0}^{\infty} (-1)^n \operatorname{erfc} \frac{(2n+1)l + x}{2\sqrt{Dt}} \tag{6.60}$$

where erfc is the complementary error function.

The total amount of the drug diffused at time t is given by integrating $-AD \int (\partial C / \partial x)_{x=l} dt$.

For a large time approximation,

$$\frac{M_t}{M_\infty} = 1 - \frac{8}{\pi^2} \sum_{n=0}^{\infty} \frac{1}{(2n+1)^2} \exp\left(-\frac{D(2n+1)^2 \pi^2}{4l^2} t\right) \tag{6.61a}$$

$$\cong 1 - \frac{8}{\pi^2} \exp\left(-\frac{D\pi^2 t}{4l^2}\right) \tag{6.61b}$$

TABLE 6.4
Fractional Release of a Slab, Cylinder, and Sphere for Dissolved Drug

Slab	$$\frac{M_t}{M_\infty} = 2\left(\frac{Dt}{\pi l^2}\right)^{1/2}$$	$0 \leq \dfrac{M_t}{M_\infty} \leq 0.6$
	$$\frac{M_t}{M_\infty} = 1 - \frac{8}{\pi^2}\exp\left(-\frac{D\pi^2}{4l^2}t\right)$$	$0.4 \leq \dfrac{M_t}{M_\infty} \leq 1.0$
Cylinder	$$\frac{M_t}{M_\infty} = 4\left(\frac{Dt}{\pi a^2}\right)^{1/2} - \frac{Dt}{a^2}$$	$0 \leq \dfrac{M_t}{M_\infty} \leq 0.4$
	$$\frac{M_t}{M_\infty} = 1 - \frac{4}{2.405^2}\exp\left(-\frac{2.405^2 Dt}{a^2}\right)$$	$0.6 \leq \dfrac{M_t}{M_\infty} \leq 1.0$
Sphere	$$\frac{M_t}{M_\infty} = 6\left(\frac{Dt}{\pi a^2}\right)^{1/2} - 3\frac{Dt}{a^2}$$	$0 \leq \dfrac{M_t}{M_\infty} \leq 0.7$
	$$\frac{M_t}{M_\infty} = 1 - \frac{6}{\pi^2}\exp\left(-\frac{D\pi^2}{a^2}t\right)$$	$0.7 \leq \dfrac{M_t}{M_\infty} \leq 1.0$

Note: l = half thickness of a slab, a = radius of a cylinder or sphere.

For a small time approximation,

$$\frac{M_t}{M_\infty} = 2\left(\frac{Dt}{l^2}\right)^{1/2}\left\{\frac{1}{\pi^{1/2}} + 2\sum_{n=1}^{\infty}(-1)^n \text{ierfc}\frac{nl}{\sqrt{Dt}}\right\} \qquad (6.61c)$$

$$\cong 2\sqrt{\frac{Dt}{\pi l^2}} \qquad (6.61d)$$

where ierfc is the inverse complementary error function.

The mathematical equations used, for the release of drug for other geometries, are shown in Table 6.4. With the exception of Equation (6.61d) for short times, one should use the nonlinear parameter estimation methods to determine the diffusivity of a drug. As shown in Table 6.4, it is recommended to use the approximation equations for long times and rearrange them into:

$$\ln\left[\frac{\pi^2}{8}\left(1 - \frac{M_t}{M_\infty}\right)\right] = -\frac{\pi^2 D}{4l^2}t \qquad (6.62)$$

The plot of the left-hand-side term vs. time gives a straight line with a slope of $\pi^2 D/l^2$. The approximate solutions, given in Table 6.4, are accurate within less than

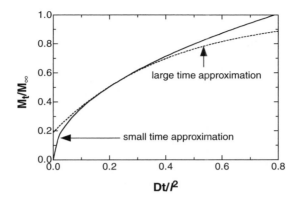

FIGURE 6.14 Fractional release profiles from a slab based on short- and long-time approximations.

1% error when compared to their corresponding exact solutions. Figure 6.14 shows the application areas of the equations for short- and long-time approximations.

Example 6.6

A contact lens has been equilibrated with an aqueous solution of pilocarpine nitrate. The total amount of the drug loaded in the lens was 1.54 mg. The following drug release data were obtained:

Time (min)	0.44	1.0	1.2	2.6	4.0	4.5	10.6	12.1	21.0
Drug released (mg)	0.15	0.23	0.44	0.72	0.85	0.95	1.32	1.37	1.42

Calculate the diffusivity of the drug. Assume the thickness of the lens is 75 µm.

Solution

First, calculate the fractional release (M_t / M_∞), and plot M_t / M_∞ vs. $\sqrt{\text{time}}$ up to M_t / M_∞ of 0.6, as shown in Figure 6.15a. The slope is then calculated as:

$$\text{Slope} = 4\left(\frac{D}{\pi l^2}\right)^{1/2} = 0.42 \text{ / hr}^{0.5}, \quad D = \left(\frac{0.42}{4}\right)^2 \pi(0.0075)^2 = 5.5\times10^{-6} \text{cm}^2 \text{ / min}$$

The fractional release data are rearranged according to Equation (6.62), and the plot of $\ln (\pi^2 / 8)(1 - M_t / M_\infty)$ vs. time is shown in Figure 6.15b. The slope is calculated as:

$$\text{Slope} = -\frac{\pi^2 D}{4l^2} = -0.165 \text{ / hr}, \quad D = \frac{0.165\times 4\times(0.0075)^2}{\pi^2} = 3.8\times10^{-6} \text{cm}^2 \text{ / min}$$

In general, the first couple of data points are not reliable because some drugs on the surface burst rapidly, and the concentration difference at a later time is very small.

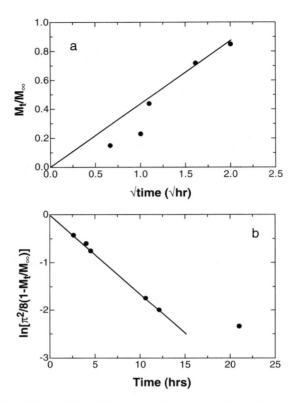

FIGURE 6.15 Calculation of drug diffusivity using short- and long-time approximations.

The dimensionless time term, (Dt / l^2 or Dt / a^2), is a valuable tool for demonstrating the effects of the design variables on drug release. When drug release experiments are carried out, one may change the size of the dosage forms along with the content composition. In order to find out whether a change in the drug release kinetics is due to the composition or the size, the time scale is normalized with the size (i.e., t / l^2). For a given content composition, the fractional release profiles are plotted against t / l^2. In this way one may estimate the size of the dosage form based on the experimental data of smaller or larger dosage forms. For example, if it takes 12 hr to release 90% of a drug in 725 μm beads, then the beads may be designed as 725 × $\sqrt{2}$ =1025 μm to release 90% of the drug in 24 hr.

A majority of oral solid dosage forms are tablets and caplets. Tablets can be handled as slabs or cylinders. More accurately, the tablet shape has both slab and cylinder features. Drug release occurs through radial and lateral surfaces, and diffusion of a solute in a tablet is expressed by:

$$\frac{\partial C}{\partial t} = D\left(\frac{\partial^2 C}{\partial z^2} + \frac{\partial^2 C}{\partial r^2} + \frac{1}{r}\frac{\partial C}{\partial r} \right) \qquad (6.63)$$

$$C = C_o \quad \text{at} \quad t = 0 \tag{6.64a}$$

$$C = 0 \quad \text{at} \quad z = l, \ r = a, \ t > 0 \tag{6.64b}$$

where r and z are the radial and lateral coordinates, respectively and a and l are the diameter and thickness of a tablet, respectively.

The solutions of Equation (6.63) under long-time and short-time approximations are given, respectively, by:

$$\frac{M_t}{M_\infty} = 1 - \frac{32}{(2.048)^2 \pi^2} \exp\left[-D\left(\frac{2.048^2}{a^2} + \frac{\pi^2}{4l^2}\right) \right] \tag{6.65a}$$

$$\frac{M_t}{M_\infty} = \sqrt{64\tau} - 4\tau - \frac{8\pi}{3}\tau^{3/2} + 4\sqrt{\frac{Dt}{\pi l^2}} - \frac{a}{l}\left[32\tau - 16\pi\,\tau^{3/2} - \frac{32\pi}{3}\tau^2 \right] \tag{6.65b}$$

where $\tau = Dt / \pi l^2$.

For an average tablet size (e.g., $a = 10$ mm and $l = 4.5$ mm) and the diffusion coefficient of 7×10^{-7} cm^2/sec, the errors of the values of fractional release at 10 hr calculated by the slab and cylinder equations are about 9 and 32%, respectively, compared with the value obtained by Equation (6.65a).

6.3.2 Dispersed Drug in Polymeric Drug Carriers

If the drugs are distributed within a polymer matrix as solid particles and the solubility of the drugs in the polymer is very low or the drugs do not dissolve rapidly in the incoming solvent (i.e., water), the incoming water moves slowly inwardly. In this case, the drug release kinetics from the matrix are completely different from those described in Section 6.3.1 and schematically illustrated in Figure 6.16. Upon contact with water, the solid drug particles in the surface layer dissolve first. Once the water moves inwardly, the remaining drugs inside the layer are completely exhausted. Under the microscope, one is able to observe the moving front separating from the dissolved and the solid drugs. In the treatment of release kinetics by Higuchi, the concentration gradient from the moving front to the outer surface of the matrix is linear (pseudo–steady-state approximation).

Fick's first law is used to describe the diffusion of drug as:

$$\text{mass flux} = J = D\frac{\partial C}{\partial \delta} = D\frac{\Delta C}{\Delta \delta} = \frac{DC_{s,m}}{x} \tag{6.66}$$

$$\frac{dM_t}{dt} = AJ = \frac{ADKC_s}{x} \tag{6.67}$$

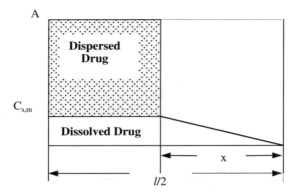

FIGURE 6.16 A schematic diagram of drug release from a dispersed matrix system.

where $C_{s,m}$ is the saturated drug concentration in the matrix and C_s is the saturated drug concentration in the water. The total amount of the drug diffused out through both sides of the slab at time t ($= 2x/l$) is given by the mass balance as:

$$\frac{2x}{l} = \frac{M_t + AxKC_s/2}{M_\infty} \tag{6.68}$$

where l is the thickness of the slab. The second numerator term in the right-hand side of Equation (6.68) is the remaining drug in the depleted region $(0 - x)$. Rearranging Equation (6.68) results in:

$$x = \frac{M_t/M_\infty}{\left(\dfrac{2}{l} - \dfrac{AKC_s/2}{M_\infty}\right)} \tag{6.69}$$

Substituting Equation (6.69) into Equation (6.67) yields:

$$\frac{dM_t}{dt} = \frac{ADKC_sM_\infty}{M_t}\left(\frac{2}{l} - \frac{AKC_s}{2M_\infty}\right) \tag{6.70}$$

Integration of Equation (6.70) gives:

$$M_t^2 = 2ADKC_s\left(\frac{2}{l} - \frac{AKC_s}{2M_\infty}\right)M_\infty t \tag{6.71}$$

Substituting $M_\infty = AC_o l/2$ into Equation (6.71) yields:

$$M_t = A\left[DKC_s t(2C_o - C_s)\right]^{1/2} \cong A\left(2DKC_sC_o t\right)^{1/2}, \quad C_o \gg C_s \tag{6.72}$$

TABLE 6.5
Fractional Drug Release and Exhaustion Time
for Dispersed Matrix Systems

	Drug Release	Exhaustion Time
Slab	$M_t = A\sqrt{2DKC_oC_st}$	$t_\infty = \dfrac{l^2C_o}{8DKC_s}$
Cylinder	$\left(1 - \dfrac{M_t}{M_\infty}\right)\ln\left(1 - \dfrac{M_t}{M_\infty}\right) + \dfrac{M_t}{M_\infty} = \dfrac{4DKC_s}{C_or_o^2}$	$t_\infty = \dfrac{C_or_o^2}{4DKC_s}$
Sphere	$\left[1 - \left(1 - \dfrac{M_t}{M_\infty}\right)^{2/3}\right] - \dfrac{2}{3}\dfrac{M_t}{M_\infty} = \dfrac{2DKC_s}{C_or_o^2}$	$t_\infty = \dfrac{C_or_o^2}{6DKC_s}$

The release rate at time t is given as:

$$\frac{dM_t}{dt} = \frac{A}{2}\sqrt{\frac{DKC_s(2C_o - C_s)}{t}} \cong \frac{A}{2}\sqrt{\frac{2DKC_sC_o}{t}} \tag{6.73}$$

The time, when the dispersed drug is exhausted, is:

$$t_\infty = \frac{l^2C_o}{8DKC_s} \tag{6.74}$$

Mathematical equations used for the amount of drug released at time t and the exhaustion time for other geometries (cylinder and sphere) are shown in Table 6.5.

Equation (6.61d) and Equation (6.72) show that the release of the dissolved and dispersed drugs is proportional to the square root of time. In dispersed drug systems, this linear relationship with $t^{1/2}$ extends all the way to t_∞, the exhaustion time of a solid drug. Meanwhile, the drug release of the dissolved drug tails off at an extended period of time after 60% release. According to Equation (6.74) (called the Higuchi equation), the release of the dispersed drug is proportional to the square root of the drug loading (C_o). The Higuchi equation is often used to show the release of a dispersed drug that has a relatively low initial drug concentration (<5%). To find out the effect of this initial drug concentration on the drug release kinetics, one should normalize the kinetics by the initial concentration (i.e., $M_t / C_o^{1/2}$). As shown in Figure 6.17, the amount of the drug released is larger than the amount calculated by Equation (6.72) when the initial drug concentration increases. The release of drug still maintains a linear relationship with the square root of time. As drug loading increases, bigger cavities or channels are created by the occupied spaces of the drug. The end result is high permeability of the drug. Assuming a random dispersion of the spherical drug particles, Equation (6.72) and Equation (6.73) are modified to:

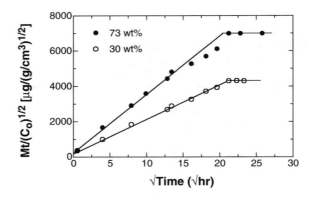

FIGURE 6.17 Normalized release of chloramphenicol from poly(ethylene-vinyl acetate) matrices. [Graph reconstructed from data by Baker et al. in *Controlled Release Pesticide Symposium,* N. Cardarelli (Ed.), University of Akron, Akron, OH, 1974, p. 40.1.]

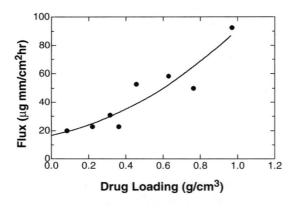

FIGURE 6.18 Comparative permeabilities of chloramphenicol from poly(ethylene-vinyl acetate) matrices. [Graph reconstructed from data by Baker et al. in *Controlled Release Pesticide Symposium,* N. Cardarelli (Ed.), University of Akron, Akron, OH, 1974, p. 40.1.]

$$M_t = A\left[2DKC_sC_ot\frac{1+2C_o/\rho}{1-C_o/\rho}\right]^{1/2} \tag{6.75a}$$

$$\frac{dM_t}{dt} = \frac{A}{2}\left[\frac{2DKC_o}{t}\frac{1+2C_o/\rho}{1-C_o/\rho}\right]^{1/2} \tag{6.75b}$$

where ρ is the density of the drug. Figure 6.18 shows the experimental and predicted permeabilities of chloramphenicol from poly(ethylene-vinyl acetate) matrices. The experimental permeabilities are calculated from the slopes of the release for each drug loading.

Release kinetic expression for a tablet (radius r_o and thickness l_o) can be developed by using Higuchi's pseudo–steady-state approximation and mass balance. With macroscopic observation of the moving boundary of a dispersed drug tablet, Equation (6.76) can be formulated by:

$$\frac{M_t}{M_\infty} = \frac{\pi r_o^2 l_o A - \pi r l A}{\pi r_o^2 l_o A} = 1 - \left(\frac{r}{r_o}\right)^2 \frac{l}{l_o} \tag{6.76}$$

where r and l are radial and lateral moving boundaries at the time t. l can be calculated by:

$$l = l_o - 2\sqrt{\frac{2DC_s t}{A}} \tag{6.77}$$

Substituting Equation (6.77) into Equation (6.76) yields:

$$\left(\frac{r}{r_o}\right)^2 = \frac{1 - M_t / M_\infty}{1 - (r_o / l_o)\sqrt{2Kt}} \tag{6.78}$$

where K is $4C_s D / A l_o^2$. The moving front of the drug-depleted area for a cylinder can be derived as:

$$\frac{1}{4}\left(r_o^2 - r^2\right) + \frac{r_o^2}{2}\ln\left(\frac{r}{r_o}\right) = \frac{DC_s t}{A} \tag{6.79}$$

Substituting Equation (6.78) into Equation (6.79) and rearranging the resulting equation yields:

$$1 + \frac{1 - M_t / M_\infty}{1 - (r_o / l_o)\sqrt{Kt}} \ln\left(\frac{1 - M_t / M_\infty}{1 - (r_o / l_o)\sqrt{Kt}}\right) - \frac{1 - M_t / M_\infty}{1 - (r_o / l_o)\sqrt{Kt}} = Kt \tag{6.80}$$

The value of D determined by Higuchi's equation was observed to be about 30% larger than that calculated by Equation (6.80).

Higuchi's approximation of the "pseudo–steady state" is no longer valid when $A \leq C_s$. Instead of assuming a linear concentration gradient within the drug-depleted layer, Fick's second law of diffusion is used to calculate the concentration profiles of the dissolved drug as:

$$\frac{\partial C}{\partial t} = D \frac{\partial^2 C}{\partial x^2} \tag{6.81}$$

The boundary conditions in the region $0 < x < \xi$ are given by:

$$C = 0 \qquad\qquad\qquad\qquad x = 0 \qquad\qquad (6.82a)$$

$$C = C_s \qquad\qquad\qquad\qquad x = \xi \qquad\qquad (6.82b)$$

and at the interface between undissolved and dissolved drugs an additional boundary condition is given by:

$$(A - C_s)\frac{\partial \xi}{\partial t} = D\frac{\partial C}{\partial x} \qquad\qquad x = \xi \qquad\qquad (6.82c)$$

The cumulative amount of drug released and the concentration profile can be obtained as:

$$M_t = \frac{2C_s}{erf(\eta)}\sqrt{\frac{Dt}{\pi}} \qquad\qquad (6.83)$$

$$C = C_s\frac{erf(\beta)}{erf(\eta)} \qquad\qquad (6.84)$$

where

$$\eta = \frac{\xi}{2\sqrt{Dt}} \quad \text{and} \quad \beta = \frac{x}{\sqrt{Dt}} \qquad\qquad (6.85)$$

The following equation must be satisfied to obtain the value of η:

$$\sqrt{\pi}\,\eta\exp(\eta^2)erf(\eta) = \frac{C_s}{A - C_s} \qquad\qquad (6.86)$$

When C approaches C_s, η is very large, $erf(\eta)$ approaches 1 and Equation (6.83) becomes:

$$M_t = AC_s\sqrt{\frac{Dt}{\pi}} \qquad\qquad (6.87)$$

which is the same equation derived for the dissolved drug systems. For $A \gg C_s$, η is small and Equation (6.86) becomes:

$$erf(\eta) = \sqrt{\frac{2C_s}{\pi(A - C_s)}} \qquad\qquad (6.88)$$

Substituting Equation (6.88) into Equation (6.83) yields:

$$M_t \cong A\sqrt{2DC_s(A - C_s)t} \qquad\qquad (6.89)$$

Equation (6.89) is identical with Equation (6.72) derived under the pseudo–steady-state approximation. The error caused by Higuchi's equation increases with decreasing values of A/C_s.

Higuchi's equation and the exact analytical equation cannot satisfactorily explain the release kinetics of a dispersed drug if the solubility of the drug and its rate of dissolution can substantially affect the release kinetics. Higuchi's equation and the exact equation assume that the drug dissolution rate is much faster than the drug diffusion rate. On the contrary, when the diffusion rate of drug is much faster than the drug dissolution rate, the release kinetics described in the above section are not consistent with the experimental results. Drug release from a matrix containing a drug with a slow dissolution rate occurs by first dissolving the drug in penetrating solvents and then diffusing out of the matrix. The relative magnitude of the two rates governs the overall drug release kinetics.

The diffusion equation describing drug dissolution and drug diffusion for a semiinfinite sheet is given by:

$$\frac{\partial C}{\partial t} = D\frac{\partial^2 C}{\partial x^2} - k_d(C_s - C)\delta(C_d - C_s) \tag{6.90}$$

with

$$\delta(C_d - C_s) = \begin{cases} 0 & C_d \le C_s \\ 1 & C_d > C_s \end{cases} \tag{6.91}$$

where k_d is the dissolution rate constant and C_d is the concentration of dissolved drug. The appropriate initial and boundary conditions for a dissolved drug are given by:

$$C = C_s \qquad 0 \le x \le l \qquad t = 0 \tag{6.92a}$$

$$C = 0 \qquad x = 0 \qquad t > 0 \tag{6.92b}$$

The fractional release can be derived as:

$$\frac{M_t}{M_\infty} = 2\frac{C_s}{C_o}\sqrt{\frac{D}{k_d l^2}}\left((k_d t + 0.5)\mathrm{erf}(\sqrt{k_d t}) + \sqrt{\frac{k_d t}{\pi}}\exp(-k_d t)\right), \qquad C_s k_d t \le C_o \tag{6.93}$$

Equation (6.93) can be simplified for large values of $k_d t$ (or small times) as:

$$\frac{M_t}{M_\infty} = 2\frac{C_s}{C_o}\sqrt{\frac{Dk_d}{l^2}}\left(t + \frac{1}{2k_d}\right) \tag{6.94}$$

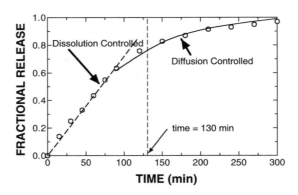

FIGURE 6.19 Release of KCl from an ethyl cellulose matrix. [Graph reconstructed from data by Gurney et al., *Biomaterials,* 3, 27 (1982).]

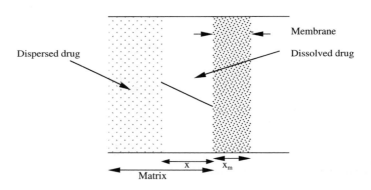

FIGURE 6.20 Drug release from a membrane–matrix system.

Equation (6.94) illustrates that zero-order release kinetics are obtained if drug dissolution controls the release kinetics. However, as soon as the last particle in the matrix dissolves, the controlling mechanism of drug release shifts to Fickian diffusion. Figure 6.19 shows the dissolution-controlled release of KCl at the early stage of release and the diffusion-controlled release at the later stage of release from an ethyl cellulose tablet.

6.4 DIFFUSION IN A MEMBRANE–MATRIX SYSTEM

A membrane–matrix device consists of a core matrix, which is dispersed with drugs, and an encapsulated membrane barrier layer. The rate of diffusion of the drug through the outer barrier is much slower than the inner matrix. One may postulate that the drug release is governed by the relative contributions of the outer membrane layer and the inner core matrix. The diffusion of the drug through a membrane layer–core matrix system is illustrated in Figure 6.20.

According to Fick's first law, the rate of diffusion through the core matrix is:

$$\frac{dM_t}{dt} = \frac{D}{x}(C_s - C_b) \qquad (6.95)$$

where C_b is the concentration at the interface of the membrane and the core matrix. The rate of permeation of the drug through the barrier membrane is expressed by Fick's first law as:

$$\frac{dM_t}{dt} = \frac{D_m}{x_m}(C_b^* - C_a) \qquad (6.96)$$

where D_m is the diffusivity in the membrane, x_m is the thickness of the membrane, C_b^* is the drug concentration at the interface of the membrane and the core matrix, and C_a is the drug concentration at the surface of the membrane (assuming the sink condition, i.e., $C_a = 0$). Substituting C_b^* of Equation (6.96) into Equation (6.95) gives:

$$\frac{dM_t}{dt} = \frac{D}{x}\left[C_s - \frac{C_s D x_m}{\dfrac{D_m x}{K_m} + D x_m} \right] \qquad (6.97)$$

where $K_m = C_b / C_b^*$ is the partition coefficient between the membrane and the core matrix. Also, the drug release rate is related to the differential moving front as:

$$\frac{dM_t}{dt} = A\frac{dx}{dt} - \frac{C_s}{2}\frac{dx}{dt} \qquad (6.98)$$

Substituting Equation (6.98) into Equation (6.97) and integrating the resulting equation yields:

$$x^2 + 2\frac{D x_m K_p}{D_m}x - 2\frac{DC_s t}{C_o - C_s / 2} = 0 \qquad (6.99)$$

The amount of drug released is given as:

$$M_t = A x C_o \qquad (6.100)$$

Solving Equation (6.99) for x and substituting it into Equation (6.100) when $C_o \gg C_s$ yields:

$$M_t = -\frac{AC_o D x_m K_p}{D_m} + A\sqrt{\left(\frac{C_o D x_m K_m}{D_m}\right)^2 + 2C_o DC_s t} \qquad (6.101)$$

TABLE 6.6
Release Kinetics of Membrane–Matrix Systems

Slab	$M_t = AxC_o$	$x^2 + 2\dfrac{Dx_mK_p}{D_m}x - 2\dfrac{DC_st}{C_o} = 0$
Cylinder	$M_t = \pi h C_o(r_o^2 - r^2)$	$\dfrac{r^2}{2}\ln\dfrac{r}{r_o} + \left(\dfrac{1}{4} + \dfrac{Dx_mK_p}{2D_mr_o}\right)(r_o^2 - r^2) - \dfrac{DC_st}{C_o} = 0$
Sphere	$M_t = \dfrac{4}{3}\pi C_o(r_o^3 - r^3)$	$1 - 3\dfrac{r}{r_o^2} + 2\dfrac{r^3}{r_o^3} + \dfrac{2Dx_mK_p}{D_mr_o}\left(1 - \dfrac{r^3}{r_o^3}\right) - \dfrac{6DC_st}{C_or_o^2} = 0$

Differentiating Equation (6.101) gives the release rate:

$$\frac{dM_t}{dt} = \frac{AC_oDC_s}{\sqrt{\left(\dfrac{C_oDx_mK_m}{D_m}\right)^2 + 2C_oDC_st}} \qquad (6.102)$$

Equation (6.102) demonstrates the relative contributions of the membrane barrier and the core matrix to drug release kinetics. If the first term of the square root (diffusion through the membrane) is much larger than the second term (diffusion through the core matrix), Equation (6.102) is reduced to:

$$\frac{dM_t}{dt} = \frac{AC_sD_m}{x_m} \qquad (6.103)$$

Equation (6.103) shows that the release rate is constant throughout the drug release time. When the second term is much larger than the first term, Equation (6.102) becomes:

$$\frac{dM_t}{dt} = A\sqrt{\frac{C_oDC_s}{2t}} \qquad (6.104)$$

In this case, the diffusion of the drug through the core matrix controls the release kinetics. Equation (6.104) is the Higuchi expression. The mathematical expressions for membrane–matrix systems of other geometries can be derived in similar fashion and are shown in Table 6.6.

Olanoff et al. studied the release of tetracycline from a trilaminate membrane device as shown in Figure 6.21. The core matrix is prepared from a copolymer of HEMA and MMA (63/37) and the membrane coating is prepared with the same polymer but tighter composition (2/98 and 14/86). As shown in Figure 6.21, Equation (6.101) predicts the experimental data. For the 2/98 coating composition, Equation

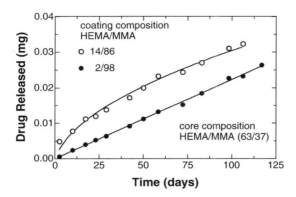

FIGURE 6.21 Release of tetracycline from trilaminate membrane–matrix devices. [Graph reconstructed from data by Olanoff et al., *J. Pharm. Sci.*, 68, 1147 (1979).]

(6.96) or Equation (6.103) can be used after changing the time scale t to t − t_{lag} for the time lag.

6.5 DIFFUSION DURING THE SWELLING OF A MATRIX

The systems described in the previous sections use polymer materials whose dimensions never change or which easily respond to a new condition. In this situation, the Fickian equation of diffusion can be applied to the penetration of solvent into a polymer. However, the glassy hydrogel system, which consists of the hydrophilic and hydrophobic polymer structure, encounters swelling upon contact with water. The swelling will continue until a new equilibrium is reached. Glassy hydrogels do not swell rapidly and it takes a long time for them to rearrange their polymer structure to the penetrating solvent molecules (i.e., polymer relaxation). Depending on the relative magnitude of the diffusion of solvent to the polymer relaxation, the diffusional transport process is characterized as:

Case II: The sorption process is governed by the polymer relaxation and the amount absorbed and the penetrating front position is linearly dependent on time.

Case I: The sorption process is dominated by the Fickian diffusion of solvent with negligible polymer relaxation.

Anomalous: The sorption process is controlled by both the Fickian diffusion of solvent and the polymer relaxation.

When water-soluble drugs are entrapped in glassy hydrogels, the release of the drugs engages simultaneously the absorption of water and desorption of drug while the hydrogels swell slowly. Drug release kinetics are governed by the rate of polymer swelling (via solvent diffusion and polymer relaxation) and the rate of drug diffusion. However, in the presence of water-soluble drugs in the glassy hydrogels, the sorption of water is enhanced at a much faster rate. Thus, drug release kinetics is determined

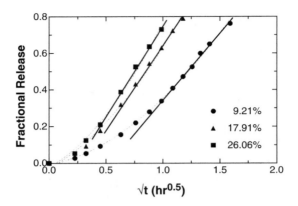

FIGURE 6.22 Release of thiamine HCl from glassy hydrogel sheets of poly(2-hydroxyethylmethacrylate). [Graph reconstructed from data by P. I. Lee, in *Controlled-Release Technology: Pharmaceutical Applications,* P. I. Lee and W. R. Good (Eds.), ACS Symp. Ser. No. 348, American Chemical Society, Washington, D.C., 1987. p. 71.]

by the polymer relaxation rate and the rate of drug diffusion. The case where polymer relaxation occurs rapidly to water as related to the rate of drug diffusion results in Fickian release kinetics as expressed by Equation (6.61d) or Equation (6.72). For example, release kinetics from fully swollen hydrogels (i.e., no polymer relaxation) are dependent on the square root of time. Figure 6.22 shows the fractional release of thiamine HCl from a glassy hydrogel sheet. As a swelling solvent (i.e., water) enters into the glassy hydrogel containing a water-soluble drug (dissolved or dispersed), the glass transition temperature of the glassy hydrogel is lowered below the experimental temperature, and the polymer chains slowly rearrange to accommodate the water molecules. Until an equilibrium state is reached, the polymer relaxation process plays a role in drug release kinetics. As shown in Figure 6.22, anomalous release kinetics are observed during the early swelling period. At the significantly or fully swollen stage, drug release kinetics become Fickian (i.e., square root of time). The duration of the anomalous release kinetics depends on the drug loading because the rate of absorption of water is a function of the amount of drug present in the glassy hydrogel.

Polymer relaxation or swelling has been taken into consideration for the diffusion of solvent and drug release. A time-dependent diffusion coefficient approach has been applied to describe anomalous sorption kinetics of penetrating solvents and various anomalous release behaviors. The diffusion coefficients of penetrant and drug in polymers are supposed to be influenced by a response of the polymer chains to the penetrant. One can imagine that the diffusion coefficient can be dependent on the polymer volume fraction. The polymer volume fraction is time dependent during the swelling process, so it is reasonable to expect a time-dependent drug diffusion coefficient.

To describe various anomalous release behaviors from glassy hydrogels, the following time-dependent drug diffusion coefficient is defined:

$$D(t) = D_i + (D_\infty - D_i)(1 - \exp(-kt)) \tag{6.105}$$

where D_i is the instantaneous drug diffusion coefficient, D_∞ is the diffusion coefficient at equilibrium swelling, and k is the polymer relaxation constant in the specific drug–solvent–polymer system. Redefining a new time variable given by:

$$dT = D(t)dt \tag{6.106}$$

where

$$T = D_\infty\left[t - \left(1 - \frac{D_i}{D_\infty}\right)\frac{1}{k}(1 - \exp(-kt))\right] \tag{6.107}$$

and substituting $D(t)$ into Equation (6.57) for the dissolved drug yields the same form of Equation (6.57) but t is replaced by T.

The exact solutions for drug release from glassy hydrogels containing dissolved and dispersed drugs can be expressed by forms similar to those of a constant diffusion coefficient by replacing Dt/l^2 with the following expression:

$$\frac{D_\infty t}{l^2} - \left(1 - \frac{D_i}{D_\infty}\right)\left(\frac{D_\infty}{kl^2}\right)[1 - \exp(-kt)] \tag{6.108}$$

For dissolved drugs ($A \leq C_s$), the exact analytical solution for drug release from glassy hydrogels is given by:

$$\frac{M_t}{M_\infty} = 1 - \sum_{n=0}^{\infty}\frac{32}{(n+0.5)^2}\exp\left\{-(n+0.5)^2\pi^2\left[\frac{D_\infty t}{l^2} - \left(1 - \frac{D_i}{D_\infty}\right)\left(\frac{D_\infty}{kl^2}\right)[1 - \exp(-kt)]\right]\right\} \tag{6.109}$$

For small time approximation, Equation (6.109) becomes:

$$\frac{M_t}{M_\infty} = \frac{4}{\sqrt{\pi}}\left\{\frac{D_\infty t}{l^2} - \left(1 - \frac{D_i}{D_\infty}\right)\left(\frac{D_\infty}{kl^2}\right)[1 - \exp(-kt)]\right\}^{1/2} \tag{6.110}$$

For dispersed drugs ($A > C_s$), the analytical solution for drug release from glassy hydrogels is given by:

$$\frac{M_t}{M_\infty} = \frac{1}{(A/C_s)\mathrm{erf}(\zeta)}\frac{2}{\sqrt{\pi}}\left\{\frac{D_\infty t}{l^2} - \left(1 - \frac{D_i}{D_\infty}\right)\left(\frac{D_\infty}{kl^2}\right)[1 - \exp(-kt)]\right\}^{1/2} \tag{6.111}$$

with

$$\sqrt{\pi}\zeta\exp(\zeta^2)\mathrm{erf}(\zeta) = \frac{C_s}{A - C_s} \tag{6.112}$$

The thickness of the diffusion moving front separating the undissolved core from the dissolved region is given by:

$$\frac{x}{l} = 2\zeta\left\{\frac{D_\infty t}{l^2} - \left(1 - \frac{D_i}{D_\infty}\right)\left(\frac{D_\infty}{kl^2}\right)[1 - \exp(-kt)]\right\}^{1/2} \tag{6.113}$$

ζ is determined by Equation (6.112).

The term D_∞ / kl^2 in the above equations is called the Deborah number, De_r, for the drug release system:

$$De_r = \frac{D_\infty}{kl^2} \tag{6.114}$$

The Deborah number relates the relative importance of polymer relaxation time (k^{-1}) and the characteristic drug diffusion time (l^2 / D_∞) and can describe various drug release kinetics in glassy hydrogels. When the Deborah number is very small, the diffusion equation becomes a Fickian behavior having the constant diffusion coefficient D_∞ because Equation (6.108) yields $D_\infty t / l^2$. Drug release from significantly or fully swollen hydrogels falls under this situation in which the drug diffusion process is slow compared to the polymer relaxation process. On the other hand, when the Deborah number is very large, $D(t) = D_i$ in Equation (6.105) and the diffusion follows the same Fickian equation except for a much smaller diffusion coefficient. It takes a very long time for the polymer to rearrange its polymer chain to a penetrant and thus there is no variation of the polymer structure during drug release. When the polymer relaxation time and the characteristic diffusion time are at comparable rates (i.e., intermediate values of the Deborah number), the diffusion coefficient is time dependent [i.e., Equation (6.105)] to approach its equilibrium value. Anomalous release kinetics will be observed. However, another parameter, D_i / D_∞, in the above equations plays a role in drug release behaviors. When $De_r \approx 1$ or > 1 (≥ 10), anomalous drug release behavior will be zero-order with $D_i / D_\infty \ll 1$. Table 6.7 shows the dependence of drug release behaviors on the Deborah number.

Figure 6.23 shows drug release behaviors of swellable polymer beads. As the ratio D_i / D_∞ is close to 1, the release kinetics become Fickian and for $D_i / D_\infty \approx 0$, the drug release follows zero-order kinetics. For most common hydrogels, anomalous release behaviors are observed, showing that the initial diffusion coefficient takes a part in the release kinetics. The release kinetics become Fickian as drug loading in glassy hydrogels increases.

TABLE 6.7
General Characteristics of Drug Release Behavior on Deborah Number

$De_r \to 0$	$D(t) \to D_\infty$	Fickian diffusion (rubbery state)
$De_r \approx 1$ or > 1		Anomalous diffusion
$De_r \approx 1$ and $D_i / D_\infty \ll 1$		Case II
$De_r \to \infty$	$D(t) \to D_i$	Fickian diffusion (glassy state)

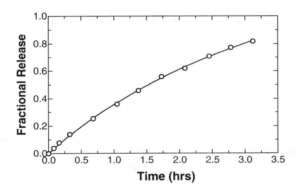

FIGURE 6.23 The release of thiamine HCl from a glassy poly(2-hydroxyethylmethacrylate) sheet. [Graph reconstructed from data by P. I. Lee, in *Controlled-Release Technology: Pharmaceutical Applications,* P. I. Lee and W. R. Good (Eds.), ACS Symp. Ser. No. 348, American Chemical Society, Washington, D.C., 1987. p. 71.]

Another parameter determining the drug release mechanism from glassy hydrogels, the swelling interface number, S_w, has been introduced as:

$$S_w = \frac{\nu \, \delta(t)}{D} \tag{6.115}$$

where ν is the moving velocity of the glassy–rubbery swelling front and $\delta(t)$ is the time-dependent swollen gel thickness. When S_w is much larger than 1, the rate of drug diffusion is much slower than the rate of swelling and thus a Fickian diffusion behavior will be observed. When S_w is much smaller than 1, the rate of drug diffusion is much faster than the swelling front advances, the release kinetics are governed by the rate of swelling (i.e., polymer relaxation) and zero-order release kinetics are expected. For intermediate values of S_w (i.e., close to 1), anomalous release behaviors are expected. The Deborah number and swelling interface number guide one to screen hydrogel materials to develop swelling-controlled systems with zero-order release kinetics.

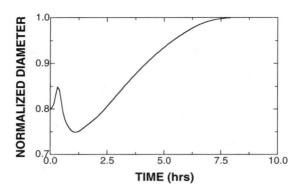

FIGURE 6.24 Experimental observation of dimensional changes during the release of oxprenolol HCl from poly(methylmethacrylate-co-methacrylic acid) beads. [Graph reconstructed from data by Kim and Lee, *Pharm. Res.,* 9, 1268 (1992).]

There is a phenomenon unique to glassy hydrogels during drug release: dimensional changes. As water penetrates into glassy hydrogels, dissolved drugs in hydrogel matrices produce great osmotic pressure and thus the swollen gel expands further while the glassy polymers swell. At the early stage of drug release, the polymer swelling does not contribute much more to the overall dimensional change than the osmotic pressure of the dissolved drug. However, as drug release continues, the osmotic pressure diminishes while the polymer swelling increases slowly to its equilibrium. These two simultaneous processes give rise to a peak dimension during drug release in glassy hydrogels. Whether the peak becomes the maximum dimensional change is dependent on the degree of the maximum swelling of the polymer. For low water-swellable hydrogels, the overall dimension reaches the maximum peak very rapidly and then falls off very slowly to completion with the tailing of drug release. Figure 6.24 shows that the peak is not the maximum because of the slow, high swelling of the polymer.

6.6   DIFFUSION IN MATRIX EROSION/DEGRADATION

The diffusion processes described in the previous sections were applied to physically and chemically stable polymer materials. It is possible to incorporate drugs into polymers that undergo physical or chemical changes during a diffusion process. The erosion/degradation of a polymer matrix enhances the rate of drug diffusion due to a decrease in the diffusion path length and/or an increase in the space of the diffusion of the drugs. There are two types of diffusion in matrix erosion/degradation processes: homogeneous and heterogeneous erosion/degradation.

6.6.1   HOMOGENEOUS EROSION/DEGRADATION

The diffusion of the drug occurs in polymer materials that are eroded or degraded throughout the entire matrix. The drug is uniformly dispersed throughout the matrix. The release rate of the drug is given by the Higuchi model:

$$\frac{dM_t}{dt} = \sqrt{\frac{A^2 DKC_s C_o}{2t}} \qquad (6.73)$$

The rate of diffusion (or diffusivity) increases with time because the polymer chains are cleaved, thus creating a larger space and allowing the drug to diffuse out of the matrix at a faster rate. The increase in the diffusivity of the drug is then:

$$\frac{D}{D_o} = \frac{N_o}{N_o - N} \qquad (6.116)$$

where D_o is the initial diffusivity in the matrix, N_o is the initial number of bonds, and N is the number of cleaved bonds. Equation (6.116) illustrates that the increase in the diffusivity of the drug is inversely proportional to the number of bonds available for cleavage. The rate of bond cleavage is assumed to be first order with respect to the number of cleavable bonds present:

$$\frac{dN}{dt} = k_c (N_o - N) \qquad (6.117)$$

where k_c is the cleavage rate constant. Integrating Equation (6.117) yields:

$$\ln\left(\frac{N_o}{N_o - N}\right) = k_c t \qquad (6.118)$$

Substituting Equation (6.116) into Equation (6.118) yields:

$$D = D_o e^{k_c t} \qquad (6.119)$$

Substituting Equation (6.119) into Equation (6.73) yields:

$$\frac{dM_t}{dt} = \sqrt{\frac{A^2 D_o e^{k_c t} KC_s C_o}{2t}} \qquad (6.120)$$

Example 6.7

The release of levonorgestrel from a biodegradable poly(ortho ester) containing 30% drug and 2.0% calcium lactate is shown in Figure 6.25. Homogeneous degradation takes place in the whole matrix because the influx of water into the matrix makes it weakly basic by calcium lactate. The weak base reacts with the slightly acidic poly(ortho ester). Calculate the cleavage rate constant.

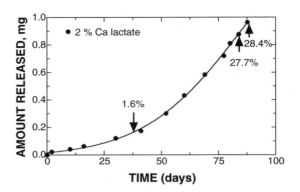

FIGURE 6.25 The release of levonorgestrel from a poly(orthoester) slab containing 30% drug and 2% calcium lactate. [Graph reconstructed from data by Heller et al. in *Controlled Release of Bioactive Materials*, R. W. Baker (Ed.), Academic Press, New York, 1980, p. 1.]

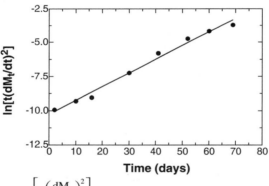

FIGURE 6.26 Plot of $\ln\left[t\left(\dfrac{dM_t}{dt}\right)^2\right]$ vs. time.

Solution

Equation (6.120) is more suited for numerical than analytical integration, using the Runge–Kutta 4th method. However, Equation (6.120) can be rearranged as:

$$\ln\left[t\left(\frac{dM_t}{dt}\right)^2\right] = k_c t + \text{constant} \qquad (6.121)$$

The data shown in Figure 6.25 are fitted with a fourth-order polynomial equation; the first derivative with respect to time (i.e., dM_t/dt) is taken. A plot of the left-hand-side term of Equation (6.121) vs. time (Figure 6.26) gives a straight line with a slope of k_c.

$$k_c = 2.8 \times 10^{-5} / \text{hr}$$

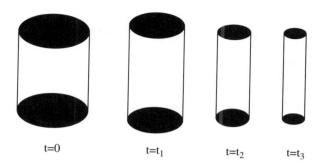

FIGURE 6.27 Heterogeneous degradation/erosion system.

6.6.2 HETEROGENEOUS EROSION/DEGRADATION

Unlike the homogeneous degradation of the polymer chains, the polymer degrades on the surface of the matrix as shown in Figure 6.27. The drug release is then dependent upon the polymer erosion/degradation. First, assume that there is no diffusion in the matrix. The amount of drug release from a cylinder with a radius r_o and a length h is given by:

$$\frac{dM_t}{dt} = 2\pi h k_e r C_o \qquad (6.122)$$

where k_e is the surface erosion/degradation rate constant and r is the radius remaining of the cylinder. The amount of drug released can be given by the mass balance as:

$$M_t = \pi h C_o (r_o^2 - r^2) \qquad (6.123)$$

Differentiating Equation (6.123) and substituting the resulting equation into Equation (6.122) yields:

$$r = r_o - k_e t \qquad (6.124)$$

Substitution of Equation (6.124) into Equation (6.123) yields:

$$\frac{M_t}{M_\infty} = 1 - \left(1 - \frac{k_e}{r_o}t\right)^2 \qquad (6.125)$$

where $M_\infty = \pi h r_o^2 C_o$. A similar approach is used to obtain the expressions for other geometries as:

$$\frac{M_t}{M_\infty} = 1 - \left(1 - \frac{k_e}{r_o (\text{or } l_o)}\right)^n \qquad (6.126)$$

where n is 1 for a slab, 2 for a cylinder, and 3 for a sphere.

Example 6.8

Drug release experiments have been carried out on a surface erosion-controlled tablet; 47.4% of the drug was released at t = 2.6 hr. The initial diameter was 11.5 mm and the initial thickness l_o was 4.5 mm. Calculate the surface erosion rate constant.

Solution

The rate of drug release from the tablet is given by:

$$\frac{dM_t}{dt} = 2\pi k_e r(r + l) \tag{6.127}$$

where l is the thickness of the remaining tablet. The time-dependent radius and the thickness of the tablet are given by Equation (6.124). Integrating Equation (6.127) after substituting Equation (6.124) for the radius and thickness yields:

$$\frac{M_t}{M_\infty} = 1 - \left(1 - \frac{k_e}{r_o} t\right)^2 \left(1 - \frac{2k_e}{l_o} t\right) \tag{6.128}$$

Therefore,

$$0.474 = 1 - \left(1 - \frac{k_e}{0.575} 2.6\right)^2 \left(1 - \frac{2k_e}{0.45} 2.6\right)$$

By trial and error, $k_e = 2.73 \times 10^{-2}$ cm / hr.

Second, the drug diffusion in the matrix and heterogeneous erosion of the matrix govern drug release kinetics. As shown in Figure 6.28, the penetration of water (or dissolution medium) into the matrix is initially much faster than the erosion of the matrix at the surface and results in the formation of a drug-depleted layer (drug diffusion layer). Upon reaching a critical level of water concentration on the surface, the polymer starts dissolving. Lee derived mathematical expressions for this drug diffusion and polymer erosion controlled system. Equation (6.57) is used to describe this diffusion of the drug in the system. However, the following initial and boundary conditions must be met:

$$D\frac{\partial C}{\partial t} = (C_o - C_s)\frac{\partial R}{\partial t} \qquad x = R \tag{6.129a}$$

$$\frac{\partial C}{\partial x} = (C_o - C_s)\left(\frac{\partial R}{\partial t} - \frac{\partial S}{\partial t}\right) \qquad x = S - R \tag{6.129b}$$

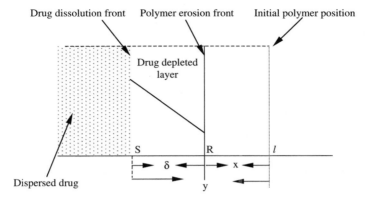

FIGURE 6.28 Schematic diagram of a drug diffusion/polymer erosion controlled system containing a dispersed drug.

$$R = l \qquad t = 0 \qquad\qquad (6.129c)$$

$$C = 0 \qquad x = S \qquad\qquad (6.129d)$$

$$C = C_s \qquad x = R \qquad\qquad (6.129e)$$

$$\left(D\frac{\partial C}{\partial x}\right)^2 + (C_o - C_s)\left(\frac{\partial S}{\partial t}\frac{\partial C}{\partial x} + D\frac{\partial^2 C}{\partial x^2}\right) = 0 \qquad x = R - S \qquad (6.129f)$$

The fractional release from the matrix is given as:

$$\frac{M_t}{M_\infty} = \delta + \left(\frac{k_e a}{D}\right)\left(\frac{Dt}{l^2}\right) - \delta\frac{C_s}{C_o}\left(\frac{1}{2} + \frac{a_3}{6}\right) \qquad (6.130a)$$

$$\frac{Dt}{l^2} = \frac{1}{12}\left[6\frac{C_o}{C_s} - 4 - a_3\right]\left[\delta - \frac{\ln(1 + 2\delta h)}{2h}\right] \qquad (6.130b)$$

$$a_3 = \frac{C_o}{C_s} + \delta h - \sqrt{\left(\frac{C_o}{C_s} + \delta h\right)^2 - 1 - 2\delta h} \qquad (6.130c)$$

$$h = \frac{1}{2}\left(1 - \frac{C_o}{C_s}\right)\frac{k_e l}{D} \qquad (6.130d)$$

where l is the half thickness of the slab and δ is the thickness of the drug-depleted layer [$= (S - R)/l$].

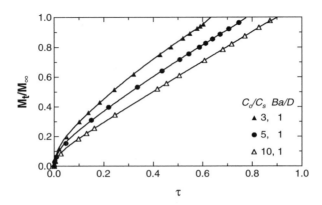

FIGURE 6.29 Effects of drug diffusion, polymer erosion, and drug loading on the drug release kinetics of drug dissolution/polymer erosion controlled systems.

Equation (6.130a) through Equation (6.130d) show that the drug release is influenced by the drug diffusion layer. When the rates of the moving drug dissolution front and the polymer erosion front are equal, the drug-depleted layer is synchronized and constant until the dry drug in the core completely dissolves. From this synchronization point, the drug release has a linear relationship with the release time as shown in Equation (6.130a). For a given ratio of $k_e l / D$, the duration of the initial Fickian release becomes shorter and a longer linear release can be obtained when the drug loading (C_o / C_s) increases, as shown in Figure 6.29. In an extreme situation (very large loading), the drug dissolution front may coincide with the polymer erosion front. Then, Equation (6.130a) is equal to Equation (6.126) for a slab. For a given drug loading, a larger $k_e l / D$ leads to a longer linear release kinetics.

When $C_o < C_s$ (i.e., dissolved state of the drug in a matrix), the release is given by:

$$\frac{M_t}{M_\infty} = \sqrt{\frac{4D}{3l^2} t} + \frac{k_e l}{D} t \qquad (6.131)$$

6.7 DIFFUSION IN A MATRIX SWELLING/EROSION

However, there are not many polymers which undergo only eroding while drugs diffuse out. Rather, polymers swell first before erosion takes place. Upon contact with water, a water-soluble polymer absorbs water, entangled polymer chains start relaxing, and then the polymer starts swelling. Once the concentration of water at the surface of the swollen polymer reaches a threshold level, the swollen polymer starts eroding. From this point on, swelling and erosion take place simultaneously. If the rate of erosion is very large so that upon absorbing water the polymer erodes, the system becomes an erosion-controlled system, as described in Section 6.5.

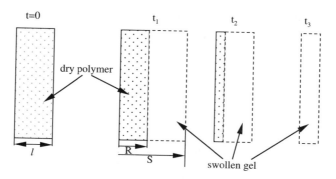

FIGURE 6.30 Swelling and erosion phenomena of a water-soluble polymer.

As soon as a polymer matrix absorbs water, drugs placed in the polymer interstices dissolve and release while the polymer undergoes the process mentioned above. If the rate of drug dissolution at the water moving (penetrating) front is fast, the swelling front and drug diffusion front are the same. However, there are two distinct fronts inside a matrix that may be observed along with the erosion front at the surface of the matrix if the drug dissolution rate at the water front is small. When the rates of swelling and erosion are equal, the two fronts (e.g., swelling front and erosion front) are synchronized so that the swollen gel thickness remains constant until the swelling front reaches the core of the matrix. Within the synchronized layer, the concentration gradient from the swelling front to the surface of the matrix becomes the same with time, and thus the drug release rate becomes constant (zero-order kinetics) with a planar geometry. However, other geometries render release nonlinearly due to the decreasing surface area both at the swelling and erosion fronts with time. Figure 6.30 schematically presents the swelling/erosion controlled system.

Drug release phenomena from swelling-and-erosion–controlled systems are much more complicated and have been described mathematically. Diffusion equations of three transporting materials (i.e., solvent, drug, and polymer) are:

$$\frac{\partial C_s}{\partial t} = D_s \frac{\partial^2 C_s}{\partial x^2} \qquad (6.132a)$$

$$\frac{\partial C_d}{\partial t} = D_d \frac{\partial^2 C_d}{\partial x^2} \qquad (6.132b)$$

$$\frac{\partial C_p}{\partial t} = D_p \frac{\partial^2 C_p}{\partial x^2} - \frac{dS}{dt} \frac{\partial C_p}{\partial x} \qquad (6.132c)$$

where the subscripts s, d, and p denote the solvent, the drug, and the polymer, respectively. Equation (6.132c) expresses the diffusion of the dissolved polymer through the swollen gel layer.

The initial and boundary conditions are:

$$C_s = C_d = 0 \qquad t = 0 \tag{6.133a}$$

$$S = l \qquad t = 0 \tag{6.133b}$$

$$C_s = C_{s,0} \qquad t = 0 \tag{6.133c}$$

$$(C_s + C_d)\frac{\partial R}{\partial t} = -\left(D_s\frac{\partial C_s}{\partial x} + D_d\frac{\partial C_d}{\partial x}\right) \qquad at \ x = R \tag{6.133d}$$

$$C_s = C_s^*, \quad C_d = C_d^*, \quad C_p = C_p^* \qquad at \ x = R \tag{6.133e}$$

$$C_s = C_{s,eq}, \quad C_d = C_{d,eq} \qquad at \ x = S \tag{6.133f}$$

The drug and polymer concentrations at the swelling front R are given by:

$$C_p^* = \frac{1/\rho_p}{\left(\dfrac{1}{\rho_p} + \dfrac{T_g - T}{\beta/\alpha_f}\dfrac{1}{\rho_s} + \dfrac{1}{\rho_d}\right)}, \quad C_d^* = \frac{1/\rho_d}{\left(\dfrac{1}{\rho_p} + \dfrac{T_g - T}{\beta/\alpha_f}\dfrac{1}{\rho_s} + \dfrac{1}{\rho_d}\right)} \tag{6.133g}$$

where α_f, β, ρ, T_g, and T are the linear expansion coefficient of the polymer, the expansion coefficient contribution of the solvent to the polymer, the density, the glass transition temperature of the polymer, and the experimental temperature, respectively.

Under the assumption that the concentration profiles of the solvent and the drug in the swollen gel layer are linear (i.e., pseudo–steady-state), the drug release can be expressed by:

$$\frac{M_t}{M_\infty} = \frac{C_d^* + C_{d,eq}}{2l}\left(\sqrt{2At} + Bt\right) \tag{6.134}$$

$$A = D_s(C_{s,eq} - C_s^*)\left(\frac{C_{s,eq}}{C_{s,eq} + C_{d,eq}} + \frac{1}{C_s^* + C_d^*}\right)$$
$$+ D_d(C_d^* - C_{d,eq})\left(\frac{C_{d,eq}}{C_{s,eq} + C_{d,eq}} + \frac{1}{C_s^* + C_d^*}\right) \tag{6.135}$$

$$B = \frac{k_d}{C_{s,eq} + C_{d,eq}} \tag{6.136}$$

where k_d is the disentanglement rate of the polymer and can be given by:

$$k_d = \frac{r_g}{t_r} \qquad (6.137)$$

where r_g and t_r are the radius of gyration of the polymer chains and the minimum time required for polymer chain entanglement, respectively.

The swollen gel thickness can be calculated by:

$$-\frac{S-R}{B} - \frac{A}{B^2}(S-R) = t \qquad (6.138)$$

When the rate of drug diffusion is much slower than the rate of polymer erosion (i.e., $B^2 \gg A$), Equation (6.134) becomes:

$$\frac{M_t}{M_\infty} = \frac{k_d}{2l}\left(\frac{C_{d,eq} + C_d^*}{C_{s,eq} + C_{d,eq}}\right)t \qquad (6.139)$$

Zero-order release kinetics expressed by Equation (6.139) agree with Equation (6.126) for heterogeneous erosion-controlled systems. However, when the rate of polymer erosion is very slow, the rate of drug diffusion through the swollen gel layer controls drug release kinetics (i.e., $B^2 \ll A$), and Equation (6.134) becomes:

$$\frac{M_t}{M_\infty} = \left(\frac{C_{d,eq} + C_d^*}{l}\right)\sqrt{\frac{At}{2}} \qquad (6.140)$$

When the rate of polymer swelling due to the absorption of solvent is synchronized with the rate of erosion, the swollen gel thickness $(S - R)$ becomes constant as given by:

$$S - R = \frac{1}{k_d}\left[\begin{array}{l} D_s(C_{s,eq} - C_s^*)\left(C_{s,eq} - \dfrac{C_{s,eq} + C_{d,eq}}{C_s^* + C_d^*}\right) \\[2ex] + D(C_{d,eq} - C_d^*)\left(C_{d,eq} - \dfrac{C_{s,eq} + C_{d,eq}}{C_s^* + C_d^*}\right) \end{array}\right] \qquad (6.141)$$

Equation (6.134) indicates that the physicochemical properties of drug, solvent, and polymer influence the overall release kinetics. The main key property governing swelling and erosion is the molecular weight of the polymer. Low-molecular-weight water-soluble polymers may provide synchronized swelling and erosion processes (e.g., polyethylene oxide $< 2 \times 10^6$). However, those properties cannot be easily

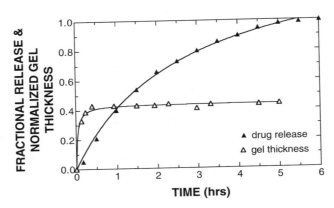

FIGURE 6.31 Swelling/erosion-controlled release of GHRH from noncross-linked PMMA/MAA beads. [Graph reconstructed from data by Kim and Lee, *Proceed. Int. Symp. Contrl. Rel. Bioact. Mater.*, 19, 208 (1992).]

obtained or time-consuming experiments are required. In this situation, Equation (6.134) can be written semiempirically as:

$$\frac{M_t}{M_\infty} = \alpha\sqrt{t} + \beta t \qquad (6.142)$$

where α and β are associated with a drug diffusion and polymer erosion, respectively.

Figure 6.31 demonstrates the validity of Equation (6.134) and Equation (6.141) via noncross-linked poly(methyl methacrylate-co-methacrylic acid) (PMMA/MAA) beads. The swollen gel thickness initially increases because the rate of erosion is slow. Then a constant gel thickness follows (i.e., synchronization of swelling rate and erosion rate) and continues until the core disappears. Afterwards, the gel thickness decreases. According to Equation (6.139), the release of peptide should be linear with time, but Figure 6.31 shows a nonlinear release profile due to the decrease of surface area of spherical geometry.

6.8 DIFFUSION WITH CHEMICAL REACTION IN A MEMBRANE

In certain situations, the diffusion process occurs concurrently with a particular reaction in the membrane. For instance, when a prodrug (i.e., estradiol acetate) diffuses through the skin, an enzyme in the viable epidermis converts the prodrug to estradiol and acetate. A diester prodrug (i.e., PNU-82, 899) diffuses across a Caco-2 cell monolayer, which extensively metabolizes the diester to a monoester.

Dynamic diffusion across a membrane in an irreversible first-order reaction is shown schematically in Figure 6.32. The diffusion process with the reaction is given as:

$$\frac{\partial C}{\partial t} = D\frac{\partial^2 C}{\partial x^2} - k_m C \qquad (6.143)$$

Diffusion

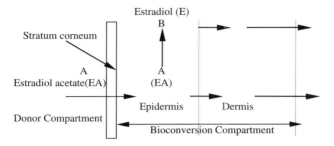

FIGURE 6.32 Schematic model for diffusion and bioreaction ($A \rightarrow B$) in a membrane.

where k_m is the bioconversion rate constant in the membrane. The initial and boundary conditions for Equation (6.143) are:

$$C = 0 \qquad\qquad x = h \qquad\qquad t = 0 \qquad\qquad (6.144a)$$

$$C = C_o \qquad\qquad x = 0 \qquad\qquad t > 0 \qquad\qquad (6.144b)$$

The solution for Equation (6.143) is written as:

$$\frac{C}{C_o} = \frac{\sinh\varphi(1 - x/h)}{\sinh\varphi} - 2\sum_{n=1}^{\infty} \frac{n\pi}{n^2\pi^2 + \varphi^2} \exp\left(-(n^2\pi^2 + \varphi^2)\frac{Dt}{h^2}\right)\sin\left(\frac{n\pi x}{h}\right) \quad (6.145)$$

where

$$\varphi^2 = \frac{h^2 k_m}{D}$$

The amount of the prodrug diffused is given as:

$$M_t = \frac{SC_o h\varphi}{\sinh\varphi}\frac{Dt}{h^2} - 2\sum_{n=1}^{\infty}\frac{(-1)^{n+1}n^2\pi^2}{(n^2\pi^2 + \varphi^2)^2}\exp\left(-\frac{(n^2\pi^2 + \varphi^2)Dt}{h^2}\right) \qquad (6.146)$$

The time lag equation yields:

$$t_{lag} = \frac{h^2}{2D}\left[\frac{\coth\varphi}{\varphi} - \frac{1}{\varphi^2}\right] \qquad (6.147)$$

At steady state (i.e., $t \rightarrow \infty$), the concentration distribution in the membrane is given by:

$$\frac{C}{C_o} = \frac{\sinh\varphi(1 - x/h)}{\sinh\varphi} \qquad (6.148)$$

The mass flux is then given by:

$$J = -D\frac{\partial C}{\partial x} = C_o\sqrt{Dk_m}\frac{\cosh\varphi(1-x/h)}{\sinh\varphi} \tag{6.149}$$

It is worthwhile to compare the flux of the reaction with the flux without the reaction in the membrane. The mass flux without reaction is given by:

$$J_{\text{no reaction}} = \frac{DC_o}{h} \tag{6.150}$$

The ratio of flux of the reaction to the flux without the reaction in the membrane is:

$$\frac{J}{J_{\text{no reaction}}} = \varphi\frac{\cosh\varphi(1-x/h)}{\sinh\varphi} \tag{6.151}$$

When the reaction in the membrane is very slow compared to diffusion ($\varphi \to 0$ or $\varphi \ll 1$), Equation (6.151) yields:

$$\frac{J}{J_{\text{no reaction}}} = 1 \quad \text{at } x = 0 \quad \text{and} \quad x = h \tag{6.152}$$

When the reaction is very fast ($\varphi \gg 1$), Equation (6.151) becomes:

$$\frac{J}{J_{\text{no reaction}}} = \varphi \gg 1 \quad \text{at } x = 0 \tag{6.153a}$$

$$\frac{J}{J_{\text{no reaction}}} = 0 \quad \text{at } x = h \tag{6.153b}$$

Equation (6.152) indicates that the effect of the reaction is negligible when the reaction rate is very slow. Equation (6.153a) and Equation (6.153b) suggest that the mass flux from the reservoir into the membrane becomes very large when the reaction rate is fast. Meanwhile, the mass flux entering the receiving site is zero because most of the prodrug is converted to metabolites.

Example 6.9

Tojo et al investigated the transdermal diffusion and metabolism of estradiol acetate in skin, as shown in Figure 6.33. The prodrug (estradiol acetate) is metabolized to estradiol in the viable epidermis. The concentration of the prodrug in the donor compartment is maintained at the saturated level. Calculate the diffusion coefficient

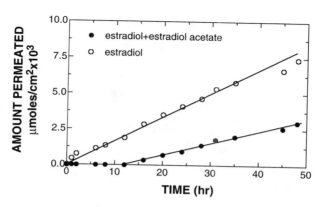

FIGURE 6.33 The diffusion of estradiol acetate and formation of estradiol by metabolism in the skin. [Graph reconstructed from data by Tojo et al., *Drug Dev. Ind. Pharm.*, 11, 1175 (1985).]

of the prodrug and the metabolism rate constant of the prodrug. Assume that the thickness of the skin is 250 μm and the solubility of the prodrug is 2×10^{-2} g/L.

Solution

From Figure 6.33, one can obtain the rate of diffusion and the time lag as:

$$\frac{dM_t}{Sdt} = \frac{\varphi C_o}{\sinh\varphi} \frac{D}{h^2} = 158 \text{ moles / cm}^2 \text{ / hr} \tag{6.154a}$$

$$t_{lag} = \frac{h^2}{2D}\left[\frac{\coth\varphi}{\varphi} - \frac{1}{\varphi^2}\right] = 0.05 \text{ hr} \tag{6.154b}$$

$$\frac{D}{h^2} = \frac{158}{63.6}\frac{\sinh\varphi}{\varphi} = \frac{1}{0.1}\left[\frac{\coth\varphi}{\varphi} - \frac{1}{\varphi^2}\right] \tag{6.154c}$$

By trial and error, $\varphi = 0.7$.
Substituting φ into Equation (6.154c) yields:

$$D = h^2 \times 0.3229 = 0.020 \text{ cm}^2 \text{ / hr}$$

The rate constant is then:

$$\varphi = h\sqrt{\frac{k_m}{D}} = 0.25\sqrt{\frac{k_m}{0.020}} = 0.7 \qquad k_m = 0.157 \text{ / sec}$$

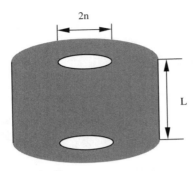

FIGURE 6.34 Schematic view of a perforated, coated tablet.

6.9 SURFACE AREA AND CONCENTRATION GRADIENT SYSTEMS

The monolithic matrix systems described in this chapter are the simplest and least expensive systems when compared to membrane–reservoir systems and others. The manufacturing process for the matrix system is generally the same as that for conventional dosage forms and highly reproducible. A major drawback is that it does not furnish zero-order release kinetics (rather, the square root of time kinetics) as suggested in the theoretical equations. This is attributed to a decrease in the release rate due to a longer diffusion length and in the drug concentration within the matrix as the drug release time progresses. This problem is much more severe for cylindrical and spherical devices because the surface area in the moving front becomes smaller with time. The decrease in the release rate with time can be overcome by modifying the matrix geometry such that the surface area increases with time. There are many examples (e.g., pie, hemisphere, or cone) for this approach. Here, we discuss a perforated, coated tablet composed of a water-insoluble drug carrier, as shown in Figure 6.34.

As in the Higuchi model, Fick's first law is applied and the flux J is:

$$J = 2\pi LD\,(n + x)\frac{dC}{dx} \qquad (6.155)$$

where x is the diffusion path length, n is the radius of the inner hole, and L is the thickness of the tablet. Integration of Equation (6.155) with respect to distance and concentration under a pseudo–steady-state approximation and sink condition yields:

$$J = \frac{2\pi LDKC_s}{\ln\dfrac{\lambda}{n}} \qquad (6.156)$$

where C_s is the drug concentration at the drug dissolution front and λ is the length between the moving front and the center of the perforated, coated tablet. The mass dissolved at time t is given by:

$$M = (\lambda^2 - n^2)L\pi\rho \tag{6.157}$$

Rearrange Equation (6.157) for λ and substitute into Equation (6.155). The resulting equation is integrated to yield:

$$t = \frac{\dfrac{1}{2}M + \left(\dfrac{M + L\pi\rho n^2}{2}\right)\ln\left(\dfrac{M}{L\pi\rho n^2} + 1\right)}{2\pi LDKC_s} \tag{6.158a}$$

or

$$t = \frac{-\dfrac{1}{2}(\lambda^2 - n^2)\rho + \lambda^2\rho \ln\dfrac{\lambda}{n}}{2DKC_s} \tag{6.158b}$$

The amount of the drug released in the sink is:

$$M_t = M - M_d \tag{6.159}$$

where M_d is the amount of the drug dissolved in the matrix and is calculated as:

$$M_d = \int_0^{\lambda-n} 2\pi L(x+n)\left(\frac{J}{2\pi DKL}\ln\left(\frac{x+n}{\lambda}\right) + C_s\right)dx \tag{6.160}$$

Substitute Equation (6.159) into Equation (6.160) and integrate the resulting equation:

$$M_t = \pi L(\lambda^2 - n^2)\left[\rho - KC_s + \frac{KC_s}{2\ln\dfrac{\lambda}{n}}\right] \tag{6.161}$$

When M_t vs. λ in Equation (6.161) is related to λ vs. t in Equation (6.158b), a drug release profile is generated. As shown in Figure 6.35, the predicted data are in agreement with the experimental data in a pie-shaped device. The pie-shaped device is a part of a perforated, coated tablet that has an angle of 2θ instead of 2π.

Example 6.10

Lipper and Higuchi investigated the release of stearic acid from a pie-shaped device. The inner hole radius is 540 μm, the thickness of the pie is 5.75 cm, the solubility of the drug in alcohol is 0.048 g/cm³, and the density of the drug is 0.94 g/cm³. The amount of drug released is 4 g at t = 300 hr. Calculate the diffusivity of the drug assuming K = 1.

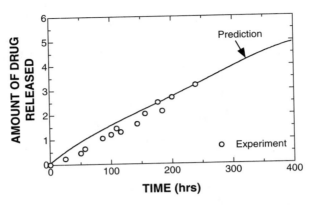

FIGURE 6.35 The release of stearic acid from a pie-shaped device. [Graph reconstructed from data by Lipper and Higuchi, *J. Pharm. Sci.*, 66, 159 (1977).]

Solution
From Equation (6.161)

$$4.0g = 0.7 \times 5.75cm(\lambda^2 - (0.054cm)^2)\left(0.94g/cm^3 - 0.048g/cm^3 + \frac{0.048g/cm^3}{2\ln\dfrac{\lambda}{0.054cm}}\right)$$

where λ can be determined by iteration. $\lambda = 1.051$.
Substituting λ into Equation (6.158b) yields:

$$300\ hr = \frac{-0.5 \times (1.051^2 - 0.054^2) \times 0.94 + 1.051^2 \times 0.94 \times \ln\dfrac{0.45}{0.054}}{2 \times 0.048D}$$

$$D = 2.47 \times 10^{-5}\ cm^2/sec$$

As shown in Equation (6.126), a controlled-release dosage form with heterogeneous erosion-controlled carriers is used to provide a constant drug release rate when the dosage form has a slab geometry. However, the common dosage forms are tablets, whose release kinetics are expressed by Equation (6.128) and deviate slightly from zero-order release kinetics. When the heterogeneous erosion-controlled carriers are employed with perforated, coated tablets, as shown in Figure 6.34, a parabolic release can be obtained from Equation (6.124) and Equation (6.127):

$$\frac{M_t}{M_\infty} = \frac{\left(n + \dfrac{k_e t}{C_o}\right)^2 - n^2}{r_o^2 - n^2} \qquad (6.162)$$

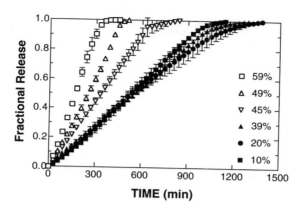

FIGURE 6.36 The release of diltiazem HCl from the perforated, coated tablets (3/16" hole size). [Graph reconstructed from data by C. Kim, *Eur. J. Pharm. Sci.,* 7, 237 (1999).]

When drug solubility is very high or drug loading is below the drug solubility, Equation (6.131) is applied to the perforated, coated tablets. Due to the diffusion term in Equation (6.131), the drug release kinetics are linear for the perforated, coated tablets. Figure 6.36 shows the release of diltiazem HCl from the perforated, coated tablets.

One of the problems associated with matrix systems is that the drug concentration in the matrix decreases with time because the initial drug loading across the cross-section of the matrix is uniform. Instead of modifying geometry to increase the surface area, which takes a special effort to make the dosage forms, a nonuniform concentration gradient in a matrix can compensate for diminishing surface area with time and increasing diffusion resistance. A nonuniform concentration gradient is constructed in which the drug concentration is small at the surface and high in the core of the matrix.

The fractional release from a matrix (planar sheet) in which the initial drug concentration distribution is $f(x)$ can be obtained by:

$$\frac{M_t}{M_\infty} = 1 - \frac{\sum_{n=0}^{\infty} \frac{(-1)^{n+1}}{2n+1} I_1(n) \exp\left(-\frac{(2n+1)^2 \pi^2 Dt}{4l^2}\right)}{\sum_{n=0}^{\infty} \frac{(-1)^{n+1}}{2n+1} I_1(n)} \qquad (6.163)$$

where

$$I_1(n) = \int_0^1 f(\zeta) \cos[(n+1)/2\pi\zeta] d\zeta \qquad (6.164)$$

Among various initial concentration distributions in a matrix, the sigmoidal drug distribution or a staircase distribution resembling a sigmoidal pattern furnishes zero-order release kinetics for the planar geometry. There are various methods to build concentration gradient matrix systems. The most convenient way to achieve the

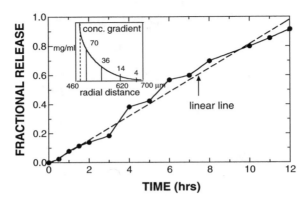

FIGURE 6.37 The release of chlorpheniramine maleate from granules with nonuniform initial drug concentration. [Graph reconstructed from data by Scott and Hollenbeck, *Pharm. Res.,* 8, 156 (1991).]

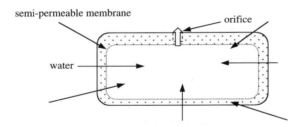

FIGURE 6.38 An elementary osmotic pump.

gradient matrix for large-scale manufacturing is that nonpareil (sugar) beads are coated by spraying different drug concentrations with different spraying times. Figure 6.37 shows the drug-release profile from granules with gradient drug concentration.

6.10 OSMOTICALLY CONTROLLED SYSTEMS

In Chapter 3, the osmosis process was described. Basically, when two different concentrations are separated by a semipermeable membrane, osmotic pressure builds up on the higher-concentration side. Several attempts have been made to use osmotic pressure as a driving force to deliver bioactive drugs. After numerous trials of osmotic pressure-driven devices, osmotic pump tablets were developed by compressing drug and excipient powders into a hard tablet followed by coating the tablet with a semipermeable membrane (e.g., cellulose acetate) and then drilling an orifice in the coating by a laser, as shown in Figure 6.38.

Upon contact with water, the semipermeable membrane of an osmotic pump tablet absorbs water, and water diffuses through the membrane and dissolves water-soluble substances, resulting in a concentrated solution and high osmotic pressure inside the membrane. This leads to drawing more water across the membrane. The flow rate of water across the membrane, dQ/dt, is given by:

$$\frac{dQ}{dt} = \frac{S}{h} L_p (\sigma \Delta \pi - \Delta P) \qquad (6.165)$$

where S and h are the surface area and thickness of the semipermeable membrane, respectively, L_p is its permeability coefficient, σ is the reflection coefficient, and $\Delta \pi$ and ΔP are the osmotic and hydrostatic pressure differences, respectively.

The rate of drug delivered through the orifice, dM/dt, is then given by:

$$\frac{dM}{dt} = \frac{dQ}{dt} \times C \qquad (6.166)$$

where C is the drug concentration inside the membrane. In general, the osmotic pressure inside the membrane is much larger than the hydrostatic pressure, and then Equation (6.166) becomes:

$$\frac{dM}{dt} = \frac{S}{h} k \pi \, C \qquad (6.167)$$

where

$$k = \sigma L_p$$

If there are solid drugs left in the osmotic pump tablet, the drug concentration becomes C_s, the solubility of the drug, and the osmotic pressure exerted by the dissolved drug is π_s. Then the rate of drug release becomes zero order as given by:

$$\left(\frac{dM_t}{dt} \right)_z = \frac{S}{h} k \pi_s C_s \qquad (6.168)$$

where $(dM_t/dt)_z$ is the zero-order release rate.

As soon as the last solid substance disappears in the osmotic tablet, the drug concentration and osmotic pressure decrease with time and the rate of drug release becomes non–zero order as given by:

$$\left(\frac{dM_t}{dt} \right)_{nz} = \frac{\left(dM_t / dt \right)_z}{\left[1 + \dfrac{1}{C_s V} \left(\dfrac{dM_t}{dt} \right)_z (t - t_z) \right]} \qquad (6.169)$$

where $(dM_t/dt)_{nz}$ is the non–zero order release rate, V is the volume of the tablet, and t_z is the total time for which the drug is delivered under zero-order release rate condition, given by:

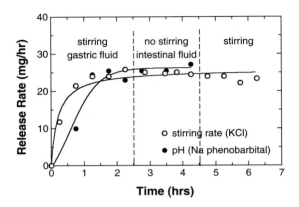

FIGURE 6.39 Effect of pH and stirring on the release of KCl from elementary osmotic pump tablets (OROS®). [Graph reconstructed from data by F. Theeuwes, *J. Pharm. Sci.*, 64, 1987 (1975).]

$$t_z = M_T \left(1 - \frac{C_s}{\rho}\right) \frac{1}{(dM_t / dt)_z} \tag{6.170}$$

where ρ is the density of the osmotic tablet and M_T is the total drug mass in the tablet ($= \rho V$). The drug concentration under a non–zero order rate is determined by:

$$C = \frac{C_s V}{V + (t - t_z) F_s} \tag{6.171}$$

where $F_s = SL_p \pi_s / h$. The amount of drug delivered at zero-order rate, M_z, is given by:

$$M_z = M_T \left(1 - \frac{C_s}{\rho}\right) \tag{6.172}$$

As presented by Equation (6.168), the zero-order release rate is independent of any other experimental conditions (e.g., pH, stirring rate, etc), as illustrated in Figure 6.39, and the percentage of zero-order release is only a function of the solubility of the drug and the density of the tablet. Thus, the less soluble the drug, the longer zero-order release kinetics can be achieved. However, the less soluble drug (i.e., smaller C_s) gives less osmotic pressure, and thus the drug release does not finish within the desired time frame. In this case, additional osmagents are incorporated into the osmotic tablet to raise the osmotic pressure and shorten the total release time. Commercial examples of the elementary osmotic pump system are Accutrim® (phenylpropanolamine HCl), Efidac 24® (chlorpheniramine), and Sudafed®24 (pseudoephedrine). The core tablet is made of the drug and NaCl as an osmagent.

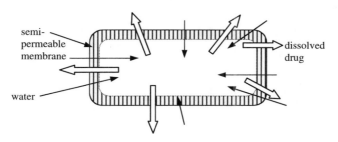

FIGURE 6.40 Microporous osmotic pump system (MPOPS).

Equation (6.172) suggests that a highly water-soluble drug generates high osmotic pressure, but the length of zero-order drug delivery is short because the concentration of drug rapidly falls below its solubility. However, there are certain drugs whose solubility is dependent on the amount of salts present in solution. For example, the solubility of salbutamol sulfate in water is 275 mg/mL whereas its solubility in saturated NaCl solution is 16 mg/mL. When salbutamol sulfate and NaCl are formulated into an osmotic pump tablet, the zero-order release of the drug is prolonged to 12 to 24 hr, which depends on the ratio of the drug to NaCl. Due to the high drug concentration at the later time of release, pulsed doses of the drug are observed. Volmax® is a commercial example of the solubility modulated osmotic pump.

Fabricating a small hole onto an osmotic pump tablet is not a common pharmaceutical process and requires a special laser drill. An elementary osmotic pump system uses a nonporous semipermeable membrane. If a microporous semipermeable membrane dresses an osmotic tablet, pore sizes are small enough for drugs and water freely to cross the membrane while exerting osmotic pressure, as presented in Figure 6.40. The microporous structure of the semipermeable membrane can be created by formulating water-soluble substances (e.g., polyethylene glycol and lactose) in the coating solution. Those water-soluble materials leach out of the coated membrane upon contact with water, leaving a microporous semipermeable morphology behind. However, one should be very careful as to the quantity of porogens to be formulated and what their molecular size should be. Otherwise, the membrane may lose its semipermeability.

Microporous osmotic pump systems (MPOPS) deliver drugs by osmotic pressure and diffusion. The rate of drug delivery is given by:

$$\left(\frac{dM_t}{dt}\right)_z = \frac{SC_s}{h}\left(k\pi_s + P\right) \tag{6.173}$$

where P is the permeability of the microporous membrane. The non–zero order release rate via osmotic pumping and diffusion is given by:

$$\left(\frac{dM_t}{dt}\right)_{nz} = \frac{F_s}{C_s}C^2 + \frac{S}{h}PC \tag{6.174}$$

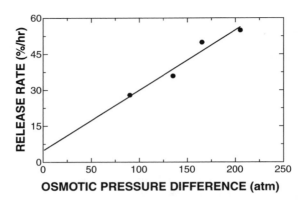

FIGURE 6.41 Effect of osmotic pressure on the release of KCl from MPOPS. [Graph reconstructed from Appel and Zentner, *Pharm. Res.*, 8, 600 (1991).]

$$-\left(\frac{dC}{dt}\right) = \frac{1}{V}\left(\frac{dM_t}{dt}\right)_{nz} \tag{6.175}$$

Substituting Equation (6.174) into Equation (6.175) and solving the resulting equation yields:

$$t - t_z = \left(\frac{Vh}{SP}\right) \ln\left[\frac{F_s\dfrac{C}{C_s} + \dfrac{SP}{h}}{\left(F_s + \dfrac{SP}{h}\right)\dfrac{C}{C_s}}\right] \tag{6.176}$$

Equation (6.173) implies that the release rate is governed by the porosity of the membrane, which influences the permeability; the polymer material, which influences the semipermeability of the membrane; the thickness and surface area of the membrane; the solubility and osmotic pressure; and the amount of drug in the core. Figure 6.41 shows the effect of osmotic pressure on the release of KCl from MPOPS. By extrapolating the linear line to zero osmotic pressure, the release rate of drug by diffusion through the microporous membrane structure can be obtained.

The OROS® and MPOPS are suited for moderately water-soluble drugs, which produce enough osmotic pressure. For a poorly water-soluble drug (<1%), the osmotic pressure generated by the drug is so small that it takes a very long time to complete drug release. To deal with this problem, "push–pull" osmotic pump tablets have been developed, as shown in Figure 6.42. The core tablet consists of two layers. The bottom layer is made of hydrophilic polymers and osmogents, whereas the top layer is composed of a drug and osmogents. As the osmogents draw water into the core tablet by osmosis, the hydrophilic polymers swell upward, and a drug suspension is produced in the top layer due to the low solubility of the drug. The bottom layer pushes the suspended drug through the orifice. Figure 6.43 shows the release of nifedipine ($C_s \approx$ 10 mg/L) from the push–pull osmotic tablet.

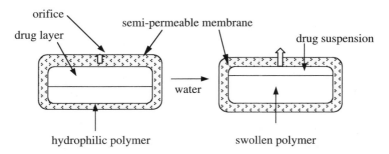

FIGURE 6.42 A push–pull osmotic pump.

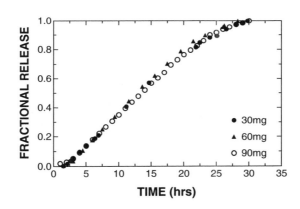

FIGURE 6.43 The release of nifedipine from Procardia XL®.

The push–pull osmotic tablet was originally designed for drugs with very low water solubility but can be used for highly water-soluble drugs. In this case, a triple-layer tablet is formed: another layer containing no drug but a water-soluble polymer sits on the double layer originally designed for the push–pull system. There is a time lag during which the water-soluble polymer in the top layer slowly dissolves and moves out through the orifice. The magnitude of the time lag is dependent on the thickness of the top layer. Commercial products based on the push–pull system are Procardia XL® (nifedipine), Glucotrol XL® (glipizide), Ditropan XL® (oxybutynin chloride), Concerta® (methylphenidate HCl), Dynacirc CR® (isradipine), Alpress™ LP (prazosin), Cardura® XL (doxazosin mesylate), IVOMEC® SR Bolus (ivermectin), and Covera-HS® (verapamil HCl).

This push–pull system has been applied to a system containing a liquid formulation (called L–OROS™). A liquid drug layer and an osmotic engine, or push layer, are encased in a hard gelatin capsule surrounded by a semipermeable membrane. However, there is a barrier layer separating the drug layer from the push layer in order to prevent any interaction between the two. A laser-drilled orifice is set in the top of the drug layer.

Example 6.11

A drug has a solubility in water of 274 mg/cm^3 and its molecular weight is 250 g/mole. An oral osmotic pump tablet of 450 mg is designed with the following properties of a semipermeable membrane:

$$S = 2.1 \text{ cm}^2 \quad h = 400 \text{ μm} \quad L_p = 2 \times 10^{-5} \text{cm}^2 / \text{atm} \cdot \text{hr} \quad \sigma = 0.97$$

Its volume is 0.27 cm^3. Calculate the oral zero-order delivery rate, the period of time (t_z) for which the drug is delivered at a zero-order delivery rate, and the delivery rate and drug concentration delivered at 1.2 t_z.

Solution

The saturated osmotic pressure is:

$$\pi_s = \frac{nRT}{V} = \frac{(450 \times 10^{-3} / 250)(0.082 \times 10^3)(310)}{0.27} = 169.5 \text{ atm}$$

$$\left(\frac{dM_t}{dt}\right)_z = \frac{S}{h} k\pi_s C_s = \frac{2.1}{400 \times 10^{-4}} (0.97 \times 2 \times 10^{-5})(169.5)(274) = 47.3 \text{ mg / hr}$$

$$t_z = M_T\left(1 - \frac{C_s}{\rho}\right) \Big/ \left(\frac{dM_t}{dt}\right)_z = \frac{450(1 - \dfrac{274}{450 / 0.27})}{47.3} = 7.95 \text{ hr}$$

$$\left(\frac{dM_t}{dt}\right)_{nz} = \frac{(dM_t/dt)_z}{\left[1 + \dfrac{1}{C_s V}\left(\dfrac{dM_t}{dt}\right)_z (t - t_z)\right]} = \frac{47.3}{\left[1 + \dfrac{47.3 \times 1.2 \times 7.95}{274 \times 0.27}\right]} = 6.66 \text{ mg / hr}$$

$$F_s = \frac{S\sigma L_p \pi_s}{h} = \frac{2.1 \times 0.97 \times 2 \times 10^{-5} \times 169.5}{400 \times 10^{-4}} = 0.173 \text{cm}^3 / \text{hr}$$

$$C = \frac{C_s V}{V + (t - t_z)F_s} = \frac{274 \times 0.173}{0.27 + 0.2 \times 7.95 \times 0.173} = 87.0 \text{ mg / cm}^3$$

SUGGESTED READINGS

1. R. W. Baker, *Controlled Release of Biologically Active Agents,* John Wiley and Sons, New York, 1987.
2. J. A. Barrie et al., Diffusion and Solution of Gases in Composite Rubber Membranes, *Trans. Faraday Soc.,* 59, 869 (1963).
3. H. S. Carslaw and J. C. Jaeger, *Conduction of Heat in Solids,* 2nd Ed., Oxford University Press, Oxford, London, 1959, Chapters 1 to 9.
4. S. K. Chandrasekran and D. R. Paul, Dissolution-Controlled Transport from Dispersed Matrices, *J. Pharm. Sci.,* 71, 1399 (1982).
5. J. Crank, *The Mathematics of Diffusion,* 2nd Ed., Oxford University Press, Oxford, London, 1975, Chapters 1 to 6.
6. T. Higuchi, Rate of Release of Medicaments from Ointment Bases Containing Drugs in Suspension, *J. Pharm. Sci.,* 50, 874 (1961).
7. C. J. Kim, *Controlled Release Dosage Form Design,* Technomic Publishing Co., Lancaster, PA, 2000.
8. A. Kyneoudis (Ed.), *Treatise on Controlled Drug Delivery,* Marcel Dekker, New York, 1992.
9. P. I. Lee, Diffusional Release of a Solute from a Polymer Matrix — Approximate Analytical Solutions, *J. Membr. Sci.,* 7, 255 (1980).
10. R. S. Langer and D. L. Wise (Eds.), *Medical Applications of Controlled Release,* Vol. I, CRC Press, Boca Raton, FL, 1984, Chapters 1 to 3.
11. B. Narashinhan and N. A. Peppas, Molecular Analysis of Drug Delivery Systems Controlled by Dissolution of the Polymer Carrier, *J. Pharm. Sci.,* 86, 297 (1997).
12. M. N. Oziak, *Heat Conduction,* John Wiley and Sons, New York, 1980, Chapters 1 to 4 and 7.
13. E. Theeuwes, Elementary Osmotic Pump, *J. Pharm. Sci.,* 64, 1987 (1975).
14. P. I. Lee, Interpretation of Drug-Release Kinetics from Hydrogel Matrices in Terms of Time-Dependent Diffusion Coefficients, in *Controlled-Release Technology: Pharmaceutical Applications,* P. I. Lee and W. R. Good (Eds.), ACS Symp. Series No. 348, American Chemical Society, Washington, D.C., 1987. p. 71.
15. P. I. Lee, Initial Concentration Distribution as a Mechanism for Regulating Drug Release from Diffusion Controlled and Surface Erosion Controlled Matrix Systems, *J. Control. Rel.,* 4, 1 (1986).
16. D. R. Paul and S. K. McSpadden, Diffusional Release of a Solute from a Polymer Matrix, *J. Membr. Sci.,* 1, 33 (1976).

PROBLEMS

1. Calculate the time required for 50% of medroxyprogesterone acetate to be released from a spherical silicone bead (0.5 cm radius). The drug loading is 30 mg/mL, the partition coefficient is 0.033, and the drug solubility in water is 3.25×10^{-3} mg/mL. The diffusion coefficient was determined to be 290 cm^2/week. Calculate the cumulative amount of drug released for 5 weeks.

2. A permeation experiment was carried out with a freshly made membrane. It was determined that the diffusion coefficient of a drug is 3.1×10^{-3} cm^2/hr, the partition coefficient is 0.15, the thickness of the membrane is 0.1 cm, the solubility of the drug is 2 mg/mL, the volume of the reservoir is 0.314 cm^2, and the total drug amount present in the reservoir is 1 mg. Calculate the cumulative amount of drug release for 30 hr.

3. A coated, perforated donut-shaped tablet was proposed to deliver a water-soluble drug for 20 hr. A water-soluble polymer was incorporated to carry the drug. The erosion rate constant of 6.6 mg/cm^2 hr was measured. The size of a tablet was 1.2 cm. Calculate the central hole size of the tablet to deliver the drug for 20 hr. Drug loading is 300 mg/cm^3.

4. Design a porous osmotic pump tablet given the following information: The solubility of the drug is 330 mg/cm^3, the drug is not ionic and its molecular weight is 87.1, surface area = 2.2 cm^2, membrane thickness = 250 μm, permeability coefficient = 3.1×10^{-6} cm^2/atm hr, reflection coefficient = 0.97, density of the drug = 2 g/cm^3, total amount of drug present in the tablet = 450 mg. Some of the drug is released from the tablet by simple diffusion through the membrane. Its permeability coefficient is 0.122×10^{-3} cm^2/hr. Calculate the zero-order delivery rate for the drug at 37°C and the time t_z. Calculate the time at which the drug release rate is 3.5 mg/hr.

5. Hydrocortisone was dispersed in a polycarprolatone tablet matrix of diameter 1.5 cm and thickness 0.17 cm. The aqueous solubility of the drug is 280 mg/L. It was observed that 60% of the drug was released from the tablet at 110 min. Calculate the diffusion coefficient of the drug through the matrix. Drug loading was 18%.

7 Polymer Science

In the medical and pharmaceutical fields, natural, semisynthetic, and synthetic polymers have made significant contributions to the improvement of human health. The drug delivery systems described in Chapter 6 are based on polymeric materials. Without them, many new or improved dosage forms would not be available for pharmaceutical applications. In general, polymers used for drug delivery systems were not originally intended for that particular purpose. For this reason, it is important to evaluate polymers carefully before using them for therapeutic applications. On the other hand, it is impossible to describe all the polymers used and investigated in drug delivery systems and pharmaceutical dosage forms. In this chapter, the basic principles of the synthesis of polymers and their characterization with respect to pharmaceutical applications will be discussed. Table 7.1 presents the various polymers that have been used or investigated for pharmaceutical applications.

7.1 CLASSIFICATION OF POLYMERS

Polymers (natural or synthetic materials) have very large molecular weights made up of repeating units (or mers) throughout their chains. Polymers are classified according to their synthesis, mechanical behavior, processing characteristics, and morphology. Examples of their synthetic classification are condensation polymers and addition (chain) polymers. In condensation polymers, monomers consisting of two functional groups (i.e., $-OH$, $-COOH$, and $-NH_2$), react with each other to form covalent bonds. For example, monomers with $-OH$ groups may react with monomers with $-COOH$ groups, thus resulting in a polymer that has an ester linkage ($-COO-$) and water as a byproduct.

As the polymerization proceeds, the number of repeating units, n, increases with time. The higher the degree of polymerization is, the higher the molecular weight will be. When monomers with bifunctional groups AA and BB are in exact proportion, the polymer molecules have infinite molecular weight.

$$-AA-BB-AA-BB-AA-BB-AA-BB-$$

TABLE 7.1
Natural and Synthetic Polymers Used for Pharmaceutical Applications

Polymer	Major Functions
Natural Polymers	
Gelatin	Binder, coacervation
Alginic acid, Na	Encapsulation
Xanthan gum, arabic gum	Matrix, binder
Chitosan	Matrix, membrane
Semisynthetic Polymers (Cellulose Derivatives)	
Methyl cellulose	Binder, coating
Ethyl cellulose	Matrix, coating
Hydroxyethyl cellulose	Binder, coating
Hydroxypropyl cellulose	Binder, coating
Hydroxyethylmethyl cellulose	Binder, coating
Hydroxypropylmethyl cellulose	Matrix, coating
Carboxymethyl cellulose sodium	Binder, disintegrant
Cellulose acetate	Membrane
Cellulose acetate butyrate	Membrane
Cellulose acetate propionate	Membrane
Cellulose acetate phthalate	Enteric
Hydroxypropylmethyl cellulose phthalate	Enteric
Synthetic Polymers	
Ion exchange resins (methacrylic acid, sulfonated polystyrene/divinylbenzene)	Matrix
Polyacrylic acid (Carbopol)	Matrix, bioadhesive
Poly(MMA/MAA)	Enteric
Poly(MMA/DEAMA)	Matrix, membrane
Poly(MMA/EA)	Membrane
Poly(vinylacetate phthalate)	Enteric
Poly(vinyl alcohol)	Matrix
Poly(vinyl pyrrolidone)	Binder
Poly(lactic acid)	Biodegradable
Poly(glycolic acid)	Biodegradable
Poly(lactic/glycolic acid)	Biodegradable
Polyethylene glycol	Binder
Polyethylene oxide	Matrix, binder
Poly(dimethyl silicone)	Matrix, membrane
Poly(hydroxyethyl methacrylate)	Matrix, membrane
Poly(ethylene/vinyl acetate)	Matrix, membrane
Poly(ethylene/vinyl alcohol)	Matrix, membrane
Polybutadiene	Adhesive/matrix
Poly(anhydride)	Bioerodible
Poly(orthoester)	Biodegradable
Poly(glutamic acid)	Biodegradable

Source: Taken from W. J. Passil, *Prog. Polym. Sci.,* 14, 629 (1989).

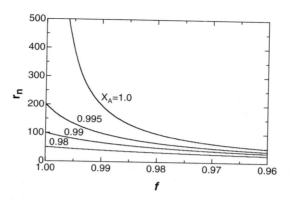

FIGURE 7.1 The effects of conversion and stoichiometric imbalance on the number average degree of polymerization.

If AA is in excess, the polymerization stops after BB is all used up. Figure 7.1 shows the relationship among the polymer chain length (or molecular weight), the stoichiometric imbalance, f, and the conversion with respect to the monomer AA groups, X_A. As f and X_A get closer to 1, the molecular weight of the condensation polymer drastically increases. Commercial condensation polymerization is carried out at $0.9 < f < 0.95$. When the same bifunctional monomers contain two reacting functional groups, the concentration of each reacting group is equimolar during the course of polymerization.

In addition (chain) polymerization, monomers containing an unsaturated (vinyl) bond polymerize in the presence of an initiator, which generates an active site at the end of the chain. Several chemical reactions take place simultaneously in the course of the polymerization. First, an initiation reaction via photo- or heat-decomposition of the initiator occurs to form the active species, which are either peroxides or azo compounds. The active species react with a monomer to generate the active site (i.e., initiation).

$$R-O-O-R \rightarrow 2RO^*$$

$$RO^* + CH_2 = CHX \rightarrow ROCH_2 - C^*HX$$

The activated monomer chain is then incorporated into another monomer, thus resulting in a growing polymer chain (i.e., propagation).

$$RO-\left[-CH_2 - C^*HX\right]_n + CH_2 = CHX \rightarrow RO-\left[-CH_2 - C^*HX\right]_{n+1}$$

Finally, the growing polymer chains with active sites are terminated when a chemical bond is formed between the two growing polymer chains (i.e., termination).

$$RO-\left[-CH_2 - C^*HX\right]_n + \left[XHC^* - CH_2 -\right]_m - OR \rightarrow$$

$$RO-\left[-CH_2 - CHX -\right]_{m+n} - OR$$

or $\qquad \rightarrow RO-\left[-CH_2-CHX-\right]_n-H \ + \ RO-\left[-CH=CHX\right]_m$

Depending on how the active species are generated, chain polymerization may be classified as:

1. Free radical polymerization
2. Anionic polymerization
3. Cationic polymerization
4. Coordination polymerization

Most polymers used in pharmaceutical applications are made via a free radical polymerization process, which will be discussed in detail in the following sections. In copolymerization, polymers are formed with more than two monomers in the polymerization process. The properties of the copolymers are influenced by the monomer type and the sequence of monomers in the chain. Random copolymers have the repeating units randomly arranged on the molecule chain. In alternating copolymers, two repeating monomer units are arranged alternatively and in an orderly fashion along the chain. Block copolymers have a chain with long sequences of each repeating unit along the main polymer chain. In grafted copolymers, the long sequences of one repeating unit are grafted onto the backbone of the other polymer. Random and alternating copolymers possess the average physiochemical properties of both polymer A and polymer B, while block copolymers possess the properties of both polymer A and polymer B.

$\left[AABAABBAABABBBAABAAA \right]$ random

$\left[ABABABABABABABABABAB \right]$ alternating

$\left[AAAABBBBBBBBAAAAABBBB \right]$ block

$$\left[\begin{array}{c} AAAAAAAAAAAAAAAAAAAA \\ | \qquad\quad | \qquad\quad | \\ B \qquad\; B \qquad\; B \\ | \qquad\quad | \qquad\quad | \\ B \qquad\; B \qquad\; B \\ | \qquad\quad | \qquad\quad | \\ B \qquad\; B \qquad\; B \end{array} \right] \qquad \text{grafted}$$

Another method of classification of polymers is based on polymer processability upon heating to obtain a final shape (product). In this way, polymers can be classified as thermoplastic or thermosetting. Thermoplastic polymers (e.g., polyethylene, polymethyl methacrylate, Eudragit®) are uncross-linked, heated to viscous flow, and extruded or molded. They are solidified upon cooling below their glass transition temperature, T_g. Thermoplastic polymers can be repeatedly heated and reformed without undergoing any changes in their physicochemical properties. Particular solvents can be used to dissolve thermoplastic polymers. On the other hand, simultaneous polymerization and fabrication steps produce thermosetting polymers (e.g., phenol/formaldehyde resins, epoxy resins). Two components, a low- or intermediate-molecular-weight polymer and a curing agent, are polymerized to a higher molecular

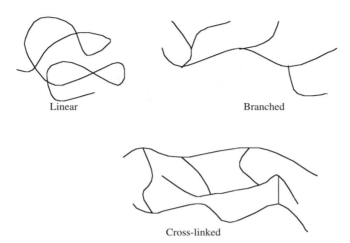

Linear   Branched

Cross-linked

FIGURE 7.2 Structural arrangement of polymers.

weight and then cross-linked at an elevated temperature. The resulting material, when cooled below T_g, is rigid (the segment lengths between cross-links are too short for random coil) and cannot be reformed (no viscous flow) upon heating because it decomposes. There is no solvent to dissolve thermosetting polymers.

The third method of classification is based on the structure or shape of the polymer molecules: linear, branched (short and long), or cross-linked, as shown in Figure 7.2. Linear chain polymers are generally randomly coiled. The occupied volume of a random coil is much larger than that of the constituent atoms. As a result, the polymer chains are deeply interpenetrated and entangled by the other chains. Some polymers have branched chains in their linear backbone chains. The branching is the result of a side reaction during polymerization. Cross-linked polymers form a network structure with monomers that have more than two functional groups during a condensation–polymerization or with cross-linking agents (di- or multivinyl monomers) during a free radical polymerization. Network polymers can never be dissolved in any solvent, as was pointed out in the description of thermosetting polymers, but they can swell in a good solvent to various extents, depending upon the degree of polymer cross-linking.

When melted polymers are cooled down or the polymers in solution are concentrated by the evaporation of the solvent, the polymer molecular structure is arranged in such a way that the polymer chain is packed as closely as possible to attain the least amount of potential energy. Certain polymers aggregate to each other regularly in an ordered manner (Figure 7.3). The polymers, which possess a long-range, three-dimensional, ordered structure, are called crystalline polymers. Their packing efficiency is not perfect, and thus the degree of crystallinity, ranging from a few percent to about 99%, is defined as the fraction of the total polymer chain in the crystalline regions. Crystalline and noncrystalline regions are intermixed in a semicrystalline polymer. In an amorphous polymer, the chains do not form an ordered arrangement and are randomly structured by a short-range order of repeating units.

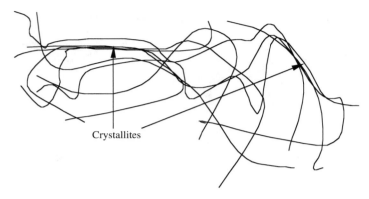

FIGURE 7.3 Crystallites of a semicrystalline polymer.

An amorphous polymer can be thought of as analogous to a bunch of worms moving constantly. An individual segment of the polymer chain moves by single rotation around the bond in the main polymer chain.

7.2 MOLECULAR WEIGHT AND MOLECULAR WEIGHT DISTRIBUTION OF POLYMERS

A simple substance has a uniform and low molecular weight. A polymer molecule, on the contrary, has high and various molecular weights (molecular weight distribution) even though it is made up of the same composition (except in the case of biopolymers, e.g., proteins). The distributed molecular weight of the polymers in a free radical polymerization occurs randomly depending on when and how the growing polymer chains are terminated. In a condensation polymerization, the polymerization is terminated due to the lack of reactive groups or other restrictions. In either case, the final product contains molecules of many different molecular weights.

The molecular weight distribution of the polymers can be represented by plotting the weight fraction of polymer chain length with respect to the polymer chain length or molecular weight, as shown in Figure 7.4. Average molecular weights of polymers are defined and used to characterize the molecular weight properties of the polymers.

The number average degree of polymerization is defined as:

$$\bar{r}_n = \frac{\sum\limits_{n=1}^{\infty} rP_r}{\sum\limits_{n=1}^{\infty} P_r} \tag{7.1}$$

where $\bar{r}_n$ is the number average chain length based on the total number of chains, and P_r is the number of the polymer molecule of chain length r per unit volume. Such quantities are referred to as moments of distribution:

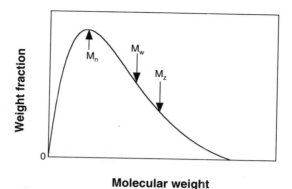

Molecular weight

FIGURE 7.4 Molecular weight distribution of polymers.

$$Q_n = n^{th} \text{ moment of distribution} = \sum_{n=1}^{\infty} r^n P_r \qquad (7.2)$$

Substituting Equation (7.2) into Equation (7.1) yields:

$$\bar{r}_n = \frac{Q_1}{Q_o} \qquad (7.3)$$

or

$$\bar{r}_n = \sum_{n=1}^{\infty} F(r)r \qquad (7.4)$$

where $F(r)$ is the number fraction that has chain length r.

The weight average degree of polymerization, $\bar{r}_w$, is defined as:

$$\bar{r}_w = \frac{\displaystyle\sum_{n=1}^{\infty} r^2 P_r}{\displaystyle\sum_{n=1}^{\infty} r P_r} = \frac{Q_2}{Q_1}, \qquad (7.5)$$

or

$$\bar{r}_w = \sum_{n=1}^{\infty} w(r)r \qquad (7.6)$$

where $w(r)$ is the weight fraction of the chain length r.

Higher average degree of polymerization (no physical meaning) is defined as:

$$\bar{r}_z = \frac{\sum_{n=1}^{\infty} r^3 P_r}{\sum_{n=1}^{\infty} r^2 P_r} = \frac{Q_3}{Q_2} \tag{7.7}$$

In general, $\bar{r}_z > \bar{r}_w > \bar{r}_n$. The polymer properties depend strongly on the molecules that make up the bulk of the weight (e.g., on $\bar{r}_w$ more than $\bar{r}_n$): $\bar{r}_w$ is a more useful parameter as a measure of the polymers. The number average molecular weight and the weight average molecular weight of polymers $\overline{M}_n$ and $\overline{M}_w$ are calculated as:

$$\overline{M}_n = M_o \bar{r}_n \tag{7.8}$$

$$\overline{M}_w = M_o \bar{r}_w \tag{7.9}$$

where M_o is the molecular weight of the repeating unit or monomer. $\overline{M}_n$ and $\overline{M}_w$ can be measured by osmometry and light scattering, respectively (see Section 7.3.2 and Section 7.3.3). It is not proper to characterize polymers with only one molecular weight. The ratio $\overline{M}_w / \overline{M}_n$ is used as a measure of the width of the molecular weight distribution. This ratio is called polydispersity; in practice, its values vary from 1 to $\approx$ 50.

7.3 CHARACTERIZATION OF POLYMERS

The most important physical properties of polymers are their molecular weight and its distribution. Many characteristics of polymers, including solubility, dissolution rate, rigidity, and tensile strength, are dependent on molecular weight. Pharmaceutical scientists should know the molecular weights of the polymers they use or determine them for quality control purposes. In this section, several methods used to determine the molecular weight of polymers will be described.

7.3.1 VISCOSITY METHOD

The viscosity method is the most common and simplest way to determine the molecular weight of a polymer based on the size of the polymer. The method actually measures the size of the polymer in a solution and then relates this size to its molecular weight through a theoretical expression.

The measurement of the size of the polymer is carried out in a capillary viscometer. The presence of polymer molecules in a solvent affects the relative motion of the solvent (i.e., solution viscosity). Even very dilute solutions of polymers are very viscous. When a dilute solution of a polymer travels along a capillary tube, as shown in Figure 7.5, there is a parabolic velocity gradient across the capillary tube with the maximum velocity at the center of the tube and a minimum velocity at the

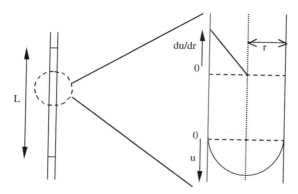

FIGURE 7.5 Capillary viscometer.

wall of the tube. It is assumed that no turbulence exists and that the fluid is a laminar Newtonian.

The volumetric flow rate of laminar Newtonian flow of a liquid through a capillary tube is expressed by Poiseuille's law as:

$$\frac{dQ}{dt} = \frac{\pi r^4 \Delta P}{8\mu L}$$ (7.10)

where dQ/dt is the volume flow rate, r is the radius of the capillary tube, L is the length of the capillary tube, ΔP is the hydrostatic pressure difference between the liquid at positions h_1 and h_2 by the acceleration of the free fall, and μ is the viscosity of the liquid. The time needed, t, for the liquid to fall from h_1 to h_2 is given as:

$$t = \frac{8\mu L}{\pi g \rho r^4} \int_{h_1}^{h_2} \frac{dQ}{h}$$ (7.11)

where ρ is the density of the liquid. For a given viscometer, the total volume of the liquid passing through the capillary tube is constant. Thus Equation (7.11) becomes:

$$t = A \frac{\mu}{\rho}$$ (7.12)

where μ/ρ is the kinematic (dynamic) viscosity, and A is a constant that can be determined by calibration with liquids of known viscosity. However, knowing this constant is not important; a more important concern is addressing the relative change in viscosity when the polymer is added to a solvent. The relative viscosity is defined as:

$$\eta_r = \frac{t}{t_o} \frac{\rho}{\rho_o}$$ (7.13a)

where the subscript o is for the pure solvent. In very dilute solutions of polymers, the density difference between the solution and the solvent is negligible, and Equation (7.13a) is then rewritten as:

$$\eta_r = \frac{t}{t_o} \tag{7.13b}$$

The term specific viscosity is commonly used rather than relative viscosity. The specific viscosity is the increment in viscosity due to the addition of the polymer as:

$$\eta_{sp} = \eta_r - 1 = \frac{t - t_o}{t_o} \tag{7.14}$$

Another term, reduced viscosity, is used to describe the ability of the polymer to increase the viscosity of the solvent ($\eta_{red} = \eta_{sp} / c$, where c is the concentration of the polymer in the solution). The reduced viscosity of a polymer solution directly results from the intermolecular interactions (polymer and solvent molecules). These effects are then eliminated by extrapolating to an infinite dilution. The dependence of the reduced viscosity on the concentration of the polymer solution is given as:

$$\left(\frac{\eta_{sp}}{c} \right) = [\eta] + \alpha c + \alpha^2 c + ... \tag{7.15}$$

where α is a constant and $[\eta]$ is the intrinsic viscosity (or limiting viscosity number) and defined as:

$$[\eta] = \lim_{c \to 0} \frac{\eta_{sp}}{c} \tag{7.16}$$

The intrinsic viscosity is determined graphically by extrapolating the reduced viscosity to zero polymer concentration (c→0), as shown in Figure 7.6.

Table 7.2 presents the equations for the extrapolation of the viscosity data to obtain the intrinsic viscosity. It is common to use the Huggins and Kraemer equations to determine the intrinsic viscosity.

For a given polymer–solvent system, the intrinsic viscosity varies with the molecular weight of the polymer. According to Flory, the intrinsic viscosity is directly proportional to the hydrodynamic volume occupied by the random coil of the polymer molecule in a solution. In addition, the hydrodynamic volume is related to the cube of the typical linear dimension of the random coil (root mean square end-to-end distance). The intrinsic viscosity is expressed as:

$$[\eta] = \Phi \frac{\left(\bar{r}^2 \right)^{3/2}}{M} \tag{7.17}$$

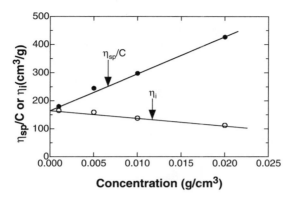

FIGURE 7.6 Determination of the intrinsic viscosity of polyvinylpyrrolidone in 70% isopropyl alcohol at 23°C.

TABLE 7.2
Equations to Determine Intrinsic Viscosity

Huggins equation	$\eta_{sp}/c = [\eta] + k[\eta]^2 c$	Most useful equation
Kraemer equation	$\ln \eta_r / c = [\eta] + k[\eta]^2 c$	Usually used in combination with Huggins equation
Martin equation	$\log(\eta_{sp}/c) = \log[\eta] + k'[\eta]c$	
Schulz–Blanscheke equation	$\eta_{sp}/c = [\eta] + \gamma \eta_{sp}[\eta]$	

Definitions for Viscosity Terms

$\eta_r = \eta/\eta_o = t/t_o,$	$\eta_{sp} = \eta_r - 1,$	$\eta_{red} = \eta_{sp}/c$
$\eta_i = (\ln \eta_r)/c,$	$[\eta] = (\eta_{sp}/c)_{c=0} = (\eta_i)_{c=0}$	

where Φ is a universal constant, M is the molecular weight of the polymer, and $(\bar{r}^2)$ is the mean square end-to-end distance. Φ is a function of the polydispersity, the solvent, and the molar mass. It has a theoretical value of $2.5 \times 10^{25} - 2.8 \times 10^{25}$ when $[\eta]$ is given in dL/g and $(\bar{r}^2)^{1/2}$ is in cm. The root mean square end-to-end radius is:

$$\left(\bar{r}^2\right)^{1/2} = \beta\left(\bar{r}_o^2\right)^{1/2} \tag{7.18}$$

where $(\bar{r}_o^2)^{1/2}$ is the unperturbed root mean square end-to-end distance and β is the linear expansion factor. The expansion factor is calculated by:

$$\beta^3 = \frac{[\eta]}{[\eta]_\Theta} \tag{7.19}$$

where $[\eta]_\Theta$ is the intrinsic viscosity measured at the theta temperature at which the polymer chain attains its unperturbed dimension.

Since $(\bar{r}_o^2)^{1/2} \propto n^{1/2} \propto M^{1/2}$, where n is the number of links in the polymer chains, $(\bar{r}_o^2)^{1/2} / M$ is independent of the environmental conditions of the system (i.e., solvent, temperature, and molecular weight) and only dependent on the chain structure (i.e., bond angles, flexibility). Equation (7.17) is written:

$$[\eta] = \Phi \left(\frac{\bar{r}_o^2}{M} \right)^{3/2} M^{1/2} \beta^3 \tag{7.20}$$

$$= KM^{1/2}\beta^3$$

where $K = \Phi(\bar{r}_o^2 / M)^{3/2}$ is a constant for a given polymer–solvent system and varies with temperature. In a theta solvent, $\beta = 1$ and Equation (7.20) becomes:

$$[\eta]_\Theta = KM^{1/2} \tag{7.21}$$

For a nontheta temperature and solvent, the expansion factor is dependent on the molecular weight:

$$\beta^5 - \beta^3 = C'M^{1/2}(1 - \Theta / T) \tag{7.22}$$

where C' is a constant and Θ is the theta temperature. When $\beta \gg 1$, $\beta^5 \gg \beta^3$ and β^3 can be approximated to $M^{0.3}$. In general,

$$\beta^3 = M^\varepsilon \tag{7.23}$$

where ε is a constant ranging from 0 for the theta temperature to 0.3 for a good solvent. Equation (7.20) can be rewritten by:

$$[\eta] = KM^a \tag{7.24}$$

where a is a constant ranging from 0.5 to 0.8. Equation (7.24) is called the Mark–Houwink equation. Typical values of K and a are shown in Table 7.3. The molecular weight obtained by the intrinsic viscosity method is more closely related to the weight average molecular weight ($\overline{M}_w$) than the number average molecular weight ($\overline{M}_n$).

7.3.2 OSMOMETRY

As shown in Figure 7.7, a semipermeable membrane, which is permeable to a solvent but impermeable to a solute, separates the two compartments. If a pure solvent is in both compartments, A and B, the chemical potentials in both compartments are

TABLE 7.3
Mark–Houwink Parameters for Polymer–Solvent Combinations

Polymer	Temperature (°C)	Solvent	a	K(mL/g) × 10⁻³
Alginic acid, Na salt	25	Aq. NaCl (0.2M)	1.0	7.97
Cellulose acetate (DS 0.49)	25	Dimethylacetamide	0.60	191
Cellulose triacetate	25	Acetone	0.82	14.9
Ethyl cellulose	25	Chloroform	0.89	11.8
Hydroxyethyl cellulose	25	Water	0.87	9.53
Methyl cellulose (DS 1.74)	25	Water	0.55	316
Na carboxymethylcellulose (DS 1.06)	25	Aq. NaCl (0.2M)	0.74	43
Polyethylene oxide	35	Water	0.82	640
Poly(vinyl acetate)	30	Acetone	0.72	12
Poly(vinyl alcohol),100%	25	Water	0.63	0.595
Poly(vinyl pyrrolidone)	25	Water	0.55	56.5

Source: Taken from J. Brandrup and E. H. Immergut (Eds.), *Polymer Handbook,* 4th Ed., John Wiley and Sons, New York, 1995.

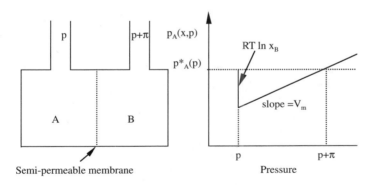

FIGURE 7.7 Osmosis.

equal (also see Chapter 3). When a small amount of the solute is added to compartment B, the chemical potential of the solvent in compartment B is reduced, and the solvent in compartment A starts moving toward compartment B through the membrane until a new equilibrium is reached, thus producing an osmotic pressure in compartment B. When equilibrium is reached, the chemical potentials of the solvent in both compartments are equal:

$$\mu_A^*(p) = \mu_A(x_A, \pi + p) \tag{7.25}$$

where π, p, and x_A are the osmotic pressure, the experimental pressure, and the solute concentration, respectively, and μ_A^* and μ_A are the chemical potentials of the pure solvent and the concentrated solution, respectively. Equation (7.25) is rewritten in terms of the pure solvent as:

$$\mu_A(x_A, \pi + p) = \mu_A^*(\pi + p) + RT \ln x_B$$
$$= \mu_A^*(p) + \int_p^{\pi+p} V_m dp \tag{7.26}$$

where R, T, and V_m are the gas constant, temperature, and volume of solvent, respectively. Therefore, one can obtain:

$$-RT \ln(1 - x_A) = \int_p^{\pi+p} V_m dp \tag{7.27}$$

For dilute solutions, $\ln(1 - x_A) = -x_A$. If the molar volume of the solvent is constant, Equation (7.27) becomes:

$$\frac{\pi}{c} = \frac{RT}{M} \tag{7.28}$$

where M and c are the molecular weight of solute and the solute concentration, respectively. Since π is dependent on the number of molecules, $\overline{M}_n$ can be calculated from Equation (7.28).

Equation (7.28) is applicable only to infinite dilution of simple molecules, as illustrated in Chapter 3. At finite polymer concentrations, the osmotic pressure can be expressed as a power series:

$$\frac{\pi}{c} = RT\left[\frac{1}{\overline{M}_n} + A_2 c + A_3 c^2 + \ldots\right] \tag{7.29}$$

where A_2 and A_3 are the second and third virial coefficients, respectively.

A plot of π/c vs. c yields a straight line with a y-intercept of $RT/\overline{M}_n$, as shown in Figure 7.8, in which one can determine the number average molecular weight of the polymer. This method can be used to determine molecular weights ranging from 10,000 to 500,000 daltons. The method is less sensitive for very high molecular weights, and very-low-molecular-weight polymers pass through the membrane.

7.3.3 LIGHT SCATTERING

When a beam of light travels through matter, light is scattered in all directions, as shown in Figure 7.9. In polymer solutions, the polymer molecules scatter more light than the solvent does. When the amplitude (intensity) of scattered light is proportional to the mass of the scattering particle, the weight average molecular weight ($\overline{M}_w$) is thus obtained. The intensity of scattered light at some angle, R_θ, is given by:

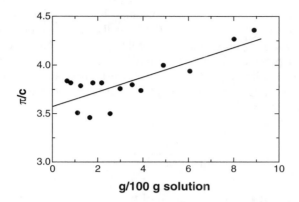

FIGURE 7.8 Determination of number average molecular weight by osmometry. [Graph reconstructed from data by Roughton and Kendrew, *Haemoglobin*, Butterworth, London, 1949, p. 197.]

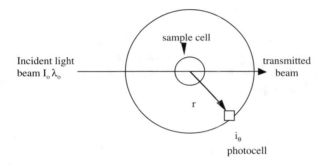

FIGURE 7.9 Rayleigh scattering.

$$R_\theta = i_\theta r^2 / I_o \tag{7.30}$$

where i_θ, I_o, and r are the scattered light intensity at angle θ, the intensity of the incidental beam, and the distance from the scattering center, respectively.

For an ideal solution of small molecules, the number of scattering centers per unit volume is related to the concentration of the solute as follows:

$$\frac{Kc}{\overline{R}_\theta} = \frac{1}{M} \tag{7.31}$$

where $\overline{R}_\theta$ is the excess Rayleigh scattering [$= R_{\theta(\text{solution})} - R_{\theta(\text{solvent})}$], M is the molar mass, and K is the optical constant:

$$K = \frac{2\pi^2 n^2}{\lambda^4 N} \left(\frac{\partial n}{\partial c}\right)^2 \tag{7.32a}$$

where n is the refractive index of the solvent, λ is the wavelength of the incidental beam, N is Avogadro's number, and $\partial n / \partial c$ is the refractive index increment.

Equation (7.31) requires the particle to be small when compared to λ (<0.05λ). However, most polymer molecules are larger than this, at least in one dimension. The size differences introduce path length and result in phase differences in different parts of the molecules (dissymmetry). This interference decreases the intensity at an angle of 0°. Equation (7.31) is modified to:

$$\frac{Kc}{\overline{R}_\theta} = \frac{1}{P(\theta)}\left[\frac{1}{M_w} + 2A_2c + 3A_3c^2 + ...\right] \tag{7.32b}$$

where A_2 and A_3 are the second and third virial coefficients, respectively, and $P(\theta)$ is the particle scattering factor describing the angular dependence of scattering:

$$\frac{1}{P(\theta)} = 1 + \frac{16\pi^2}{3\lambda^2} <s^2> \sin^2(\theta/2) \tag{7.33}$$

where $<s^2>$ is the radius of gyration of the polymer molecule. In general, $P(\theta)$ is difficult to estimate and depends on the shape of the particles (e.g., random coil, rod, disc). If $P(\theta) = 1$, there is no interference. Combining Equation (7.32) and Equation (7.33) yields:

$$\frac{Kc}{\overline{R}_\theta} = \frac{1}{M_w}\left[1 + \frac{16\pi^2}{3\lambda^2} <s^2> \sin^2(\theta/2)\right] + 2A_2c \tag{7.34}$$

The excess Rayleigh intensity is dependent on the concentration of the polymer and the angle. To determine the weight average molecular weight of the polymer, a Zimm plot can be used, as shown in Figure 7.10. From the grid points, extrapolate to zero concentration first and then, to zero angle. This results in $(Kc/\overline{R}_\theta)_{c=\theta=0} = 1/\overline{M}_w$. The k in the x-coordinate ($\sin^2\theta/2 + kc$) is an arbitrarily assigned number to maintain reasonable space between the points. The radius of gyration and the second virial coefficient are obtained from the zero concentration extrapolation and the zero angle extrapolation lines, respectively. When the low angle (θ) gets closer to 0° (about <5°), the sine term is very close to 0, and Equation (7.34) becomes:

$$\frac{Kc}{\overline{R}_\theta} = \frac{1}{M_w} + 2A_2c \tag{7.35}$$

If a light scattering instrument provides very low angle measurements (low angle laser light scattering photometer, LALLSP), it avoids the extrapolation of light scattering data to zero angle. For low polymer concentrations (i.e., less than 10^{-4} g/mL), the term with the second virial coefficient is negligible. Equation (7.34) then becomes:

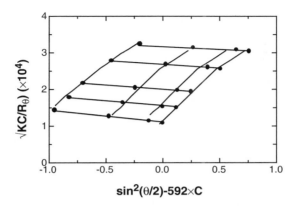

FIGURE 7.10 Zimm plot for a berry-starch. [Graph reconstructed from data by Wyeth Corporation, Application Brochure (Biopolymers), 1999.]

$$\frac{Kc}{R_\theta} = \frac{1}{M_w}\left[1 + \frac{16\pi^2}{3\lambda^2} <s^2> \sin^2(\theta/2)\right] \qquad (7.36)$$

Equation (7.36) is known as the Debye plot. Figure 7.11a and Figure 7.11b show the excess Rayleigh scattering intensities of polyacrylamide from MALLSP (multi angle laser light scattering photometer) and LALLSP, respectively.

7.3.4 SIZE EXCLUSION CHROMATOGRAPHY (SEC)

The methods described in the previous sections determine the average values of the polymer molecular weight in a dilute solution. The properties of the polymer depend on the distribution of molecular weight and molecular average. Size exclusion chromatography (SEC) is a method in which the polymer molecules in a dilute solution flow through packed porous beads and are separated according to their size. The large molecules do not penetrate the inner pores of the beads and are eluted before the smaller molecules, as shown in Figure 7.12. However, the exact molecular weights of the separated polymers are unknown since the polymers are being separated by their size (not their molecular weight). To find out the molecular weight, one should calibrate the SEC. Assume the molecular weight calibration curve, M(v), is given by

$$M(v) = D_1 \exp(-D_2 v) \qquad (7.37)$$

where D_1 and D_2 are the intercept and the slope of the calibration curve, respectively, and v is the retention volume.

The molecular weights and the molecular weight distributions of the samples can be determined as follows:

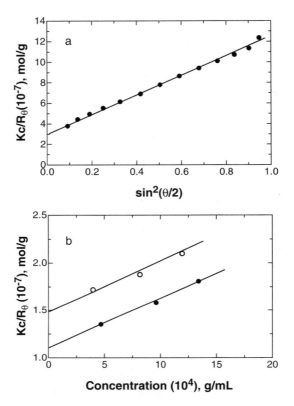

FIGURE 7.11 Excess Rayleigh scattering intensities of a polyacrylamide from (a) MALLSP and (b) LALLSP. [Graphs reconstructed from data by Wyeth Corp. and Kim, Ph.D. dissertation, McMaster University, Hamilton, Ontario, 1984.]

1. A standard calibration curve is constructed by injecting standards or samples of known molecular weight (most likely molecular weight at a peak retention volume), as shown in Figure 7.13a.
2. The chromatogram of the unknown sample is obtained as shown in Figure 7.13b. If the detector response, $F_c(v)$, is independent of molecular size, then the response is proportional to concentration:

$$F_c(v) \propto C(v) \tag{7.38}$$

The weight fraction of polymer in $v - (v + dv)$ is $F(v)dv$, and given as:

$$F(v)dv = \frac{C(v)dv}{\int_{V_A}^{V_B} C(v)dv} = \frac{F_c(v)dv}{\int_{V_A}^{V_B} F_c(v)dv} = \frac{F_c(v)}{\sum F_c(v)}, \quad \int F(v)dv = 1 \tag{7.39}$$

where $F(v)$ is the normalized detector response.

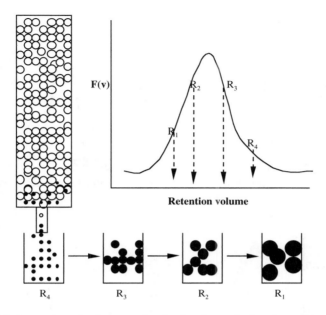

FIGURE 7.12 Separation of polymer molecules by size exclusion chromatography.

3. Converting the weight fraction in v – (v + dv) to a weight fraction in M – (M + dM) or ln M – (ln M + dln M) gives:

$$-F(v)\, dv = W(M)\, dM = W(\ln M)\, d\ln M$$

or

$$W(M) = -\frac{F(v)}{dM/dv}; \qquad W(\ln M) = -\frac{F(v)}{d\ln M/dv} \qquad (7.40)$$

Figure 7.13c shows the transformed chromatogram of W(ln M) vs. ln M. The cumulative weight in range M at the retention volume V_B is given by:

$$\mathrm{cumW(M)} = \int_{V_B}^{V} F(v)\, dv \qquad (7.41)$$

The molecular averages are determined as:

$$\overline{M}_i(\mathrm{uc}) = \frac{\int F(v) M(v)^{i-1}\, dv}{\int F(v) M(v)^{i-2}\, dv} \qquad (7.42)$$

where $\overline{M}_i(\mathrm{uc})$ is the *i*th average molecular weight of the whole polymer that is uncorrected for the imperfect resolution due to instrumental spreading.

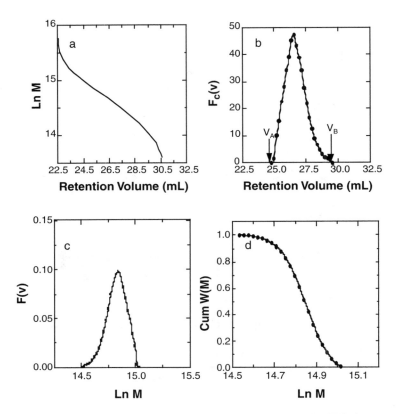

FIGURE 7.13 Analysis of SEC chromatogram: (a) calibration curve; (b) SEC chromatogram; (c) molecular weight distribution; (d) cumulative molecular weight distribution.

The corrected (true) detector response for an imperfect resolution, W(y), can be written as:

$$F(v) = \int_0^\infty W(y)\, G(v, y)\, dy \tag{7.43}$$

where G(v,y) is the instrumental spreading function. The molecular averages are expressed as:

$$\frac{\overline{M}_i(uc)}{\overline{M}_i(c)} = \frac{\displaystyle\int_0^\infty F(v)M(v)^{i-1}\,dv \,/\, \int_0^\infty F(v)M(v)^{i-2}\,dv}{\displaystyle\int_0^\infty W(v)M(v)^{i-1}\,dv \,/\, \int_0^\infty W(v)M(v)^{i-2}\,dv} \tag{7.44}$$

where $\overline{M}_i(c)$ is the ith molecular weight average corrected for imperfect resolution. Substituting Equation (7.37) into Equation (7.44) and taking the Laplace transform of the resulting equation yields:

$$\frac{\overline{M}_i(uc)}{\overline{M}_i(c)} = \frac{\overline{F}(-D_2(i-1))\overline{W}(-D_2(i-2))}{\overline{W}(-D_2(i-1))\overline{F}(-D_2(i-2))} \tag{7.45}$$

where $\overline{W}$ and $\overline{F}$ are the bilateral Laplace transforms of W and F, respectively. When the instrumental spreading function is Gaussian and has a variance of σ^2, Equation (7.45) becomes:

$$\frac{\overline{M}_i(uc)}{\overline{M}_i(c)} = \exp[(2i-3)(D_2\sigma)^2 / 2] \tag{7.46}$$

The right-hand-side term of the above equation is the correction factor for the ith molecular weight average due to the instrumental spreading. Once the slope of the calibration curve and the variance of the instrumental spreading function are known, the corrected molecular averages can be determined from Equation (7.46). There are several methods for the calibration of size exclusion chromatography in order to obtain the true molecular weight distribution and the molecular weight averages, as follows.

7.3.4.1 Effective Linear Calibration Method without Peak Broadening Correction

This method requires a broad molecular weight standard with known $\overline{M}_n$ and $\overline{M}_w$. It is very simple and assumes that there is no peak broadening:

$$F(v) = W(v) \tag{7.47}$$

where $F(v)$ and $W(v)$ are the uncorrected and corrected detector responses for peak broadening, respectively. Therefore,

$$\overline{M}_i(uc) = \overline{M}_i(c) \tag{7.48}$$

Then,
$$\overline{M}_n(c) = \left(\int_0^\infty F(v)M(v)^{-1}dv \right)^{-1} \tag{7.49}$$

and
$$\overline{M}_w(c) = \int_0^\infty F(v)M(v)dv \tag{7.50}$$

Incorporating Equation (7.37) into Equation (7.49) and Equation (7.50) leads to:

$$\frac{\overline{M}_w(c)}{\overline{M}_n(c)} = \left(\int_0^\infty F(v)M(v)dv \right)\left(\int_0^\infty F(v)M(v)^{-1}dv \right) \tag{7.51}$$

There is one unknown (D_2) in Equation (7.51), which can be determined by a single-variable search technique. Once D_2 is known, the intercept of the calibration curve, D_1, is determined by:

$$\overline{M}_n(c) = D_1\left(\int_0^\infty F(v)e^{D_2 v}dv\right)^{-1} \tag{7.52a}$$

or

$$\overline{M}_w(c) = D_1\int_0^\infty F(v)e^{-D_2 v}dv \tag{7.52b}$$

However, both $\overline{M}_n$ and $\overline{M}_w$ are unknown for most broad molecular weight standards and either $\overline{M}_n$ or $\overline{M}_w$ is known. When using two broad molecular weight standards with known $\overline{M}_n$ or $\overline{M}_w$, D_2 is determined from Equation (7.53):

$$\frac{\overline{M}_{n_1}(c)}{\overline{M}_{n_2}(c)} = \frac{\int_0^\infty F_2(v)e^{D_2 v}dv}{\int_0^\infty F_1(v)e^{D_2 v}{}_1dv} \quad or \quad \frac{\overline{M}_{w_1}(c)}{\overline{M}_{w_2}(c)} = \frac{\int_0^\infty F_1(v)e^{-D_2 v}dv}{\int_0^\infty F_2(v)e^{-D_2 v}dv} \tag{7.53}$$

Then, D_1 is obtained:

$$\overline{M}_{n_1}(c) = D_1 / \int_0^\infty F_1(v)e^{D_2 v}dv \qquad \overline{M}_{n_2}(c) = D_1 / \int_0^\infty F_2(v)e^{D_2 v}dv \tag{7.54a}$$

or

$$\overline{M}_{w_1}(c) = D_1\int_0^\infty F_1(v)e^{-D_2 v}dv \qquad \overline{M}_{w_{21}}(c) = D_1\int_0^\infty F_2(v)e^{-D_2 v}dv \tag{7.54b}$$

Example 7.1.
Determine the number and the weight average molecular weights of the data (first and second columns) in Table 7.4.

Solution
$M(v) = 4.742 \times 10^{13} \exp(-1.37v)$ was used for the molecular weight calibration curve. The second column has been normalized according to Equation (7.39). The number average and the weight average molecular weights are given as:

$$\overline{M}_n = \left(\int F(v)/M(v)dv\right)^{-1} \qquad \overline{M}_w = \int F(v)M(v)dv$$

From fourth and fifth columns, $\overline{M}_n = 5.81\times10^5$ and $\overline{M}_w = 2.01\times10^6$. The polydispersity ($=\overline{M}_w/\overline{M}_n$) is 3.46.

TABLE 7.4
Molecular Weight Calculation

Volume	F(v)	M(v)	F(v)/M(v)	F(v)×M(v)
10.917	0.0041	15,154,000	2.76e–10	63,300
11.083	0.0125	12,071,470	1.04e–09	151,000
11.249	0.0161	9,615,964	1.67e–09	155,000
11.416	0.0245	7,649,457	3.20e–09	187,000
11.583	0.0317	6,085,109	5.21e–09	193,000
11.749	0.0394	4,847,314	8.13e–09	191,000
11.916	0.0478	3,856,017	1.24e–08	184,000
12.083	0.0502	3,067,444	1.64e–08	154,000
12.249	0.0573	2,443,484	2.35e–08	140,000
12.416	0.0645	1,943,780	3.32e–08	125,000
12.582	0.0711	1,548,388	4.59e–08	110,000
12.748	0.0759	1,233,425	6.15e–08	93,600
12.915	0.0777	981,183	7.92e–08	76,200
13.082	0.0759	780,527	9.72e–08	59,200
13.249	0.0687	620,906	1.11e–07	42,700
13.415	0.0639	494,605	1.29e–07	31,600
13.582	0.0538	393,456	1.37e–07	21,200
13.748	0.0466	313,421	1.49e–07	14,600
13.915	0.0358	249,325	1.44e–07	8,930
14.082	0.0287	198,337	1.45e–07	5,690
14.248	0.0203	157,992	1.28e–07	3,210
14.415	0.0125	125,682	9.95e–08	1,570
14.581	0.0077	100,117	7.76e–08	778
14.748	0.0047	79,642	6.00e–08	381
14.915	0.0041	63,355	6.60e–08	265
15.081	0.0030	50,468	5.92e–08	151
15.248	0.0012	40,147	2.96e–08	48
	1.000		1.72e–06	2.01e+06
	↑		↑	↑
	$\sum F(v)$		$\sum F(v)/M(v)$	$\sum F(v) \times M(v)$

7.3.4.2 Effective Linear Calibration Method with Peak Broadening Correction

This method requires two broad molecular weight standards with known $\overline{M}_n$ and $\overline{M}_w$. The method (1) described above does not provide the true calibration curve but it does provide an effective one. This method allows the determination of D_1, D_2, and σ. It is assumed that the variance of the peak broadening, σ, is independent of the molecular weight (or retention volume). Combining Equation (7.37), Equation (7.42), and Equation (7.46) yields:

$$\overline{M}_{n_1}(c) = D_1 \exp\left[\frac{(D_2\sigma)^2}{2}\right] \bigg/ \int_0^\infty F_1(v)e^{D_2 v}dv \qquad (7.55a)$$

$$\overline{M}_{n_2}(c) = D_1 \exp\left[\frac{(D_2\sigma)^2}{2}\right] \bigg/ \int_0^\infty F_2(v)e^{D_2 v}dv \qquad (7.55b)$$

$$\overline{M}_{w_1}(c) = D_1 \exp\left[-\frac{(D_2\sigma)^2}{2}\right] \times \int_0^\infty F_1(v)e^{-D_2 v}dv \qquad (7.55c)$$

$$\overline{M}_{w_2}(c) = D_1 \exp\left[-\frac{(D_2\sigma)^2}{2}\right] \times \int_0^\infty F_2(v)e^{-D_2 v}dv \qquad (7.55d)$$

When Equation (7.55a) through Equation (7.55d) are cross–multiplied, they yield Equation (7.56):

$$\frac{\overline{M}_{w_1}(c)\overline{M}_{n_2}(c)}{\overline{M}_{n_1}(c)\overline{M}_{w_2}(c)} = \frac{\int_0^\infty F_1(v)e^{-D_2 v}dv \int_0^\infty F_1(v)e^{D_2 v}dv}{\int_0^\infty F_2(v)e^{-D_2 v}dv \int_0^\infty F_2(v)e^{D_2 v}dv} \qquad (7.56)$$

The parameter D_2 is obtained by a single-variable search technique as determined from Equation (7.51). Then, σ is obtained by:

$$\frac{\overline{M}_{w_1}(c)}{\overline{M}_{n_1}(c)} = \exp\left[-(D_2\sigma)^2\right] \int_0^\infty F_1(v)e^{-D_2 v}dv \int_0^\infty F_1(v)e^{D_2 v}dv \qquad (7.57)$$

D_2 and σ are substituted into one equation of Equation (7.55a) through Equation (7.55d) to obtain D_1.

7.3.4.3 Universal Calibration Method

Since size exclusion chromatography separates polymer molecules by their size (especially hydrodynamic size), plotting the molecular size vs. the retention volume should be universal, regardless of the polymer molecular weight. The universal calibration curve is given as:

$$J(v) = [\eta](v)M(v) \qquad (7.58)$$

where $J(v)$ and $[\eta](v)$ are the hydrodynamic volume of the polymer molecules in the eluent solvent and the intrinsic viscosity at the retention volume v, respectively. The universal calibration curve is constructed with a narrow molecular weight distribution (MWD) of polystyrene standard in most cases. If the Mark–Houwink equation of the polymer in question is known, the molecular weight calibration curve is determined as follows:

$$J_{ps}(v) = [\eta]_{ps}(v)M_{ps}(v) = J_x(v) = [\eta]_x(v)M_x(v) \tag{7.59}$$

where the subscripts ps and x denote the polystyrene and the polymer in question, respectively. The molecular weight calibration curve of the polymer is:

$$M_x(v) = \left(\frac{[\eta]_{ps}(v)M_{ps}(v)}{K} \right)^{\beta} \tag{7.60}$$

where $\beta = 1/(a + 1)$ and a and K are the Mark–Houwink constants for the polymer.

If the Mark–Houwink constants of the polymer are unknown, then the two broad MWD standards method, with known $\overline{M}_n$ and $\overline{M}_w$, is used. The molecular weight averages of the two polymer standards are expressed as:

$$\overline{M}_{n_1}(c) = \alpha \, \exp\left[\frac{(D_2\sigma_1)^2}{2} \right] \left[\int_0^{\infty} F_1(v)J(v)^{-\beta} dv \right]^{-1} \tag{7.61a}$$

$$\overline{M}_{w_1}(c) = \alpha \, \exp\left[-\frac{(D_2\sigma_1)^2}{2} \right] \left[\int_0^{\infty} F_1(v)J(v)^{-\beta} dv \right] \tag{7.61b}$$

where σ_1 is the variance of the peak broadening for standard 1 and $\alpha = K^{-\beta}$. Combining Equation (7.61a) and Equation (7.61b) eliminates the term $(D_2\sigma_1)$:

$$\overline{M}_{n_1}(c)\overline{M}_{w_1}(c) = K^{-2\beta} \left[\int_0^{\infty} F_1(v)J(v)^{\beta} dv \Big/ \int_0^{\infty} F_1(v)J(v)^{-\beta} dv \right] \tag{7.62}$$

Likewise, one can obtain a similar equation for standard 2, which eliminates the term K and yields:

$$\frac{\overline{M}_{n_1}(c)\overline{M}_{w_1}(c)}{\overline{M}_{n_2}(c)\overline{M}_{w_2}(c)} = \frac{\displaystyle\int_0^{\infty} F_1(v)J(v)^{\beta} dv \int_0^{\infty} F_2(v)J(v)^{-\beta} dv}{\displaystyle\int_0^{\infty} F_2(v)J(v)^{\beta} dv \int_0^{\infty} F_2(v)J(v)^{-\beta} dv} \tag{7.63}$$

β is obtained from Equation (7.63) by a single-variable search technique. Then, substituting β into Equation (7.62) gives K. $D_2\sigma_1$ and $D_2\sigma_2$ are calculated from Equation (7.61b) and the similar equation for standard 2, respectively. Once K and β (or a) are known, the slope of the calibration curve, D_2, is obtained from Equation (7.60). If the universal calibration based on polystyrene standards is expressed as:

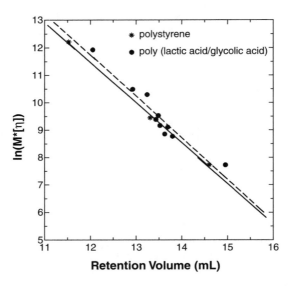

FIGURE 7.14 Universal calibration curve in tetrahydrofuran. [Graph reconstructed from data by Kenley et al., *Macromolecules,* 20, 2403 (1987).]

$$\log\left\{ [\eta]_{ps}(v)M_{ps}(v)\right\} = A + Bv \tag{7.64a}$$

then
$$D_2 = -2.303B\,\beta \tag{7.64b}$$

and
$$D_1 = 10^{A\beta}K^{-\beta} \tag{7.64c}$$

Figure 7.14 shows the universal calibration curve in tetrahydrofuran.

7.3.4.4 Multiple Detector System (e.g., Concentration and Light-Scattering Detectors)

The methods described so far use a single concentration detector, which may be an ultraviolet (UV) detector or a differential refractometer (DRI). A calibration curve is required to obtain the average molecular weights and the molecular weight distribution. When a concentration detector (e.g., UV or DRI) is used with an absolute detector (e.g., light scattering), the true molecular weight average is:

$$\overline{M}_w(c) = \int_0^\infty F(v)\overline{M}_w(v, uc)dv \tag{7.65}$$

where $\overline{M}_w(v, uc)$ is the weight average molecular weight measured by SEC using a DRI (or UV) and a light-scattering detector (LALLSP or MALLSP) with no peak broadening at the retention volume v. $\overline{M}_n(v, uc)$ is calculated using Equation (7.66):

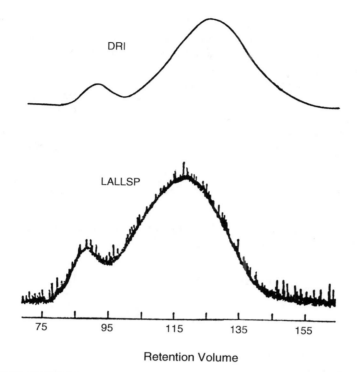

DRI

LALLSP

| | | | | |
| 75 | 95 | 115 | 135 | 155 |

Retention Volume

FIGURE 7.15 SEC/DRI/LALLSP chromatograms of dextran T150. [Reprinted from Kim, Ph.D. dissertation, McMaster University, Hamilton, Ontario, 1984.]

$$\overline{M}_n(v, uc) = \overline{M}_w(v, uc) \frac{F(v)^2}{F\left(v + D(v)\sigma(v)^2\right)F\left(v - D(v)\sigma(v)^2\right)\exp[-(D(v)\sigma(v))^2]} \quad (7.66)$$

Then,

$$\overline{M}_n(c) = \left(\int_0^\infty F(v)\overline{M}_n(v, uc)^{-1}dv\right)^{-1} \quad (7.67)$$

Figure 7.15 shows SEC/DRI/LALLSP chromatograms of dextran T150 in water at the mobile phase. It has been demonstrated that an online light-scattering detector can easily detect the effects of protein aggregation whereas the trimer peak is not easily detected by the single DRI or UV detector alone.

7.4 POLYMER SYNTHESIS

7.4.1 ADDITION HOMO-POLYMERIZATION (FREE-RADICAL HOMO-POLYMERIZATION)

The free radical addition polymerization process is commonly used to synthesize polymers for pharmaceutical applications. In this type of polymerization, four reactions take place simultaneously: initiation, propagation, chain transfer, and termination. In the initiation reaction, a monomer molecule is activated by a primary radical, which is formed by the decomposition of the initiator. This initiator is either a peroxide or an azo compound.

or

$$P - N = N - P \rightarrow 2P - N^* \tag{7.68}$$

$$I \rightarrow 2R_c^* \tag{7.69}$$

where I is the initiator and R_c^* is the primary radical. The primary radicals formed react with the monomer M (i.e., initiation).

$$R_c^* + CH_2 = CHX \rightarrow R_c - CH_2 - C^*HX$$

$$R_c^* + M \rightarrow R_1^* \tag{7.70}$$

where R_1^* is the growing radical with one monomer unit.

The rate of initiation R_I is:

$$R_I = k_{pc}[R_c^*][M] \tag{7.71}$$

where k_{pc} is the initiation rate constant. The change of the primary radical generated from the initiator is:

$$\frac{d[R_c^*]}{dt} = 2k_d[I] - k_{pc}[M][R_c^*] \tag{7.72}$$

where k_d is the initiator decomposition rate constant. However, the rate of change of the concentration in the primary radical is very small and set to 0 (stationary-state hypothesis; Figure 7.16). Then,

$$2k_d[I] = k_{pc}[M][R_c^*] \quad \text{or} \quad [R_c^*] = \frac{2k_d[I]}{k_{pc}[M]} \tag{7.73}$$

The decomposition of the initiator in a free-radical polymerization is assumed to be a first-order rate:

$$I = [I]_o e^{-k_d t} \tag{7.74}$$

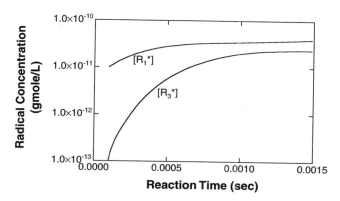

FIGURE 7.16 Stationary-state condition of free-radical concentration. (60% styrene, 0.1% AIBN, and 65°C). [Graph reconstructed from A. Hamielec, *Polymer Reaction Engineering: An Intensive Short Course on Polymer Production Technology,* McMaster University, Hamilton, Ontario, 1980.]

where $[I]_o$ is the initial initiator concentration. However, every mole of primary radical formed from the initiator does not produce a growing polymer chain. Substituting Equation (7.73) and Equation (7.74) into Equation (7.71) yields:

$$R_I = 2f\,k_d[I]_o\,e^{-k_d t} \tag{7.75}$$

where f is the initiator efficiency factor. It describes the reaction of a radical with a monomer to form a polymer radical.

In the propagation reaction, a monomer is added to the growing polymer radical (this is a chain growth step):

$$[CH_2 - C^*HX]_r + CH_2 = CHX \rightarrow [CH_2 - C^*HX]_{r+1}$$

$$R_r^* + M \rightarrow R_{r+1}^* \tag{7.76}$$

The rate of propagation (or rate of polymer production), R_p, is:

$$R_p = -\frac{d[M]}{dt} = k_p[M]\sum_{r=1}^{\infty}[R_r^*] \tag{7.77}$$

where k_p is the propagation rate constant and R_r^* is the growing polymer radical with r repeating units. If k_p is 500 *l*/mole/sec and [M] is 10 mole/*l*, then 5000 monomers are added per second. Based on how the growing polymer radical reacts with the monomer (such as head to head or head to tail), three types of structural tacticity can be formed: isotactic, syndiotactic, and atactic. In a free-radical polymerization, atactic polymers are often formed. Stereoregular polymers (syndiotactic or isotactic) can be formed using special catalysts (e.g., Ziegler-Natta polymerization). The propagation reaction is highly exothermic (≈ 20 kcal/mole). This must be taken into consideration when designing a polymer reactor.

The growing polymer chain may react with stable molecules present in the polymerization system: initiator, solvent, monomer, polymer, and chain transfer agent. In chain transfer reactions, the growing polymer chain loses the radicals to the other molecules to form the shorter polymer chains (i.e., dead polymers). For a chain transfer to monomer,

$$-CH_2 - C^*HX + CH_2 = CHX \rightarrow -CH = CHX + CH_2 - C^*HX$$

or
$$R_r^* + M \rightarrow P_r + R_1^* \tag{7.78}$$

The rate of chain transfer to monomer, R_{fm}, is given as:

$$R_{fm} = k_{fm}[R_r^*][M] \tag{7.79}$$

where k_{fm} is the rate constant of chain transfer to monomer. Similarly, the rate of chain transfer to other molecules such as solvent (R_{fs}), initiator (R_{fi}), transfer agent (R_{fa}), and polymer (R_{fp}) can be expressed as:

$$R_r^* + S \rightarrow P_r + S^*$$

$$R_p = k_p[R_r^*][S] \tag{7.80a}$$

$$R_r^* + I \rightarrow P_r + I^*$$

$$R_{fi} = k_{fi}[R_r^*][I] \tag{7.80b}$$

$$R_r^* + A \rightarrow P_r + A^*$$

$$R_{fa} = k_{fa}[R_r^*][A] \tag{7.80c}$$

$$R_r^* + P_s \rightarrow P_r + P_s^*$$

$$R_{fa} = k_{fp}[R_r^*][P_s] \tag{7.80d}$$

where k_{fs}, k_{fi}, k_{fa}, and k_{fp} are the rate constants for chain transfer to solvent, initiator, transfer agent, and polymer, respectively.

The growing polymer chains (radicals) are terminated by a bimolecular coupling reaction between two radicals. There are two possible terminations: combination and disproportionation. In combination, two radicals react to form a single bond by pairing the electrons:

$$R_r^* + R_s^* \rightarrow P_{r+s}$$

$$R_{tc} = k_{tc}[R_r^*][R_s^*] \tag{7.81}$$

where R_{tc} and k_{tc} are the rate of termination by combination and the rate constant, respectively. In disproportionation, a hydrogen is transferred from one growing chain to another and a double bond is formed in the chain that loses the hydrogen:

$$R_r^* + R_s^* \rightarrow P_r + P_s$$

$$R_{td} = k_{td}[R_r^*][R_s^*] \tag{7.82}$$

where R_{td} and k_{td} are the rate of termination by disproportionation and the rate constant, respectively. Relative importance of the termination by combination or by disproportionation can be seen from the molecular weight distribution and polydispersity of the polymer formed. If there is no distinction between the terminations by combination and disproportionation, the rate of termination (R_t) is expressed as:

$$R_r^* + R_s^* \rightarrow P$$

$$R_t = k_t[R_r^*][R_s^*] \tag{7.83}$$

where $k_t = k_{tc} + k_{td}$.

Equations (7.75), (7.77), (7.79), (7.80a) to (7.80c), (7.81), and (7.82) are used to calculate the rate of polymer production and the molecular weight distribution (and average molecular weight) of the polymer, assuming that:

1. The rate constants are independent of growing radical size $k_{p1} = k_{p2} = \ldots\ldots\ldots = k_{pr} = k_p$. k_{tc} and k_{td} are independent of values of r and s.
2. If the polymers have long chains, then the consumption of the monomer in polymerization, other than propagation, is negligible (long chain approximation):

$$R_p = -\frac{d[M]}{dt} = k_p[M]\sum_{r=1}^{\infty}[R_r^*] \tag{7.84}$$

3. The stationary-state approximation is applicable to all radical species:

$$\frac{d[R_1^*]}{dt} = \frac{d[R_2^*]}{dt} = \cdots\cdots\cdots = \frac{d[R_r^*]}{dt} = 0 \qquad (7.85)$$

4. There is no chain transfer to the polymer (no branching).

The change of each radical concentration in the polymerization is:

$$\frac{d[R_1^*]}{dt} = R_I + \{k_{fm}[M] + k_{fs}[S] + k_{fi}[I]\}\sum_{r=1}^{\infty}[R_r^*] - \{k_p[M] + k_t[R_r^*]\}[R_1^*] = 0 \qquad (7.86a)$$

$$\downarrow \qquad\qquad \downarrow \qquad\qquad\qquad \downarrow \qquad\qquad \downarrow$$

$$\frac{d[R_r^*]}{dt} = k_p[M][R_{r-1}^*] - \{k_p[M] + k_{fm}[M] + k_{fs}[S] + k_{fi}[I] + k_t\sum_{r=1}^{\infty}[R_r^*]\}[R_r^*] = 0 \quad (7.86b)$$

The summation of all the equations for each radical yields:

$$R_I - k_t[R^*]^2 = 0 \qquad (7.87)$$

$$[R^*] = \sum_{r=1}^{\infty}[R_r^*] = \text{ the total radical concentration at steady state; then,}$$

$$[R^*] = \left(\frac{R_I}{k_t}\right)^{1/2} \qquad (7.88)$$

The consumption rate of the monomer (or production rate of polymer) is expressed by substituting equation (7.88) into equation (7.77):

$$R_p = k_p[M]\left(\frac{R_I}{k_t}\right)^{1/2} \propto [M][I]_o^{1/2} \qquad (7.89)$$

If the initiator concentration is constant during the polymerization, the monomer conversion is:

$$\ln[1-X] = -k_p\left(\frac{2fk_d}{k_t}\right)^{1/2}[I]_o^{1/2}t \qquad (7.90)$$

$$X = \frac{[M]_o - [M]}{[M]}$$

where $[M]_o$ is the initial monomer concentration. Figure 7.17 shows the plot of $\ln[1-X]$ vs. time.

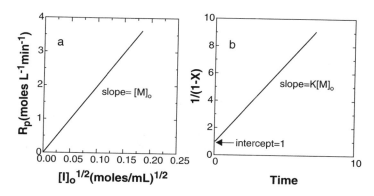

FIGURE 7.17 Conversion vs. polymerization time (a) and rate vs. initial initiator concentration (b).

The molecular weight distribution and the average molecular weight in a free-radical polymerization can be calculated from kinetics. The kinetic chain length v is defined as the average number of monomers consumed per number of chains initiated during the polymerization. It is the ratio of the propagation rate to the initiation rate (or the termination rate with a steady-state approximation):

$$v = \frac{R_p}{R_I} = \frac{R_p}{R_t} = \frac{k_p[M]}{k_t^{1/2}R_I^{1/2}} = \frac{k_p^2[M]^2}{k_t R_p} \tag{7.91}$$

where the chain transfer reaction is not involved in the polymerization and v is related to $\bar{r}_n$ as follows:

for the termination by combination: $\bar{r}_n = 2v$

for the termination by disproportionation: $\bar{r}_n = v$

When the chain transfer reaction is important:

$$\bar{r}_n = \frac{R_p}{R_t + \sum R_f} \tag{7.92a}$$

$$\frac{1}{\bar{r}_n} = \frac{k_t R_p}{k_p[M]^2} + \frac{k_{fm}}{k_p} + \frac{k_{fs}[S]}{k_p[M]} + \frac{k_{fi}[I]}{k_p[M]} \tag{7.92b}$$

All the transfer reactions cause a decrease in $\bar{r}_n$.

The change of a polymer radical with one repeating unit, as shown in equation (7.88), can be rewritten as:

$$[R^*] = \sum [R_r^*] = \left(\frac{R_I}{k_{tc} + k_{td}} \right)^{1/2} = \frac{R_p}{k_p[M]} \qquad (7.93a)$$

$$\sum_{r=2}^{\infty} [R_r^*] = [R^*] - [R_1^*] \qquad (7.93b)$$

$$\frac{d[R_1^*]}{dt} = 0 \qquad (7.94a)$$

$$[R_1^*] = \left(\frac{\tau + \beta}{1 + \tau + \beta} \right) \frac{R_p}{k_p[M]} \qquad (7.94b)$$

where

$$\tau = \frac{k_{td} R_p}{k_p^2[M]^2} + \frac{k_{fm}}{k_p} + \frac{k_{fs}[S]}{k_p[M]} + \frac{k_{fi}[I]}{k_p[M]} \qquad (7.95a)$$

and

$$\beta = \frac{k_{tc} R_p}{k_p^2[M]^2} \qquad (7.95b)$$

When $r \geq 2$,

$$[R_r^*] = \varphi[R_{r-1}^*] = \varphi^{r-1}[R_1^*] \qquad (7.96)$$

where $\varphi = \dfrac{1}{1 + \tau + \beta}$.

The rate expression for a dead polymer is:

$$\frac{1}{V} \frac{dN_r}{dt} = \frac{dP_r}{dt} = (k_{fm}[M] + k_{fs}[S] + k_{fi}[I] + k_{td}[R^*])[R_r^*] + \frac{1}{2} k_{tc} \sum [R_s^*][R_{r-s}^*] \qquad (7.97)$$

$$\frac{dP_r}{dt} = R_p(\tau + \beta) \, (\tau + \frac{1}{2}\beta(\tau + \beta)r) \, \exp(-(\tau + \beta)r) \qquad (7.98)$$

$$\varphi^r \cong \exp(-(\tau + \beta)r) \qquad (7.99)$$

The instantaneous differential molecular weight distribution is given by:

$$\omega(r,x) = \frac{d(rP_r)/dt}{R_p} = (\tau+\beta)\left\{\tau+\frac{1}{2}\beta(\tau+\beta)r\right\}r\exp\{-(\tau+\beta)r\} \qquad (7.100)$$

The number and weight average molecular weights of the polymer produced in the total polymerization time are calculated by:

$$\overline{M}_n = \frac{M_m}{\displaystyle\sum_{r=1}^{\infty}\frac{\omega(r,x)}{r}} = \frac{M_m}{\tau+\beta/2} \qquad (7.101a)$$

$$\overline{M}_w = M_m\sum_{r=1}^{\infty}r\,\omega(r,x) = \frac{2M_m(\tau+3\,\beta/2)}{(\tau+\beta)^2} \qquad (7.101b)$$

Examples of pharmaceutical homopolymers:

7.4.1.1 Polyvinylpyrrolidone (PVP) and Its Copolymers

PVP   P(VP-co-VAc)

One half of an aqueous solution of vinylpyrrolidone (VP) is added to the reactor while the other half is added in portions during the polymerization. The polymerization is initiated when hydrogen peroxide and ammonia are added to the reaction mixture. The ammonia serves as a buffer in the solution in order to provide an alkaline condition, thus preventing the splitting off of the acetaldehyde from the monomer during the reaction. The rate of the peroxide-initiated polymerization is expressed as:

$$R_p = k[H_2O_2]^{1/2}[NH_3]^{1/4}[VP]^{3/2} \qquad (7.102)$$

The rate of polymerization is less sensitive to pH changes ranging from 7 to 12. The polymerization is completed in 2 to 3 hr.

The molecular weight of PVP is directly dependent on monomer concentration, which goes up to about 30%. Beyond 30% monomer concentration, the molecular weight is inversely proportional to the peroxide concentration. There are five commercially available viscosity grades such as K-15, K-30, K-60, K-90, and K-120, whose number average molecular weights are about 10,000, 40,000, 160,000,

300,000, and 1,000,000, respectively. The values of K correspond to the weight average molecular weights and are related to the relative viscosity (η_r) in the Fikentsher formula:

$$\frac{\log \eta_r}{c} = \frac{75k^2}{1+1.5kc} + k \tag{7.103}$$

where c is the concentration of PVP in g/100 ml solution and k is a constant related to the molecular weight ($K = k \times 1000$).

PVP is used in diverse pharmaceutical applications, such as a tablet binder, granulating agent, and thickening agent. PVP forms a soluble complex with iodine, and increases the solubility of iodine tenfold. The PVP/iodine complexes have excellent antibacterial properties with low toxicity and without staining. PVP also forms complexes with a number of drugs such as aspirin, acetaminophen, sulfathiazole, and benzocaine and the complexes may be used for sustained-release formulations for topical use. PVP also forms coprecipitates with less-water soluble drugs in a solid dispersion, enhancing their solubility. PVP has excellent properties for the formation of clear, transparent, hard films.

Copolymers of vinyl pyrrolidone and vinylacetate (PVP-co-VAc) are of interest, especially in the cosmetic industry because by reducing the hydroscopicity of PVP, they increase their adhesiveness.

Crospovidone, which is slightly cross-linked with bifunctional monomers (e.g., 1-vinyl-3-ethylidenepyrrolidone, ethylene-bis-3-(N-vinyl-pyrrolidone), is obtained by popcorn polymerization. It has been used as a disintegration agent for tablets.

7.4.1.2 Polyvinylacetate and Its Derivatives

PVAc   PVA   PVAcP

Polyvinylacetate (PVAc) has not been used in the pharmaceutical field until recently. During the polymerization, especially at high conversion, free radicals are transferred to dead polymers, resulting in the formation of branched polymers. These branched polymers are susceptible to deterioration. Because the PVAc latex particles are produced by an emulsion polymerization technique, this provides a good process for the water-based dispersion in film coatings. The main purpose of this polymer is the film coating of sustained release dosage forms. The polymer is used as a precursor in the production of polyvinylalcohol (PVA), which cannot be prepared directly by polymerization due to the unstable, isomeric monomer of acetaldehyde.

PVA is produced indirectly by saponification of PVAc in concentrated alcohol solution in the presence of a base catalyst (e.g., NaOH). PVA is amorphous. However, it can be made into a crystalline structure by freeze and thaw processes because the functional OH group easily fits into the crystal lattice. PVA is used as a thickening and suspending agent, especially in ophthalmic formulations, due to its nonionic nature. There are a variety of PVA grades available commercially, classified by the molecular weight (9,000 – 100,000) and by the degree of hydrolysis (80 to 99⁺%). Attempts were made in vain to use it as a sustained-release drug carrier after cross-linking with glutaraldehydes.

PVA is further modified to obtain polyvinylacetatephthalate (PVAcP), which is used in enteric coatings. PVAcP is prepared from the reaction of partially hydrolyzed polyvinyl alcohol, sodium acetate and phthalic anhydride. It consists of 55 to 62% of phthalyl groups. The PVA used is a low molecular weight grade with 87 to 89 mole% hydrolyzed. Since only vinyl alcohol portions of the partially hydrolyzed PVA are phthalated, the acetyl content remains constant before and after the reaction.

7.4.1.3 Polyvinylchloride (PVC)

$$\left[\!\!\!-CH_2\!-\!\!\!\begin{array}{c}CH\\ |\\ Cl\end{array}\!\!\!-\right]_n$$

PVC

The majority of PVC is produced by free-radical suspension polymerization of vinyl chloride. PVC is available in a number of grades and forms rigid or flexible resins. A flexible resin is obtained by incorporating plasticizers into the resins.

The main use of PVC is for intravenous bags. However, PVC has been used in the controlled release of volatile insecticides, herbicides, pheromones, and perfumes by diffusion through a PVC membrane of multilaminated stripes. A monolithic matrix device of PVC can be prepared by mixing PVC particles with a suitable plasticizer and an active agent, followed by heating of the mixture in a mold. A solid PVC matrix is obtained from the subsequent cooling.

7.4.1.4 Polyisobutylene (PIB)

$$\left[\!\!\!-CH_2\!-\!\!\!\begin{array}{c}CH_3\\ |\\ C\\ |\\ CH_3\end{array}\!\!\!-\right]_n$$

Polyisobutylene

PIB is prepared by the cationic polymerization at low temperature, giving the head-to-tail configuration. The glass transition temperature of PIB is about $-70°C$ and amorphous in its normal state. As its molecular weight increases, the physical properties vary. For example, low molecular weight PIBs are viscous liquids and very high molecular weight PIBs are elastic solids. PIBs are used as pressure–sensitive adhesives (PSA), which are materials that adhere even with a finger pressure, are permanently sticky, and leave no residue when being removed from a surface. PIB PSAs normally are made of a blend of low- and high-molecular-weight fractions.

The final uses of the polymer blend are determined by incorporating various compounding ingredients such as fillers, processing aids, plasticizers, and curing agents. Among those ingredients, fillers are the most important ones that influence dynamic properties. Carbon black, used as a reinforcing filler, may enhance abrasion resistance and tensile strength because it alters polymer chain dynamics. Colloidal silicon dioxide is used as a filler in the Catapres–TTS® containing clonidine.

7.4.2 FREE-RADICAL COPOLYMERIZATION

The polymerization described so far is homo-polymerization based on single monomers. Some polymers used in pharmaceutical applications are copolymers. They have properties that each homo-polymer does not exhibit. For example, the copolymer of hydroxyethyl methacrylate and methyl methacrylate is synthesized in order to obtain a polymer exhibiting a hydrophilic/hydrophobic balance. A variety of copolymers (alternating, block, random) can be formed from two different monomers. Special processes produce alternating and block copolymers, while random copolymers are produced by free-radical copolymerization of two monomers. The polymerization steps, such as initiation, propagation, and termination, are the same as in free-radical homo-polymerization. Copolymerization kinetics are depicted as follows:

Initiation:

$$I \rightarrow 2\ R_c^* \quad \text{(initiator decomposition)}$$

$$\left.\begin{aligned} R_c^* + A &\rightarrow X_1^* \\[1em] R_c^* + B &\rightarrow Y_1^* \end{aligned}\right\} \tag{7.104}$$

where X_1^* is a radical with an A-end containing one unit of monomer A and zero units of B. A similar definition is applied to Y_1^*.

A rate expression for the initiation reaction is:

$$R_{IA} = k_{i1}[R_c^*][A], \quad R_{IB} = k_{i2}[R_c^*][B] \tag{7.105a}$$

$$\frac{d[R_c^*]}{dt} = 2f_{kd}[I] - k_{i1}[R_c^*][A] - k_{i2}[R_c^*][B] \tag{7.105b}$$

$$[R_c^*] = \frac{2fk_d[I]}{k_{i1}[A] + k_{i2}[B]} \quad \text{(stationary-state approximation)} \quad (7.105c)$$

The total initiation rate is given by:

$$R_I = 2f\,k_d[I] \tag{7.106}$$

Propagation:

$$\left. \begin{array}{c} X_j^* + A \;\rightarrow\; X_{j+1}^* \\[1.5em] X_j^* + B \;\rightarrow\; Y_{j+1}^* \\[1.5em] Y_j^* + A \;\rightarrow\; X_{j+1}^* \\[1.5em] Y_j^* + B \;\rightarrow\; Y_{j+1}^* \end{array} \right\} \tag{7.107}$$

For the above reactions, it is assumed that the reactivity of the propagating radical is dependent only on its terminal radical unit. However, the rate of addition of a monomer to the growing radical depends on the type of monomer in the penultimate position. The importance of the penultimate effects has not been widely investigated. As a result, it is assumed that the simple copolymerization equations given above are valid.

The instantaneous rates of copolymerization for monomers A and B are given as:

$$R_{PA} = k_{p11}[A]X_T + k_{p21}[A]Y_T \tag{7.108a}$$

$$R_{PB} = k_{p12}[B]X_T + k_{p22}[B]Y_T \tag{7.108b}$$

$$R_P = R_{PA} + R_{PB} \tag{7.108c}$$

where

$$X_T = \sum_{j=1}^{\infty} [X_j^*], \quad Y_T = \sum_{j=1}^{\infty} [Y_j^*] \tag{7.108d}$$

Under the stationary-state approximation,

$$R_{PA} = R_{PB} = 0 \tag{7.109a}$$

$$k_{p21}[A]Y_T = k_{p12}[B]X_T \qquad (7.109b)$$

$$Y_T = \frac{k_{p12}[B]}{k_{p21}[A]} X_T \qquad (7.109c)$$

Termination (only the disproportionation reaction is considered):

$$
\left.
\begin{array}{c}
X_i^* + X_j^* \rightarrow P_i + P_j \\[2ex]
X_i^* + Y_j^* \rightarrow P_i + P_j \\[2ex]
Y_i^* + Y_j^* \rightarrow P_i + P_j
\end{array}
\right\}
\qquad (7.110)
$$

The rate of termination is written as:

$$R_t = k_{t11}X_T + k_{t12}X_T Y_T + k_{t22}Y_T^2 \qquad (7.111)$$

where k_{t12} is the cross-termination rate constant estimated by:

$$\varphi = \frac{k_{t12}}{2(k_{t11}k_{t22})^{1/2}} \qquad (7.112)$$

For free-radical polymerization,

$$R_I = R_t \qquad (7.113a)$$

where

$$R_I = X_T^2 \varphi \qquad (7.113b)$$

and

$$\varphi = k_{t11} + 2k_{t12}\frac{k_{p12}}{k_{p21}}\frac{[B]}{[A]} + k_{t22}\left[\frac{k_{p12}}{k_{p21}}\frac{[B]}{[A]}\right]^2 \qquad (7.113c)$$

The rate of copolymerization is then:

$$R_p = \frac{-d([A]+[B])}{dt} = \frac{R_t^{1/2}(r_1[A]^2 + 2[A][B] + 2r_2[B]^2)}{\left[r_1^2\delta_A^2[A]^2 + 2\varphi r_1 r_2 \delta_A \delta_B[A][B] + r_2^2\delta_B^2[B]^2\right]^{1/2}} \qquad (7.114)$$

TABLE 7.5
Reactivity Ratios of Monomers

Monomer 1	Monomer 2	r_1	r_2
Vinyl pyrrolidone	Vinyl acetate	3.3	0.20
Methyl methacrylate	Ethyl acrylate	2.04	0.22
Methyl methacrylate	Methacrylic acid	0.78	0.33
Ethylene	Vinyl acetate	1.0	1.0
Methyl methacrylate	Vinyl pyrrolidone	5.0	0.02

Source: Taken from Brandrup et al (Eds.), *Polymer Hand-book,* 4th Ed., John Wiley and Sons, New York, 1995.

where δ_A and δ_B represent the termination/propagation constant ratios:

$$\delta_A = \frac{k_{t11}^{1/2}}{k_{p11}} \qquad \delta_B = \frac{k_{t22}^{1/2}}{k_{p22}} \qquad (7.115a)$$

and r_1 and r_2 are the reactivity ratios.

$$r_1 = \frac{k_{p11}}{k_{p12}} \qquad r_2 = \frac{k_{p22}}{k_{p21}} \qquad (7.115b)$$

The tendency of two monomers A and B to copolymerize can be predicted by their r values. When $r > 1$, the radical X^* prefers A over B. If $r < 1$, the radical X^* prefers B over A. Some of the reactivity ratios of the monomers are given in Table 7.5.

Dividing Equation (7.108a) by Equation (7.108b) gives:

$$\frac{d[A]}{d[B]} = \frac{[A]r_1[B]+[B]}{[B][A]+r_2[B]} \qquad (7.116)$$

Equation (7.116) is called the copolymer composition equation and can be written in terms of the mole fraction in both the feed and the copolymer:

$$F_1 = 1 - F_2 = \frac{r_1f_1^2 + f_1f_2}{r_1f_1^2 + 2f_1f_2 + r_2f_2^2} \qquad (7.117)$$

where F_1 and f_1 represent the mole fractions of monomer A in the increment of polymer formed at any instant and in the monomer feed composition, respectively. Equation (7.116) then becomes:

$$F_1 = \frac{d[A]}{d[A]+d[B]} \qquad f_1 = 1 - f_2 = \frac{[A]}{[A]+[B]} \qquad (7.118)$$

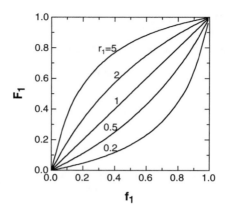

FIGURE 7.18 Instantaneous copolymer composition vs. feed composition for an ideal copolymerization with values of $r_1 = 1/r_2$.

Equation (7.113b) gives the instantaneous copolymer composition in terms of the feed composition and the reactivity ratio. Figure 7.18 shows the copolymer composition for an ideal copolymerization ($r_1 r_2 = 1$). In this case, the copolymer composition equation becomes:

$$F_1 = \frac{r_1 f_1}{f_1 (r_1 - 1) + 1} = \frac{r_1 f_1}{r_1 f_1 + f_2} \tag{7.119a}$$

and
$$r_1 = 1 / r_2 \quad \text{or} \quad k_{11} / k_{12} = k_{21} / k_{22} \tag{7.119b}$$

Figure 7.18 shows that the reactivity ratios should be very similar in order to obtain a copolymer containing appreciable quantities of both monomers. For $r_1 > 1$ and $r_2 < 1$, since one monomer (e.g., A) is more reactive than the other (e.g., B), the copolymer will contain more monomer units of A in the polymer chain and vice versa for $r_2 > 1$ and $r_1 < 1$. When $r_1 = r_2 = 1$, the copolymer composition is identical to the feed composition (i.e., $F_1 = f_1$).

When $r_1 = r_2 = 0$, each copolymer radical reacts only with the other monomer so that a monomer unit is added to the polymer chain alternatively regardless of the feed composition (i.e., $F_1 = 0.5$). An alternating copolymer is produced. If there is an excess amount of monomer initially, then one monomer is used up and the polymerization will be stopped. When $r_1 > 1$ and $r_2 > 1$, each radical has the same preference to add its own monomer. As a result, the same monomer is added to the polymer chain until the other monomer is given a chance. A block copolymer is obtained. Figure 7.19 shows the curves for the various reactivity ratios in the case of a nonideal copolymerization. Curve B crosses the diagonal line, and its point of intersection with this diagonal line is called the azeotropic composition. At this point, a copolymer will have the same composition as the monomer composition over an entire conversion range. The critical composition $(f_1)_c$ is given as:

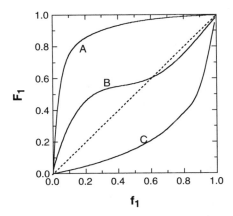

FIGURE 7.19 Instantaneous copolymer composition vs. monomer feed composition: Curve A, $r_1 = 20$, $r_2 = 0.01$; Curve b, $r_1 = 0.5$, $r_2 = 0.1$; Curve C, $r_1 = 0.1$, $r_2 = 5$.

$$\left(f_1\right)_c = \frac{1 - r_1}{2 - r_1 - r_2} \qquad (7.120)$$

As seen in Equation (7.118), the copolymer and the feed compositions vary with the conversion during the polymerization process. The drift of a feed composition with the conversion favors the less reactive monomer. To obtain F_1 at different conversions, it is necessary to integrate the copolymer composition equation. Assume that the system contains a total of M moles of monomers and $F_1 > f_1$. After dM moles of monomers have been polymerized, the copolymer contains $F_1 dM$ moles of M_1. The feed then contains $(M - dM)(f_1 - df_1)$ moles of M_1, where the first term is the total monomer concentration and the second term is the mole fraction of M_1 in the feed. The mass balance of M_1 reacted in the system is given by:

$$Mf_1 - (M - dM)(f_2 - df_1) = F_1 dM \qquad (7.121)$$

If we rearrange Equation (7.121) and neglect the second-order differential term, integrating the resulting equation yields:

$$\ln \frac{M}{M_o} = \int_{f_{10}}^{f_1} \frac{df_1}{F_1 - f_1} \qquad (7.122)$$

where M_o and f_{10} are the initial moles of monomers and the initial feed composition of M_1, respectively. Substituting Equation (7.117) into Equation (7.122) gives:

$$X = 1 - \left(\frac{f_1}{f_{10}}\right)^\alpha \left(\frac{1 - f_1}{1 - f_{10}}\right)^\beta \left(\frac{f_{10} - \delta}{f_1 - \delta}\right)^\gamma \qquad (7.123)$$

where

$$\alpha = \frac{r_2}{1-r_2}, \quad \beta = \frac{r_1}{1-r_1}, \quad \gamma = \frac{1-r_1 r_2}{(1-r_1)(1-r_2)}, \quad \text{and} \quad \delta = \frac{1-r_2}{2-r_1-r_2} \qquad (7.124)$$

When the termination reaction is a diffusion-controlled (a single k_t) process, the isothermal copolymerization is derived as:

$$\ln\left[\left(\frac{f_1}{f_{10}}\right)^a \left(\frac{1-f_1}{1-f_{10}}\right)^b \left(\frac{f_{10}-\delta}{f_1-\delta}\right)^c\right] = (mk_{p22} - k_{p21})\int_0^t \sqrt{\frac{R_I}{k_t}}\, dt \qquad (7.125)$$

where

$$m = \frac{k_{p11} - k_{p21}}{k_{p12} - k_{p22}}, \quad a = \alpha(1-m)+1$$

$$b = \beta(1-m)-m, \quad c = \gamma(1-m) \qquad (7.126)$$

Example 7.2

A vinyl monomer M_1 (1 mole) is copolymerized with another monomer M_2 (2 moles). The reactivity ratios are $r_1 = 0.6$ and $r_2 = 1.66$. Determine the mole fraction of monomer M_1 in the initially formed copolymer. What is the mole fraction of monomer M_1 in the polymer being formed when two moles of the monomers are converted to a copolymer? Draw the graph of the cumulative and the instantaneous copolymer compositions vs. the conversion.

Solution

$$f_{10} = 1/(1+2) = 0.33$$

$$F_1 = \frac{r_1 f_1^2 + f_1 f_2}{r_1 f_1^2 + 2f_1 f_2 + r_2 f_2^2} = \frac{(0.6)(0.33)^2 + (0.33)(0.67)}{(0.6)(0.33)^2 + 2(0.33)(0.67) + 1.66(0.67)^2} = 0.23$$

When two moles of the monomers are consumed,

$$\alpha = \frac{r_2}{1-r_2} = \frac{1.66}{1-1.66} = -2.52, \quad \beta = \frac{r_1}{1-r_1} = \frac{0.6}{1-0.6} = 1.5, \quad \gamma = \frac{1-r_1 r_2}{(1-r_1)(1-r_2)} \approx 0$$

The conversion is:

$$X = \frac{2}{3} = 1 - \left(\frac{f_1}{f_{10}}\right)^\alpha \left(\frac{1-f_1}{1-f_{10}}\right)^\beta \left(\frac{f_{10}-\delta}{f_1-\delta}\right)^\gamma = 1 - \left(\frac{f_1}{0.33}\right)^{-2.52} \left(\frac{1-f_1}{1-0.33}\right)^{1.5}$$

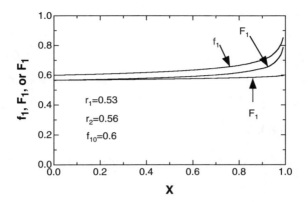

FIGURE 7.20 The cumulative and the instantaneous copolymer compositions vs. the conversion.

By trial and error, $f_1 = 0.455$ and then $F_1 = 0.334$.

Similarly, the cumulative copolymer composition, $\overline{F}_1$, is plotted against the conversion, as shown in Figure 7.20, and calculated by a mass balance equation:

$$f_{10}M_o = \overline{F}_1(M_o - M) + f_1 M \qquad (7.127a)$$

or

$$\overline{F}_1 = \frac{f_{10} - f_1(1-X)}{X} \qquad (7.127b)$$

Examples of pharmaceutical copolymers include:

7.4.2.1 Eudragit® and Kollicoat® series:

Eudragit® E

Eudragit® L or S

Eudragit® RL or RS   Eudragit® NE or Kollicoat® EMM

Kollicoat® MAE

Eudragit polymers have a methylmethacrylate backbone with other functional monomers, which provide the special application areas. All
Eudragits are used for film coatings and are available as powders, pel-
lets, and aqueous dispersions. Eudragit E has a pendant tertiary amine
group in the chain and is insoluble in the neutral medium of saliva. However, it quickly dissolves at low pH (e.g., in the stomach) because the pendant group is protonated. Eudragit E is used for taste masking. With
carboxymethylcellulose, Eudragit E is used as a rapid disintegrating film.
Eudragit L and S contain a carboxylic acid group and are insoluble at low
pH. However, they are soluble in the neutral to weakly alkaline medium
of the gastrointestinal tract. Eudragit L dissolves at pH 5.5 to 6.5 while
Eudragit S dissolves above pH 7 (lower section of the intestine).
Eudragit L and S have different ratios of methacrylic acid to methyl
methacrylate, as shown in Table 7.6. Eudragit L and S are used in enteric coatings to avoid any incompatibilities of drugs in the stomach.
Kollicoat MAE employs ethylacrylate instead of methyl methacrylate
(1:1 mole ratio composition).
Eudragit RL and RS are not soluble at any pH because the quaternary
amine fraction is very small when compared to that of methyl methacrylate. Since the functional group is quaternary amine, the polymer swells in
water, regardless of pH. As a result, water and drug molecules permeate in

TABLE 7.6
A Survey of the Composition and Function of Eudragit®

Eudragit	L	S	E	RL	RS	NE
Methacrylic acid	46.0 to 50.6	27.6 to 30.7				
Dimethylaminoethyl methacrylate			20.8 to 25.5			
Trimethylaminoethyl methacrylate				8.9 to 12.0	4.5 to 6.8	
Ethyl acrylate						0.3
Methyl methacrylate	49.4 to 56.0	69.3 to 72.4	74.5 to 79.2	88.0 to 91.1	93.2 to 95.5	0.7

and out of the swollen polymer. The degree of permeability of the polymer films depends on the composition of the amounts of quaternary amine. Eudragit® NE and Kollicoat® EMM are neutral, insoluble in water, and used for film coatings as a membrane barrier with a water-soluble excipient.

7.4.2.2 Ion Exchange Resins:

Sulfonated P(ST-co-DVB)   Quaternized P(ST-co-DVB)

The resins are prepared first by copolymerizing styrene (ST) and divinylbenzene (DVB), resulting in a cross-linked polystyrene. Usually, they are produced in the form of spherical beads. These beads are sulfonated with sulfuric acid for anionic resins and methylated with chloromethyl ether followed by quaternization with trimethylamine for cationic resins. Two types of resins exist: gel and microporous. The microporous beads are used to remove ionic substances quickly while the gel-type beads are used for sustaining drug release over a long period of time.

The ability of an ion exchange resin to exchange its mobile ions with the counter ions is dependent on the affinity for the counter ions and the concentration. The selectivity coefficient K:

$$K = \frac{[B^+]_{resin}[A^+]_{solution}}{[A^+]_{resin}[B^+]_{solution}}$$

Various sustained-release dosage forms have been developed based on resins that form complexes with ionic drugs. Upon contact with the hydrogen or chloride ions in the stomach, the bound drug in the resins dissociates and diffuses out of the resin matrix. In the intestine, the cations or the anions in the intestinal fluid are exchanged with the ionic drug bound to the resin. Drug-free resins are employed when the removal of undesirable ionic substances in the gastrointestinal tract is needed (i.e., use of cholestyamine to lower cholesterol).

7.4.2.3 Carbopol® or Carbomer®

Cross-linked Poly(acrylic acid)

Carbopol resins are very-high-molecular-weight poly(acrylic acid)s (pK$_a$ 6.5) loosely cross-linked with vinyl glycol, allyl sucrose, allyl methacrylate, or allyl penaerythritol. Their aqueous dispersions are very mildly acidic. Due to the cross-linked structure, Carbopol resins partially swell (about 1000 times) but do not dissolve in water. Upon neutralization with an alkali, the resins expand extensively like a gel-like structure and their viscosity increases drastically, thus forming an aqueous mucilage. As a result, the dispersion becomes thickened. The presence of electrolytes in aqueous solutions reduces the viscosity of the solutions, and thus high concentrations of Carbopol should be used in aqueous solutions where ionic drugs are employed. When Carbopol resins are neutralized with amine bases (e.g., triethanolamine), a transparent gel structure is formed, which is used as a lubricating gel in many cosmetic formulations. Ephedrine-free base is employed as an amine base to obtain nasal jelly for decongestion.

Carbopol resins also have been used in controlled-release dosage forms. Especially, the resins Noven AA-1 USP and Carbopol 934P NF are being extensively developed in bioadhesive drug delivery systems for topical, bucal or nasal, ocular, and rectal applications (e.g., Fentanyl®). Noven CA-1 USP and CA-2 USP are used as oral laxative and antidiarrheal products in swallowable and chewable tablets.

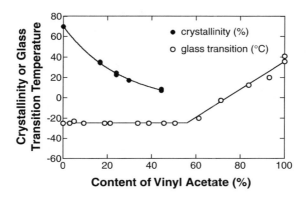

FIGURE 7.21 The effect of vinyl acetate content on the crystallinity and glass transition temperature of PEVAc. [Graph reconstructed from Johnson and Nachtrab, *Ange. Macrom. Chem.*, 7, 134 (1969) and Reding et al., *J. Polym. Sci.*, 57, 483 (1962).]

7.4.2.4 Poly(ethylene-co-vinyl acetate) (PEVAc)

PEVAc

PEVAc has been used as a rate-controlling barrier in controlled-release dosage forms (e.g., Transderm®-Nitro, Transderm®-Scop, Estraderm®, Ocusert®) because its permeability can be changed with the vinyl acetate content of the polymer. As the vinyl acetate content increases, the degree of crystallinity decreases due to the disruption of the regularity of the polymer chain, and the glass transition temperature increases due to the increase in amorphousness, meaning a decrease in the mobility of the polymer chain (Figure 7.21). The solutes diffuse easily through the amorphous area of the polymer and thus the permeability increases.

The polymer exhibits good biocompatibility, inertness, physical stability, and ease of processability. PEVAc containing 30 to 50% wt vinyl acetate content is used for drug delivery systems.

7.4.2.5 Poly(vinyl alcohol-grafted-ethylene glycol) (Kollicoat® IR)

Kollicoat® IR

Kollicoat IR is a unique polymer for pharmaceutical applications prepared by a graft polymerization process of polyethylene glycol (25%) with polyvinyl alcohol (75%). Kollicoat IR dissolves quickly in water and aqueous solutions of acid and alkali and reduces the surface tension of aqueous solutions to allow the solutions to have high spray rates. The polymer film is very flexible, not tacky, and easily colored. The polymer can be used as instant release coating, pore former, binder, protective colloid, etc.

7.4.3 STEP POLYMERIZATION (CONDENSATION POLYMERIZATION)

There are numerous ways of synthesizing polymers through step polymerization processes. Unlike addition polymerization polymers, the polymers produced by step polymerization processes are susceptible to linkage breakdown (i.e., biodegradation). This property is important in developing biodegradable polymers for drug delivery systems. Two important aspects of condensation polymerizations are that two monomers are involved in the reaction and a monomer has two reactive functional groups (i.e., hydroxyl, carboxylic acid, amine). The general reaction between two monomers, designated as A–A and B–B, is as follows:

$$nA - A + nB - B \rightarrow -[-AABB-]_n -$$

where A and B are the functional groups such as –COOH and –OH (which produce a polyester) or –COOH and –NH$_2$ (which produce a polyamide). A typical polyesterification reaction is given as:

The above equilibrium process is driven to completion by the removal of H_2O (e.g., run at 150°C under vacuum). The reaction is considered an irreversible process.

7.4.3.1 Acid-Catalyzed Esterification Polymerization of A–A and B–B

Assumptions in the kinetic analysis may be made as follows:

1. The reactivities of both functional groups in a difunctional monomer are equal (e.g., both carboxyls in a diacid).
2. The reactivity of the functional groups is independent of the size of molecule to which they are attached.

$$\underset{\text{—COH}}{\overset{\overset{\text{O}}{\|}}{}} \quad + \quad HA \quad \underset{k_2}{\overset{k_1}{\rightleftharpoons}} \quad \underset{\text{—C⁺-OH}}{\overset{\text{OH}}{|}} \quad (P) \qquad (7.128a)$$

$$\underset{\text{—C⁺-OH}}{\overset{\text{OH}}{|}} \quad + \quad HO— \quad \overset{k_3}{\longrightarrow} \quad \underset{\text{—C—O—}}{\overset{\overset{\text{O}}{\|}}{}} \quad + \quad H_2O \quad (7.128b)$$

where HA is a catalyst (acid). The protonation of carboxyl groups is very fast. Thus, the reaction shown in Equation (7.128a) is at constant equilibrium. When the byproduct (water) of the reaction shown in Equation (7.128b) is removed, this reaction is regarded as an irreversible one. The rate of polymerization is given by:

$$\frac{d[COOH]}{dt} = \frac{d[OH]}{dt} = -k_3[C^+OOH_2][OH] = -k_3[P][OH] \qquad (7.129)$$

where [COOH], [OH], and [C⁺OOH$_2$] are the concentrations of the carboxylic acid, the hydroxyl, and the protonated carboxylic acid groups present in the molecules, respectively.

At instantaneous equilibrium, Equation (7.128a) yields:

$$k_1[COOH][HA] = k_2[P][A^-]$$

or
$$[P] = \left(\frac{k_1}{k_2}\right)\frac{[COOH][HA]}{[A^-]} \qquad (7.130)$$

Substituting Equation (7.130) into Equation (7.129) yields:

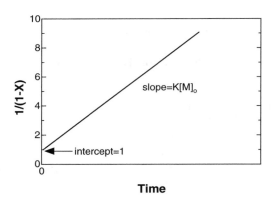

FIGURE 7.22 The conversion vs. time for condensation polymerization.

$$\frac{d[COOH]}{dt} = -k_3 \left(\frac{k_1}{k_2}\right)\left(\frac{[HA]}{[A^-]}\right)[COOH][OH]$$

$$= -\left(\frac{k_1 k_3 [H^+]}{k_2 K_{HA}}\right)[COOH][OH] = -K[COOH][OH]$$

$$(7.131a)$$

where

$$K_{HA} = \frac{[H^+][A^-]}{[HA]} \quad \text{and} \quad K = \frac{k_1 k_3 [H^+]}{k_2 K_{HA}} \qquad (7.131b)$$

If an equimolar mixture (stoichiometric equivalence) is used, then [COOH] = [OH] = [M]. Equation (7.131) is given by:

$$\frac{d[M]}{dt} = -K[M]^2 \qquad (7.132)$$

Integration of Equation (7.132) (by simple second-order reaction) yields:

$$\frac{1}{[M]} - \frac{1}{[M_o]} = Kt \quad \text{or} \quad \frac{1}{1-X} = K[M_o]t + 1 \qquad (7.133)$$

where $[M_o]$ and X are the initial monomer concentration and the conversion of monomer, respectively. Figure 7.22 shows the conversion vs. time.

7.4.3.2 Self-Catalyzed Condensation Polymerization

Here, one of the monomers acts as a catalyst for the condensation polymerization:

$$
\begin{array}{c}
\text{O} \\
\parallel \\
\text{—COH}
\end{array}
\quad
\underset{k_2}{\overset{k_1}{\rightleftharpoons}}
\quad
\text{H}^+ +
\begin{array}{c}
\text{O} \\
\parallel \\
\text{—C—O}^-
\end{array}
\qquad (7.134a)
$$

$$
\begin{array}{c}
\text{O} \\
\parallel \\
\text{—COH}
\end{array}
\quad + \quad \text{H}^+
\quad \rightleftharpoons \quad
\begin{array}{c}
\text{OH} \\
\mid \\
\text{—C}^+\text{—OH}
\end{array}
\quad (\text{X})
\qquad (7.134b)
$$

$$
\text{X} \quad + \quad \text{—OH} \quad \longrightarrow \quad
\begin{array}{c}
\text{O} \\
\parallel \\
\text{—C—O}^-
\end{array}
+ \text{H}^+ + \text{H}_2\text{O}
\qquad (7.134c)
$$

The reactions shown in Equation (7.134a) and Equation (7.134b) are at equilibrium and occur very fast. During reactions, the charge balance must be neutral:

$$[X] + [H^+] = [-COO^-] \qquad (7.135a)$$

$$K_1 = \frac{k_1}{k_2} = \frac{[H^+][-COO^-]}{[-COOH]} \qquad (7.135b)$$

$$K_2 = \frac{k_3}{k_4} = \frac{[X]}{[-COOH][H^+]} \qquad (7.135c)$$

Substituting Equation (7.135b) and Equation (7.135c) into Equation (7.135a) yields:

$$[X] = \frac{K_2 K_1^{1/2}[-COOH]^{3/2}}{(1 + K_2[-COOH])^{1/2}} \qquad (7.136)$$

Then, the rate of polymerization is given by:

$$\frac{d[-COOH]}{dt} = \frac{d[-OH]}{dt} = -\frac{k_5 K_2 K_1^{1/2}[-COOH]^{3/2}[-OH]}{(1 + K_2[-COOH])^{1/2}} \qquad (7.137)$$

When $[H^+] \gg [X]$, Equation (7.135a), Equation (7.135b), and Equation (7.135c) give $K_2[-COOH] \ll 1$. Then, Equation (7.137) becomes:

$$\frac{d[-COOH]}{dt} = \frac{d[-OH]}{dt} = -k_5 K_2 K_1^{1/2}[-COOH]^{3/2}[-OH] \qquad (7.138)$$

$$= -k[-COOH]^{3/2}[-OH]$$

For an equimolar mixture (i.e., $[-COOH] = [-OH] = [M]$), Equation (7.138) becomes:

$$\frac{d[M]}{dt} = -k[M]^{5/2} \tag{7.139a}$$

or

$$\left([M]_o^{-3/2} - [M]^{-3/2}\right) = -3/2 \ kt \tag{7.139b}$$

7.4.3.3 Molecular Weight Control

The molecular weight of polymers is dependent on the time of the reaction or the conversion of the monomer. If precise stoichiometric quantities of monomers A–A and B–B are used, then the polymer molecules will have both types of end groups, one A and one B. Further polymerization yields an unstable molecular weight polymer (in principle one molecule of infinite molecular weight). To overcome this problem, a few approaches must be applied:

7.4.3.3.1 The Use of a Stoichiometric Imbalance

Instead of using an equimolar mixture, one may use a slight stoichiometric imbalance of one monomer. At some point in the polymerization, the deficient reactant is used up and the molecules have two end groups with the same functional groups (i.e., those of the monomer in excess).

Let us consider two monomers, A–A and excess B–B. The conversion of monomer A, X_A, is expressed as:

$$X_A = \frac{N_{Ao} - N_A}{N_{Ao}} = \frac{N_{Bo} - N_B}{N_{Bo}} = \frac{1}{f} + \frac{N_B}{N_{Ao}} \tag{7.140}$$

where N_{Ao} and N_{Bo} are the initial number of A and B functional groups, respectively, and N_A and N_B are the number of A and B functional groups at time t, respectively, and f is the stoichiometric imbalance given by:

$$f = \frac{N_{Ao}}{N_{Bo}} \tag{7.141}$$

where $N_A = N_{Ao}(1 - X_A)$ and $N_B = N_{Ao}(1/f - X_A)$.

The total number of molecules initially present, N_{To}, is written as:

$$N_{To} = \frac{1}{2}(N_{Ao} + N_{Bo}) = \frac{1}{2}N_{Ao}(1 + \frac{1}{f}) \tag{7.142}$$

The total number of molecules present at time t, N_T, is given by:

$$N_T = \frac{1}{2}(N_A + N_B) = \frac{1}{2}N_{Ao}(1 + \frac{1}{f} - 2X_A) \tag{7.143}$$

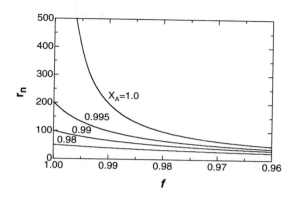

FIGURE 7.23 Conversion vs. number average degree of polymerization.

Dividing Equation (7.142) by Equation (7.143) yields:

$$\bar{r}_n = \frac{\text{initial total number of monomer units}}{\text{total number of monomer units at time } t} = \frac{(1+1/f)}{(1+1/f-2X_A)} \quad (7.144)$$

Let us examine the limiting cases. First, for the complete conversion ($X_A = 1$), Equation (7.143) reduces to:

$$\bar{r}_n = \frac{1+f}{1-f} \quad (7.145)$$

Equation (7.145) provides the upper limit on the polymer molecular weight. Second, for the equimolar mixture ($f = 1$), Equation (7.145) becomes:

$$\bar{r}_n = \frac{1+X_A}{1-X_A} \quad (7.146)$$

Equation (7.146) gives the infinite molecular weight of the polymer at $X_A = 1$. In practice, the polymer is produced when $f = 1$ and $X_A > 0.98$ or when $X_A = 1$ and $f > 0.95$ so that the number average degree of polymerization ($\bar{r}_n$) is greater than 50. Figure 7.23 shows the number average degree of polymerization vs. monomer imbalance ratio in a conversion.

7.4.3.3.2 The Addition of a Monofunctional Compound

The monofunctional compound (e.g., ----B) acts as a chain terminator since it produces molecules with unreactive ends. Let us consider A–A and B–B with BX. The initial total number of molecules is given by:

$$N_{To} = \frac{1}{2}(N_{Ao} + N_{Bo}) + N_{BXo} \quad (7.147)$$

where N_{BXo} is the initial number of molecules BX and is expressed as:

$$N_{BXo} = N_X + 2N_{X^2} \qquad (7.148)$$

where N_X and N_{X^2} are the number of molecules with one X group end (i.e., A——X and B——X) and two X group ends (X——X) at any time t, respectively. The total number of molecules at any time t is given as:

$$N_T = \frac{1}{2}(N_A + N_B - N_X) + N_X + N_{X^2} = \frac{1}{2}(N_A + N_B + N_{BXo}) \qquad (7.149)$$

The number average degree of polymerization then becomes:

$$\bar{r}_n = \frac{N_{Ao} + N_{Bo} + 2N_{BXo}}{N_A + N_B + N_{BXo}} = \frac{1 + (N_{Bo} + 2N_{BXo})/N_{Ao}}{(N_A/N_{Ao}) + (N_B + N_{BXo})/N_{Ao}}$$

or

$$\bar{r}_n = \frac{1+f}{1+f-2fX_A} \qquad (7.150)$$

Examples of pharmaceutical condensation polymers include:

7.4.3.4 Polyanhydrides

Polyanhydride

Historically, polyanhydrides were synthesized for engineering materials. Because of their hydrolytical instability, these polyanhydrides have never been commercialized for engineering purposes. This instability has a beneficial aspect in drug delivery systems since the implant incorporated with an active drug does not need to be retrieved. The anhydride has a labile bond in the main chain of the polymer. This labile bond then breaks down into two carboxylic acid groups.

Several combinations of monomers used to prepare polyanhydrides are classified as aliphatic, aromatic, aliphatic–aromatic, amine-based, and fatty acid-based polyanhydrides. The structures of these monomers determine the final properties of the polyanhydride (i.e., especially hydrolysis and molecular weight). Thus, the proper selection of the monomers is a key element in the development of pharmaceutically and biomedically useful polymers.

Many synthetic methods have been unsuccessfully employed to produce high-molecular-weight polyanhydrides, with the exception of melt condensation polymerization. Melt polycondensation occurs in two steps. First, the prepolymers are prepared by refluxing the dicarboxylic acid monomers with acetic anhydride. These purified prepolymers have degrees of polymerization from 1 to 20 and are polymerized further at high temperature under vacuum to remove the acetic anhydride byproduct. The resulting polymers will have degrees of polymerization from 100 to over 1000. Polyanhydrides consisting of p-(carboxyphenoxy) propane and sebacic acid (pCPP/SA) have been widely studied.

Polyanhydrides give more controllable dosage forms than polylactic acid-based ones. Polyanhydrides undergo surface erosion-controlled kinetics. This type of kinetics controls the water penetration in such a way that only at the surface of the matrix are the labile bonds of polyanhydride broken down and eroded from the outside. As expected, the rate of polymer degradation is dependent on polymer composition. As a result, drug release is linear with respect to time and the percentage of drug release is equal to the percentage of polymer eroded. Aliphatic acid groups (e.g., SA) degrade much faster than aromatic acids (e.g., CPP). Compression molding or solvent casting techniques have been used to form drug-loaded polyanhydrides because of their high melting points. Figure 7.24 shows the release of drugs from compression-molded polyanhydrides.

Recently, a new polyanhydride, poly(fatty acid–sebacic acid), has been synthesized. This polyanhydride uses hydrophobic dimers of erucic acid. Some of its physical properties relevant to the fabrication of drug delivery devices are also improved over those of the other anhydrides based on CPP: lower melting temperature, higher solubility in solvents, and higher mechanical strength. The erosion of the polymers is dependent on

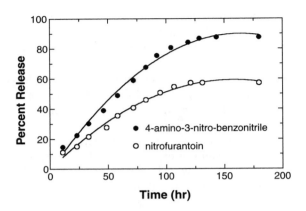

FIGURE 7.24 Release of drugs from compression-molded poly(CPP/SA:20/80) in 0.1 M, pH 7.4 phosphate buffer at 37°C. [Graph reconstructed from data by Erfan et al., *Proceed. Int. Symp. Control. Rel. Bioact. Mater.*, 25, 723 (1998).]

the number of alkyl units in the fatty acid. The shorter the alkyl chain, the shorter the erosion time. An erosion byproduct, fatty acid dimers, tends to remain on the surface of the matrices, which in turn act as a diffusion barrier layer for the release of drugs from polymer matrices.

poly(fatty acid dimer–sebacic acids)

Polyanhydrides have been modified by incorporating amino acids into imide bonds. The imide with the terminal carboxylic acids is activated with acetic anhydride and copolymerized with sebacic acid or CCP. Poly(anhydride–imides) increase the mechanical properties of the polyanhydrides. Degradation of poly(anhydride–imide)s is similar to that of polyanhydrides (i.e., surface erosion). Two different cleavable bonds (anhydride and ester) in the polymer chains have been included in polyanhydrides. Carboxylic acid-terminated ε-caprolactone oligomers or carboxylic acid-terminated monomers (e.g., salicylic acid) have been polymerized with activated monomers (e.g., SA).

Poly(anhydride – ester) containing salicylic acid

The Mark–Houwink constants for polyanhydrides [P(CPP-SA, 20/80)] in chloroform in the range of MW of 14,000 to 245,000 are given by:

$$[\eta]_{Clf}^{PA} = 3.88 \times 10^{-7} M_w^{0.658} \qquad (7.151)$$

A commercial product based on polyanhydrides is Gliadel® wafer containing carmustine, an antitumor agent. The wafer, 1.45 cm in diameter and 1 mm thick, is made of poly[bis-(*p*-carboxyphenoxy) propane: sebacic acid] in an 80:20 molar ratio.

7.4.3.5 Poly(orthoesters)

Polyorthoester

Attempts to make polymers that lead to a surface erosion-controlled dosage form and inhibit drug diffusion in the polymers lead to the development of polyorthoesters. There are several families of polyorthoesters depending on the monomers used. Recently, a semisolid polyorthoester of molecular weight of about 30,000 has been developed for specific applications. These high-molecular-weight polymers are produced almost instantaneously when polyols are reacted with a diketene acetal in the presence of a small amount of acid. Unlike transesterification reactions, which take longer reaction times at elevated temperature under vacuum, the polymerization is completed in 1 hr. Dense cross-linked polymers are the only products of this polymerization. However, the addition of a small quantity of iodine (a catalyst) in pyridine results in a linear polyorthoester due to competing cationic polymerizations. The polymer structure of 3,9-diethylidene-2,4,8,10-tetraoxaspiro[5,5] undecane (DETOSU)–based poly(orthoesters) contains an acidlabile linkage.

Degradation of poly(orthoesters) based on
3,9-bis(ethylidene-2,4,8,10-
tetraoxaspiro[5,5] undecane) (DETOSU)

The hydrolysis of polyorthoesters is controlled by the incorporation of acidic or basic materials because these polymers possess an acid-sensitive linkage in the polymer main chain. The addition of acidic ingredients increases the hydrolysis rate whereas basic ingredients decrease the rate of hydrolysis. The poly(orthoesters) break down to pentaerythritol dipropionate and diols. However, the hydrolysis is not acid specific and undergoes general acid-catalyzed process. The rate of the hydrolysis is dependent on the buffer concentration and the chemical nature of the buffer. Change in the diol portions in the polymer structure allows control of their mechanical properties. In addition, pH-sensitive poly(orthoesters) have been synthesized by incorporating a tertiary amine (e.g., N-methyldiethanolamine). Tertiary amine-containing poly(orthoesters) incorporated with the enzyme glucose oxidase have been used to deliver insulin. The enzyme oxidizes glucose, and the environmental pH becomes acidic. The acidic pH increases the hydrolysis rate of poly(orthoester), and embibed insulin releases. Auto-catalyzable poly(orthoesters) have been developed by inclusion of a glycolide sequence that can be hydrolyzed without introducing acidic excipients. Once glycolic acid chains are hydrolyzed, the produced glycolic acids catalyze breaking of ortho-ester bonds. Figure 7.25 shows the release of propionic acid and the weight loss of poly(orthoester) consisting of lactic acid moiety.

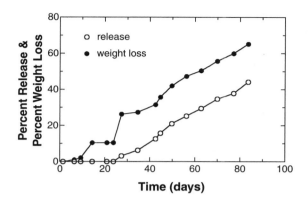

FIGURE 7.25 Release of propionic acid and weight loss of poly(orthoester) containing lactoyl–lactic dimers (PEO95LAC5). [Graph reconstructed from data by Schwach-Abdellaoui et al., *Proceed. Int. Symp. Control. Rel. Bioact. Mater.*, 25, 713 (1998).]

7.4.3.6 Poly(amino acids)

From the viewpoint of polylactic acid and polyglycolic acid, byproducts of which are chemicals naturally present in body, the development of poly(amino acids) is genuine. However, the antigenic nature of the poly(amino acids) that contain three or more amino acids inhibits their widespread use. Besides, the cleavage of the amide bond depends on enzymes, resulting in poor *in vivo* controlled release. Poly(amino acids) have been used mainly to deliver drugs from implants in animals.

Poly(amino acids) are usually copolymers due to the difficulty of producing polyamide sequences: poly(glutamic acid–glutamate). The degradation of poly(glutamic acid–glutamate) is dependent on the copolymer ratio, as shown in Figure 7.26, which controls the hydrophilicity of the polymer.

Poly(amino acids) are insoluble in common solvents, are difficult to fabricate due to high melting point, and absorb a significant amount of water when their acid content reaches over 50 mol%. To solve these problems, polyesters derived from amino acids and lactic acids [e.g., poly(lactic acid-co-lysine) PLAL] are developed. The PLAL system is further modified by reaction with lysine *N*-carboxyanhydride derivatives. Another modification of poly(amino acids) includes poly(iminocarbonates), which are derived from the polymerization of desaminotyrosyl tyrosine alkyl esters. These polymers are easily processable and can be used as support materials for cell growth due to a high tissue compatibility. Mechanical properties of tyrosine-derived poly(carbonates) are in between those of poly(orthoesters) and poly(lactic acid) or poly(glycolic acid). The rate of degradation of poly(iminocarbonates) is similar to that of poly(lactic acid).

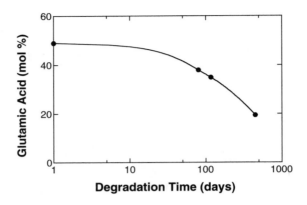

FIGURE 7.26 Degradation of poly(glutamic acid–glutamate). [Graph reconstructed from data by Sidman et al., *J. Memb. Sci.,* 7, 277 (1980).]

Poly(lactic acid - co - amino acid)

7.4.3.7 Silicone polymers

Silicone polymers are one of the most widely used types of polymer within the medical and pharmaceutical industries. Silicone polymers are inorganic polymers with no carbon atoms in the backbone chain, which is a chain of alternating silicon and oxygen atoms. Silicone polymers are highly biocompatible, easily fabricated, and highly permeable to many important drugs. Besides, they can be sterilized by heat, which is an important aspect for implantable devices. The physical properties of the polymers vary with their molecular weight, the number and type of organic groups attached to the silicone, and the configuration of the molecular structure (i.e., linear, cross-linked, cyclic).

$$\left(\!\begin{array}{c} R \\ | \\ -Si-O- \\ | \\ R \end{array}\!\right)_n$$

Silicone polymers

Common silicone polymers are polydimethylsiloxane, polymethylphenyl-siloxane, and polydiphenylsiloxane. Most silicone polymers are synthesized by the condensation polymerization of purified chlorosilane and water. Dimethicones are liquid polymers having the general form of $CH_3(Si(CH_3)_2O)_nSi(CH_3)_3$. The dimethicones are prepared over a wide range of viscosity grades. The polymers have been used as a lubricant for artificial eyes and joints and as water repellants in lotions and creams. Polymethylphenylsiloxanes are used as a lubricant for syringes. Glassware coated with silicone polymers is rendered so hydrophobic that water drains easily from such containers. Activated dimethicones are a mixture of silicone oil and finely divided silica. The activated dimethicones enhance the antifoaming activities of the silicone polymers. Liquid silicone polymers are very often used as an inert drug carrier medium in controlled release systems (e.g., Progestasert®, Tranderm®-Nitro, Nitrodisc®).

$$(n+1)\left(\!\begin{array}{c} R \\ | \\ Cl-Si-Cl \\ | \\ R \end{array}\!\right) + nH_2O \longrightarrow Cl-\underset{\underset{R}{|}}{\overset{\overset{R}{|}}{Si}}-O\left(\!\underset{\underset{R}{|}}{\overset{\overset{R}{|}}{Si}}-O\!\right)_{n-1}\underset{\underset{R}{|}}{\overset{\overset{R}{|}}{Si}}-Cl + 2nHCl$$

Silicone polymers commonly have cross-linked network structures created by reacting a reactive prepolymer with a cross-linking agent. For example, a hydroxy-terminated polydimethylsiloxane is cross-linked with a methoxy-substituted silane and a catalyst as follows:

$$HO-\underset{\underset{CH_3}{|}}{\overset{\overset{CH_3}{|}}{Si}}\left(\!O-\underset{\underset{CH_3}{|}}{\overset{\overset{CH_3}{|}}{Si}}\!\right)_n OH + CH_3O-\underset{\underset{CH_3}{|}}{\overset{\overset{CH_3}{|}}{Si}}-OCH_3 \longrightarrow$$

$$\cdots\!-\underset{\underset{CH_3}{|}}{\overset{\overset{CH_3}{|}}{Si}}-O-\underset{\underset{O}{|}}{\overset{\overset{CH_3}{|}}{Si}}-O-\underset{\underset{CH_3}{|}}{\overset{\overset{CH_3}{|}}{Si}}-\cdots + CH_3OH$$

$$CH_3-\underset{|}{\overset{}{Si}}-CH_3 \ \cdots$$

The cross-linking reaction can take place at room temperature and thus these silicone polymers are useful for the fabrication of monolithic matrix systems for thermosensitive drugs.

Another example is the polymer formed with an acetoxy-terminated prepolymer and water as a curing agent. However, water is not directly incorporated but moisture is absorbed from air. The reaction is completed in 24 hr, and these polymers are used as adhesives and sealants.

A vinyl-terminated silicone prepolymer reacts with active hydrogen in another silicone prepolymer. The two separately stored liquid prepolymers are mixed together, and the mixture can be cast or molded. There is no byproduct; hence, these polymers are preferably used in biomedical applications.

Due to the liquid state of the silicone prepolymer, silicone polymers are prepared as preformed sheets and tubing or any other shape by first mixing the drug with the silicone polymer and a catalyst (e.g., stannous octoate). Then, the mixture is cast as a sheet or in a mold followed by curing overnight. For example, Norplant® is a set of flexible, closed cylindrical capsules (2.4×34 mm) of Silastic silicone polymer containing levonorgestrel for fertility control for 5 years. The capsules are inserted under the skin of the upper arm.

7.4.4 RING-OPENING POLYMERIZATION

7.4.4.1 Polylactic Acid, Polyglycolic Acid, and Polycaprolactone

$$\left[O-\underset{\underset{CH_3}{|}}{CH}-\underset{\underset{O}{||}}{C} \right]_n \qquad \left[O-CH_2-\underset{\underset{O}{||}}{C} \right]_n \qquad \left[O-(CH_2)_5-\underset{\underset{O}{||}}{C} \right]_n$$

Polylactic acid   Polyglycolic acid   Polycaprolactone

$$\left[O-\underset{\underset{CH_3}{|}}{CH_2}-\underset{\underset{O}{||}}{C} \right]_x \left[O-CH_2-\underset{\underset{O}{||}}{C} \right]_y$$

Poly(lactic acid-co-glycolic acid)

Ring-opening polymerization is different from the addition and condensation polymerizations described so far. It does not produce byproducts (e.g., water) as polycondensation does, and there is no unsaturated double bond in the monomers to lead to additional polymerization. However, some similarities do exist. Ring-opening polymerization is initiated by the opening of a cyclic structure in the monomers and followed by polyaddition. As a result, a linear polymer with a chemical composition identical to that of the monomer is obtained.

A number of polymers produced by ring-opening polymerization are used for pharmaceutical applications: some are biodegradable (e.g., lactic acid, glycolic acid, and caprolactone), while others are nonbiodegradable (e.g., ethylene oxide and propylene oxide). Biodegradable polymers, such as polylactic acid, polyglycolic acid, and poly(lactic acid-co-glycolic acid), are prepared by a direct polycondensation process and have a low molecular weight. This is attributed to more than 99.3% dehydration of the higher-molecular-weight products during the polymerization and the presence of impurities, which leads to stoichiometric imbalance. To obtain a molecular weight higher than 10,000, the cyclic dimers of these acids (latide and glycolide) must be used.

Ring-opening polymerization of lactide, glycolide, and caprolactone is initiated by metal compounds (e.g., tin, zinc, lead, antimony). However, stanneous octoate $[Sn^{II}(CO_2CH(^{n}Bu)(Et))_2]$ is the more acceptable initiator because it has been approved by government regulatory agencies as a food stabilizer. Here the monomer used is lactide, but one can apply this polymerization to other monomers (e.g., glycolide and lactone). The mechanism of the ring-opening polymerization of lactide is depicted as shown in Figure 7.27, even though the true mechanism is unclear. When the cyclic ring opens up, one end forms an ester group while the other end has a cationic character. Further addition of lactide propagates the polymerization.

Poly(esters) are the best defined widely used biodegradable and biocompatible materials. There are a number of different grades of poly(lactic acid) (PLA), poly(glycolic acid) (PGA), and copolymers of lactic and glycolic acids (PLAGA) with respect to molecular weights and compositions. One of the major advantages

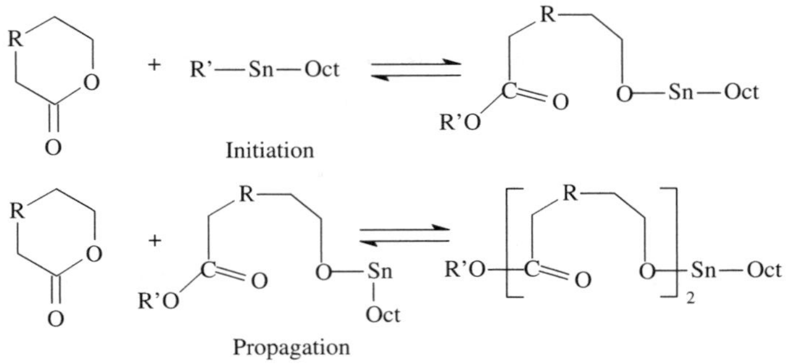

FIGURE 7.27 Initiation and propagation mechanism of Sn(Oct)$_2$-catalyzed polymerization of lactide.

of using PLA, PGA, PLAGA, and polycarprolactone (PCL) is that the byproducts of the biodegradation are lactic and glycolic acids, which are chemical compounds naturally found in the human body. As a result, these polymers are biocompatible, have been used for surgical sutures, and are adapted to pharmaceutical applications (especially, controlled release of proteins and peptides).

Lactic acid has an asymmetric α-carbon and exists as D and L enantiomers. L-Lactic acid occurs naturally, and thus poly(L-lactic acid) (PLLA) is thought to be more biocompatible than polyglycolic acid. Poly(D-lactic acid) (PDLA) and PLLA are crystalline (37% crystallinity), and the racemic PDLLA is amorphous and has a lower melting temperature and forms a better film than other PLAs do. Therefore, the amorphous PDLLAs are more prone to hydrolytic degradation than the crystalline PDLA and PLLA. On the other hand, PGA is a linear aliphatic poly(ester) and a semicrystalline polymer (50% crystallinity) with a high melting temperature. Thus, PGA is not soluble in common solvents. Absence of the methyl group in the polymer structure makes the PGAs able to be hydrolyzed faster and makes them more hydrophilic than PLAs. Random copolymers of lactic acid and glycolic acid ranging from 25 to 75% mole glycolic acid have reasonable physical properties such as easy processability and solubility.

PCL is semicrystalline, and its crystallinity decreases with an increase in its molecular weight. It is easily soluble in common solvents. However, PCL degrades at a slower rate than PGA and PLAGA do. Copolymers of caprolactone with other hydroxyl acids (e.g., lactic acid and glycolic acid) render a variety of polyesters having a wide range of biodegradability. The easy blendability of PCL creates various permeabilities and mechanical properties useful for drug delivery applications.

The degradation mechanism of polylactic acid and glycolic acid is due to the hydrolysis of the ester linkage. Unlike polyanhydrides and poly(orthoesters), poly-lactic acids and polyglycolic acids undergo bulk erosion. This means that the degradation may take place anywhere in the matrix. PGAs degrade faster than PLAs do, due to the their crystallinity and steric hindrance of the side pendant group of PLA. However, the degradation mechanisms of the poly(esters) are complex. The results of several studies have suggested that the degradation rate is size dependent, so that smaller particles will degrade slower than larger ones, and that the degradation

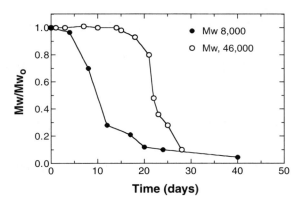

FIGURE 7.28 Erosion profiles of poly(lactic acid-co-glycolic acid) at pH 7.4. [Graph reconstructed from data by Gopferich and Burkersroda, *Proceed. Int. Symp. Control. Rel. Bioact. Mater.*, 24, 128 (1997).]

may be autocatalyzed by acidic byproducts formed during degradation. Figure 7.28 shows the effect of molecular weight of PLAGA on the erosion profiles.

The Mark–Houwink constants for PLAGA (60/40) in tetrahydrofuran have been obtained:

$$[\eta]_{\text{Thf}}^{\text{PLAGA}} = 1.07 \times 10^{-4} M_v^{0.761} \tag{7.152}$$

There are a few parenteral controlled-release products based on biodegradable polyesters, including Lupron Depot® and Zoladex®. Lupron Depot is a microparticle dosage form containing luprolide acetate, luteinizing hormone-releasing hormone, in a poly(D,L-lactic acid-co-glycolic acid). Microparticles are mixed with water before the injection. Zoladex is a thin poly(D,L-lactic acid-co-glycolic acid) cylinder containing goserelin acetate in a disposable syringe, and there is no premixing.

7.4.4.2 Polyethylene Glycol (PEG), Polyethylene Oxide (PEO), and Block Copolymers of Ethylene Oxide and Propylene Oxide (PEOPO)

Other important examples of ring-opening polymerizations are the synthesis of polyethylene oxide and the block copolymer of ethylene oxide and propylene oxide. Polyethylene oxide, also known as polyethylene glycol (PEG), is commonly produced by anionic polymerization and has a low molecular weight of less than 20,000.

$$\text{HO} -\!\!\left[\text{CH}_2\text{CH}_2\text{O} \right]_n\!\!- \text{H}$$

Polyethylene glycol or Polyethylene oxide

The polymerization is initiated when ethylene oxide reacts with alkali hydroxide to produce an anionic ethylene glycol:

$$\text{KOH} \ + \ \underset{\triangle}{\overset{O}{\triangle}} \quad \xrightarrow{\ \Delta\ } \quad \text{HOCH}_2\text{CH}_2\text{O}^-\,\text{K}^+$$

This nucleophilic anionic ethylene glycol attacks another monomer and the chain length is increased:

$$\text{HOCH}_2\text{CH}_2\text{O}^-\,\text{K}^+ \ + \ n\,\underset{\triangle}{\overset{O}{\triangle}} \quad \xrightarrow{\ \text{propagation}\ } \quad \text{H(OCH}_2\text{CH}_2)_{n+1}\!-\!\text{O}^-\,\text{K}^+$$

The reaction is terminated by the dehydration of the end group:

$$\text{H(OCH}_2\text{CH}_2)_{n+1}\!-\!\text{O}^-\,\text{K}^+ \quad \xrightarrow{\ \text{termination}\ } \quad \text{H(OCH}_2\text{CH}_2)_n\!-\!\text{CH=CH}_2 \ + \ \text{KOH}$$

The regenerated KOH works as a catalyst once again. If alkali alkoxides are used as catalysts instead of alkali hydroxides, the exchange of protons between the growing polymer and the dead polymer is:

$$\text{R(OCH}_2\text{CH}_2)_n\!-\!\text{O}^-\,\text{Na}^+ + \text{R(OCH}_2\text{CH}_2)_m\text{OH} \ \rightleftharpoons \ \text{R(OCH}_2\text{CH}_2)_n\text{OH} + \text{R(OCH}_2\text{CH}_2)_m\text{O}^-\,\text{Na}^+$$

High-molecular-weight polymers of polyethylene oxide of MW > 100,000 are prepared by a coordination polymerization with alkali earth metal compounds. These catalysts activate the epoxide ring by forming complexes with the oxygen in the oxide with the alkali earth metal:

$$\text{ROM} \ + \ \underset{\triangle}{\overset{O}{\triangle}} \quad \rightleftharpoons \quad \underset{\triangle}{\overset{O}{\triangle}}\!\!-\!\text{M}\!-\!\text{OR}$$

In chain propagation, nucleophilic attack of the alkoxide on the ethylene oxide yields:

$$\underset{\triangle}{\overset{O}{\triangle}}\!\!-\!\text{M}\!-\!\text{OR} \ + \ n\,\underset{\triangle}{\overset{O}{\triangle}} \quad \longrightarrow \quad \underset{\triangle}{\overset{O}{\triangle}}\!\!-\!\text{MO(C}_2\text{H}_4\text{O)}_n\text{R}$$

A number of different grades of polyethylene glycols and polyethylene oxides are available for pharmaceutical applications. For example, PEG 300, 400, and 600 are viscous liquids. PEG 900, 1000, and 1450 are waxy soft solids. PEG 3350, 4600, 8000, and 20,000 are hard waxy solids (Figure 7.29). PEGs with molecular weights of about 400 are 98% excreted in humans. PEGs are used as gelling agents, lubricants, binders for tablets, solubilizers, and plasticizers and for other purposes.

PEG's hydrophilicity yields water molecules to form hydrogen bonds with the polymer chains so that protein molecules are excluded or inhibited from being

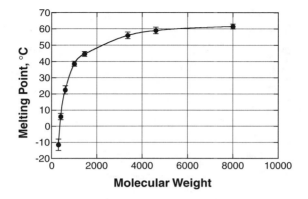

FIGURE 7.29 Molecular weight vs. melting points of PEGs. [Graph reconstructed from data in Dow Chemical's Carbowax Brochure.]

adsorbed onto solid materials. PEG has hydroxyl terminal end groups that provide the modification of the polymer. Depending on the nature of the hydroxyl end groups, diblock PLA–PEG or triblock PLA/PEG/PLA can be obtained. The hydroxyl end groups of PEG provide the initiating role for the ring-opening polymerization of lactide. Polymers containing PEG blocks have an improved property that is able to resist protein adsorption in water, and thus the adsorption of proteins onto the polymer surface is inhibited and cell–polymer interactions can be hindered. For example, PLA–PEG copolymers have lengthened blood circulation time in the body compared to PLA. In the fabrication process of PLA–PEG microparticles by the double emulsion method, PEG arranges the surface due to the hydrophilicity of the PEG block.

High-molecular-weight polyethylene oxides are used for controlled-release drug carriers, suspending agents, water-soluble coatings for tablets, flocculants, etc. The range of molecular weights is 0.1×, 0.2×, 0.3×, 0.4×, 0.6×, 0.9×, 1.0×, 2.0×, 4.0×, 5×, 7.0×, and 8.0 × 10^6. Polyethylene oxides (PEO) of molecular weights larger than 6000 are crystalline (approximately 95% crystallinity). As a result, water-soluble PEOs are resistant to absorption of atmospheric moisture, compared to other water-soluble polymers. The higher-molecular-weight PEOs have a good bioadhesive property. PEOs of molecular weights smaller than 2.0 × 10^6 provide synchronized phenomena between swelling and erosion rates during drug release (Figure 7.30) and thus nearly zero-order release kinetics are obtained, as shown in Figure 7.31. Drug diffusion plays a key role for highly water-soluble drugs due to the rapid

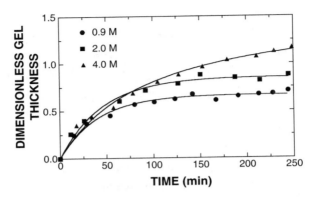

FIGURE 7.30 Dimensionless gel thickness of drug-free PEO tablets. [Graph reconstructed from data by Kim, *J. Pharm. Sci.,* 84, 303 (1995).]

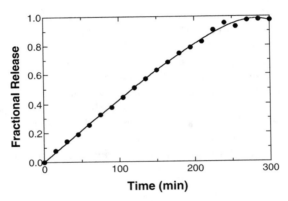

FIGURE 7.31 Release of hydroxyethyltheophylline in water from a PEO slab ($M_w = 0.6 \times 10^6$). [Graph reconstructed from data by Apicella et al. in *Polymers in Medicine: Biomedical and Pharmaceutical Applications,* R. M. Ottenbrite and E.M.O. Chiellin (Eds.), Technomic Publishing Co., Lancaster, PA, 1992, p. 23.]

penetration of water into the polymer matrix even before the swelling of the polymer. PEOs with molecular weights of 4.0×10^6 or higher exhibit anomalous release behavior because of the slower erosion rate. In addition, PEOs are good thickening agents and show pseudoplastic properties (i.e., shear thinning) whereas the oxygen in PEOs forms strong hydrogen bonds with various polar compounds such as poly(carboxylic acids), ureas, lignin, gelatin, etc.

The Mark–Houwink equations of polyethylene oxide in water are given in Table 7.7.

Block copolymers of ethylene oxide and propylene oxide, known as Pluronic® or Polaxomer®, are produced by anionic ring-opening polymerization. These block copolymers are used as nonionic surfactants, gelling agents, etc. The range of their molecular weights is 2000 to 14,600. The composition ratio of ethylene oxide to propylene oxide is 12 to 101 for a and 20 to 56 for b in the following block polymer structure:

TABLE 7.7
Mark–Houwink Constants for Polyethylene Oxide

Solvent	Temperature (°C)	$K \times 10^{-5}$	α	Approximate MW
Water	25	11.92	0.76	5 to 40 $\times 10^5$
Water	35	6.4	0.82	10^4 to 10^7
Water	45	6.9	0.81	10^4 to 10^7
0.45 M K$_2$SO$_4$	35	130	0.5	10^4 to 10^7
0.39 M MgSO$_4$	45	100	0.5	10^4 to 10^7
Benzene	25	39.7	0.686	8 to 500 $\times 10^4$

Source: From M. Grayson and D. Eckroth, *Kirk–Othmer Encyclopedia of Chemical Technology,* 3rd Ed., Vol. 18, Wiley Interscience, New York, 1982. p. 619.

$$HO\left(CH_2CH_2O\right)_a\left(\begin{matrix}CH_2CHO\\ | \\ CH_3\end{matrix}\right)_b\left(CH_2CH_2O\right)_a H$$

Pluronic copolymers with molecular weight of 11,500 have been used as a viscosity modifier and form a clear gel at 20 to 25% w/w in water. A solution of Pluronic undergoes a thermal gelation process in which a mixture of the polymer and water forms a clear solution at low temperature and then becomes a gel when raised to room temperature (above 21°C). A blend of Pluronic and lecithin is sold as Organogel for topical gel formulations.

7.4.4.3 Polyphosphazene (PPP)

Poly(phosphazenes) are also synthesized by a ring-opening polymerization of the cyclic trimer followed by substituting the chlorines with nucleophiles as shown below:

The hydrolytic breakdown of PPPs with hydrolytic labile substituents occurs in the side groups attached to the phosphorus. Due to the active site of phosphorus, PPPs provides coordinate and covalent binding with other chemical moieties (e.g., polyethylene glycol). Biodegradable PPPs are water insoluble until the side groups are hydrolyzed. For example, the PPPs substituted with alkylamino groups (i.e., $-NHCH_3$, $-NHC_2H_5$, and $-NHC_3H_7$) have hydrophilic and hydrophobic side groups. The hydrophilic side groups make the polymer water soluble when they are broken down hydrolytically, while the hydrophobic side groups make the polymer water insoluble. Through the hydrophilic side groups, the PPPs break down into nontoxic products such as phosphate, amino acids, ammonium salts, and ethanol, which are innocuous, extractable or metabolizable small molecules.

7.5 NATURAL POLYMERS AND THEIR MODIFICATION

Another way to achieve desirable polymer properties is the modification of pre-formed polymers. This modification may take place on the reactive sites of the polymer chain through alkylation, hydrolysis, sulfonation, esterification, and other various reactions of polymers. Examples of natural polymers and their modifications are cellulose and its derivatives, chitin and chitosan, and polysaccharides. These are still to this day very important polymers for pharmaceutical applications.

7.5.1 CELLULOSE

Cellulose

Cellulose is a polysaccharide; it is a natural polymer that forms the fibrous tissue of cotton and wood. It is also the most abundant of organic materials. It consists of glucose repeating units, bridged with oxygen. Each repeating unit has three hydroxyl groups per molecule of glucose. Its high crystallinity results from the strong hydrogen bonding of the hydroxyl groups along with stiff cyclic structures of the repeating units of cellulose. As a result, cellulose does not melt or dissolve. Due to its physicochemical structure, ingested cellulose passes unchanged through the digestive tract. To be used with raw materials, native cellulose is chemically modified by NaOH and CS_2 followed by H_2SO_4 to produce a "regenerated" cellulose from which films or fibers can be made. Native cellulose is derivatized to break down the hydrogen bonds, resulting in its solubility in various solvents.

Another form of cellulose, microcrystalline cellulose, has been used for pharmaceutical applications. Microcrystalline cellulose is a nonfibrous form of cellulose in which the cellulose fibers are fragmented into particle forms ranging in size from submicrons to a few hundred microns. The raw material for microcrystalline cellu-lose is a high α-purified wood cellulose. Two types of applications of microcrystal-line cellulose are dry powders and aqueous dispersions. The dry forms of the microcrystalline cellulose are used for pharmaceutical applications as fillers, binders, disintegrants, lubricants, and flow aids.

Microcrystalline cellulose is a good candidate for fillers because it is chemically inert, free from organic and inorganic contaminants, and compatible with other active drugs and excipients. The particle size distribution of microcrystalline cellulose assists in the uniform distribution of the active ingredients upon mixing. Microcrys-talline cellulose has the property of being a pressure-sensitive adhesive and thus it is a good dry binder for the formation of tablets. The hardness of the formed tablets, under a given compression pressure, is very high. Although it initially forms a very hard tablet, the formed tablet rapidly disintegrates as the hydrogen bonding forces are broken. The ratio of the hardness to the disintegration time of the tablet (kg/min) is high (5 to 10) when compared to 0.1 to 1 for most tableting excipients. Because microcrystalline cellulose has extremely low friction during tablet compression, the amount of lubricant is reduced and tablet disintegration and instant release of active ingredients are enhanced. Microcrystalline cellulose flows well in tablet or capsule mixtures so that even poorly flowing active ingredients can be formed into tablets with low weight variation.

Aqueous dispersion of microcrystalline cellulose yields white, opaque creamy gels due to the formation of elongated cellulose microcrystal aggregates, ranging in size from a few submicrons to a few microns. At concentrations greater than 1%, microcrystalline cellulose is highly thixotropic with high yield values. At concen-trations less than 1%, colloidal pseudoplastic dispersions are formed. These pseudo-plastic or thixotropic properties make a microcrystalline cellulose dispersion a well-structured suspending vehicle by itself or in combination with other hydrocolloids. Microcrystalline cellulose is compatible with water-soluble polymers (i.e., hydro-colloids) so that the mixed systems provide the best of both kinds of suspending agents, with the elasticity and yield value of the suspension. Upon adding a small amount of electrolyte, microcrystalline cellulose is flocculated. The flocculated microcrystalline cellulose prevents suspension formulations from forming hard packed cakes.

7.5.2 CELLULOSE DERIVATIVES

Cellulose derivatives

Cellulose Derivatives	R
Cellulose acetate	–H, –CO–CH$_3$
Cellulose acetate butyrate	–H, –CO–CH$_3$, –CO–CH$_2$–CH$_2$–CH$_2$–CH$_3$
Cellulose acetate phthalate	–H, –CO–CH$_3$, –CO–C$_6$H$_4$–COOH
Cellulose acetate propionate	–H, –CO–CH$_3$, –CO–CH$_2$–CH$_2$–CH$_3$
Ethyl cellulose	–H, –CH$_2$–CH$_3$
Hydroxyethyl cellulose	–H, –CH$_2$–CH$_2$–OH
Hydroxypropyl cellulose	–H, –CH$_2$–CH(OH)–CH$_3$
Hydroxyethylmethyl cellulose	–H, –CH$_3$, –CH$_2$–CH$_2$–OH
Hydroxypropylmethyl cellulose	–H, –CH$_3$, –CH$_2$–CH(OH)–CH$_3$
Hydroxypropylmethyl cellulose acetate succinate	–H, –CH$_3$, –COCH$_3$, –CO–CH$_2$–CH$_2$COOH, –CH$_2$–CH(OH)–CH$_3$, –CH$_2$–CH–CH$_3$, –OCOCH$_3$, –OCO–CH$_2$–CH$_2$–COOH
Hydroxypropylmethyl cellulose phthalate	–H, –CH$_3$, –CO–C$_6$H$_4$–COOH, –CH$_2$–CH–CH$_3$ –CH$_2$–CH(OH)–CH$_3$, –O–CO–C$_6$H$_4$–COOH
Methyl cellulose	–H, –CH$_3$
Na Carboxymethyl cellulose	–H, –CH$_2$COONa

Derivatization (or substitution) occurs on the reactive sites of the three hydroxyl groups on the glucose ring. Reaction of these hydroxyls by etherification or esterification gives cellulose ethers or cellulose esters, respectively, which are soluble in solvents and can be cast in useful forms. The distribution of the substituents of the three hydroxyls is dependent on their relative reactivity. The degree of substitution (DS) is used to express the average number of substituent groups attached to the anhydroglucose unit. The DS can vary from 0 to 3. If all three hydroxyls are substituted, the DS is equal to 3.

The cellulose derivatives can be produced by various processes. Cellulose ethers (methyl cellulose, ethyl cellulose, and carboxymethyl cellulose) are prepared by the condensation of sodium cellulose (obtained by the reaction of NaOH on cellulose) with the corresponding methyl halide (or methyl sulfate), ethyl halide (or ethyl sulfate), and carboxymethyl chloride, respectively. Hydroxyethyl and hydroxypropyl celluloses are prepared by reacting slurried cellulose with ethylene oxide and propylene oxide, respectively. A secondary hydroxyl of the hydroxyalkyl cellulose reacts again with another alkyl oxide so that the average number of moles of alkyl oxide attached to each anhydroglucose unit (i.e., moles of substituent combined, or MS) is greater than 1. For example, hydroxyalkyl cellulose with an MS = 2.5 and a DS = 1.5 contains five hydroxyalkyl groups per two units of anhydroglucose ring and three hydroxyls substituted per two units of anhydroglucose ring. However, the weight percent of the substituents in the cellulose ether is frequently expressed rather than the MS and DS. Table 7.8 shows the degree of substitution for some major cellulose derivatives. Hydroxyalkyl methyl cellulose is produced by the alkylation of hydroxyalkyl cellulose with a methyl halide. The hydroxyalkyl methyl cellulose possesses various ratios of methyl and hydroxyalkyl substituents, which govern the solubility and thermal gelation temperature of the aqueous solution. Except for ethyl cellulose, methyl cellulose, hydroxyalkyl cellulose, and hydroxyalkyl methyl cellulose are water soluble; they have been used for pharmaceutical applications, including tablet coatings, granulations, emulsions, suspensions, and extended release matrix tablets. Low-substituted hydroxypropyl cellulose is water insoluble but swells

TABLE 7.8
Degree of Substitution of Cellulose Derivatives

Cellulose Derivatives	Substitution
Cellulose acetate	32 to 44.8% acetyl
Cellulose acetate butyrate	12 to 24% acetyl, 35 to 39% butyryl
Cellulose acetate phthalate	19 to 36% acetyl, 20 to 35% phthalyl
Cellulose acetate propionate	2 to 9% acetyl, 40 to 49% propionyl
Ethyl cellulose	40 to 48% ethoxyl
Hydroxyethylcellulose	MS = 2.5 hydroxyethyl
Hydroxyethyl methylcellulose	4 to 15% ethoxyl, 20 to 26% methoxyl
Hydroxypropyl cellulose	53.4 to 77.5% hydroxypropyl
Hydroxypropyl methylcellulose acetate succinate	5 to 14% acetyl, 20 to 26% methoxyl, 5 to 10% hydroxypropoxyl, 4 to 18% succinoyl
Hydoxypropyl methylcellulose phthalate	18 to 24% methoxyl, 5 to 10% hydroxypropoxyl, 21 to 35% phthalyl
Methyl cellulose	27 to 31% methoxyl

in water. Thus, it has been used as a tablet disintegrant. Ethyl cellulose, on the other hand, is water insoluble and heat stable and has high impact strength. Ethyl cellulose is used in a number of pharmaceutical applications, including tablet or bead coatings, extended-release matrix tablets, microencapsulations for controlled-release systems, taste maskings, granulations, and tablet bindings.

An aqueous solution of water-soluble cellulose derivatives (e.g., methylcellulose, hydroxypropyl methylcellulose) is converted into a gel by raising its temperature, as known as "thermal gelation." The gel reverts to the solution again by cooling. The gelation behavior is affected by the concentration of the water-soluble derivatives and the rate of heating. Figure 7.32 shows the hysteresis of thermal gelation of hydroxypropyl methylcellulose.

Cellulose esters (e.g., cellulose triacetate, cellulose diacetate, cellulose propionate, and cellulose butyrate) are prepared by initially treating cellulose with glacial acetic acid (or propionic acid and butyric acid) followed by the corresponding acid anhydride with a trace of strong acid as a catalyst in chlorinated hydrocarbon. Complete esterification reactions result in the formation of a triester, which undergoes water hydrolysis to form a diester. Cellulose acetate alone or in combination with cellulose triacetate or cellulose butyrate is used as a semipermeable membrane for osmotic pumping tablets, primarily in controlled release systems. The permeability of the membrane can be further modulated by adding water-soluble excipients to the cellulose esters.

Water-soluble hydroxypropylmethyl cellulose and water-insoluble cellulose acetate are further treated with phthalic anhydride or succinic anhydride to yield hydroxypropyl methylcellulose phthalate, cellulose acetate phthalate, and hydroxypropylmethylcellulose acetate succinate. These polymers are used as enteric materials and are water soluble or insoluble above or below a specific pH, respectively.

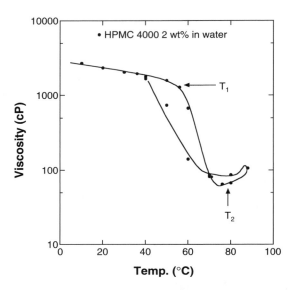

FIGURE 7.32 Thermal gelation of hydroxypropyl methylcellulose 60SH (2 wt%) in water: T_1 = the temperature at which viscosity starts decreasing; T_2 = the temperature at which viscosity starts increasing. [Graph reconstructed from data by Shin-Etsu Chemical, METO-LOSE, 1993.]

7.5.3 Chitosan

Chitosan is a useful derivative of chitin, which is the second most plentiful natural polymer, behind only cellulose. Chitin is a naturally occurring polysaccharide consisting of amino sugars. It is a natural polymer formed of repeating monomer units of β-(1-4)-2-acetamido-2-deoxy-D-glucose, resembling cellulose, except that the hydroxyl groups in position 2 have been substituted by acetylamino groups. However, about 16% of the hydroxyl groups in position 2 are deacetylated. Chitin is found in crustacean shells (e.g., crab, shrimp, and cuttlefish), insect exoskeletons, fungal cell walls, microfauna, and plankton and is associated with proteins and minerals such as calcium carbonate.

Most commercial applications use the deacetylated derivative, chitosan, which is a polysaccharide formed of repeating monomer units of beta-(1-4) 2-amino-2-deoxy-D-glucose. In general, about 20% of the repeating units are acetylated, with the remaining 80% deacetylated, and these percentages can vary with the sources of chitin and processing methods. Amino and hydroxyl groups in chitosan readily react to produce varieties of chitosan derivatives to modify its properties to meet various application requirements.

Chitin   Chitosan

Chitosan can be produced in a variety of ways including a thermal deacetylation method, an isolation method from chitosan raw materials, and a bioconversion method. Presently, commercial chitosan is produced by thermal deacetylation of chitin. Under vigorous alkaline conditions at high temperature, acetamide linkages undergo *N*-deacetylation, and about 75% of acetyl groups can be removed. However, *trans* related hydroxyl groups cannot be deacetylated. Prolonged treatment of chitin in hot alkaline solution (e.g., NaOH) provides complete *N*-deacetylation but the polymer is severely degraded to very-low-molecular-weight polymers. Extended acid treatment of chitin or chitosan results in depolymerization. The degree of deacetylation and molecular weight of chitosan are dependent on the chitin raw material, and the preparation processes of chitosan, including their temperature and duration. Thermochemical deacetylation in air yields chitosan of lower molecular weight than deacetylation in an inert atmosphere does. Higher temperature or extended time increases the degree of deacetylation but yields low molecular weight and may cause further depolymerization. Generally, more than 80% deacetylation cannot be achieved without depolymerization and shortening of the polymer chains.

The isolation of chitosan from *Mucor rouxii* cell wall gives certain desirable properties not obtainable by the commercial thermochemical method. The isolation method involves a culture growth followed by an extraction process. The chitosan yield ranges from 5 to 10% of total dry biomass weight and its molecular weight varies from 2.0×10^5 to 1.4×10^6, which depends on incubation time, medium composition, and the type and concentration of acid. The chitosan obtained from the fungal cell wall gives a much higher degree of deacetylation (i.e., 60 to 92%).

Another route of obtaining chitosan includes the enzymatic bioconversion of chitin by chitin deacetylase to chitosan by deacetylation of *N*-acetylglucosamine residues. The longer the oligosaccharide, the higher the rate of the deacetylation. The enzyme requires at least four chitin-repeating units. The enzyme appeared to show very specific action on *N*-acetylglucosamine homo polymers and an effective conversion of chitosan to more deacetylated products without degradation.

Chitosan and its derivatives have been applied to enhance the absorption of proteins (e.g., insulin) and polypeptides (e.g., buserelin). *N*-Trimethyl chitosan chloride exhibits opening of the tight junctions of the intranasal and intestinal epithelial cells so that the transport of hydrophilic compounds is increased through the paracellular transport pathway. The absorption-enhancing effect was concentration dependent and reversible and dependent on the integrity of the intercellular cell contact zone.

Chitosan and hydroxypropylchitosan were found to be enzymatically degraded so that they can be used for implantable controlled-release dosage forms. Due to the moieties of chitosan (i.e., amine and hydroxyl groups), chitosan can be cross-linked or complexed with citric acid, EDTA, or glutaraldehyde, and the cross-linked or complexed chitosans have been applied to drug delivery systems.

In addition to the novel applications mentioned above, chitosan and chitin have been exploited in numerous areas such as wound dressing, cholesterol control, food stabilization, hair/skin care, and cell/enzyme immobilization.

7.5.4 POLYSACCHARIDES

Polysaccharides are biomacromolecules consisting of monosaccharide-repeating units. Their sequences, the linkages between them, their configuration, and the presence of any other substituents cause the differences in physicochemical properties among polysaccharides. Numerous polysaccharides are employed in pharmaceutical applications; the common ones are listed below.

Acacia, known as gum arabic, is widely used in pharmaceutics as an emulsifier and a viscosity modifier. It is produced from acacia trees in which large nodules seal wounds in the bark during "gummosis." Acacia is composed of alkali and alkali earth salts of arabic acid. An aqueous solution of arabic acid is strongly acidic having a pH of 2.2 to 2.7. Acacia is an effective emulsifier, and it stabilizes emulsions by forming a firm multi-layer film around the dispersed phase as a mechanical barrier to resist rupture and coalescence. Emulsions prepared with the salt forms of arabic acid (HLB 8.0) (e.g., Mineral Oil Emulsion USP) are more stable than those obtained with arabic acid even though the latter gives a higher viscosity than the former. One of the reasons for the high viscosity of aqueous solutions of acacia is related to the branched structure of the polymer chains. Because it is an anionic polymer, acacia is incompatible with positively charged compounds including preservatives, in addition to phenolic compounds (e.g., phenol, cresols, thymol).

Tragacanth is widely used as a natural emulsifier in conjunction with acacia and is an effective viscosity modifier for suspension formulations. It contains a variety of methoxylated acids that upon contact with water become a gel. At around pH 5, it renders the maximum stable viscosity due to aging even though the maximum viscosity occurs at pH 8 with the freshly prepared solution.

Xanthan gum is an anionic, water-soluble polysaccharide obtained from a pure culture fermentation of *Xanthomonas camprestris*. It consists of a 1,4-β-D-glucose backbone and trisaccharide branches comprised of a glucuronic acid residue and two mannose residues. Due to this substance's anionic nature, like those of acacia and tragacanth, it is not compatible with cationic compounds (e.g., benzalkonium chloride), but it is moderately compatible with divalent cations. It has been used to develop sustained-release dosage forms because the high-molecular-weight gum dissolves slowly in water. Xanthan gum is less gelling but used as the viscosity modifier due to weak-gel shear-thinning properties. The solution properties of xanthan gum are not affected by ionic strength, pH (1 to 13), shear, or temperature.

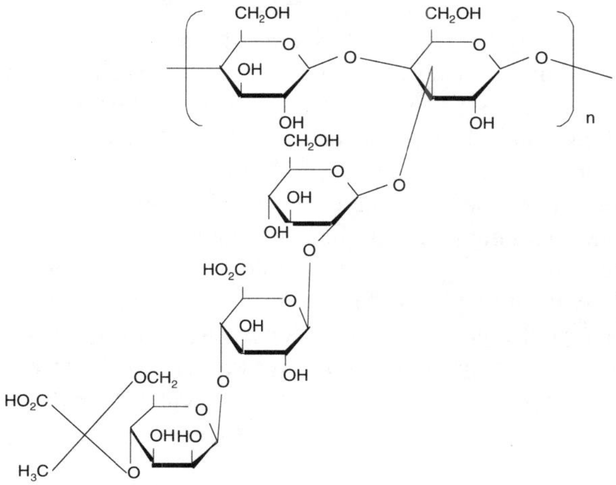

Xanthan gum

Pectin is a partially methoxylated polygalacturonic acid extracted from the skin of apple, citrus, and sugar beet fruits. It may be obtained as amidated forms (i.e., sodium or ammonium salts). It has excellent gelling properties, which are dependent on the degree of methoxylation of the carboxylic acid groups. The high methoxylation causes weak gelation in the presence of inorganic cations (e.g., Ca^{+2}) through calcium-cation bridging between adjacent twofold helical chains comprised of $-COO^-$, whereas in the absence of inorganic cations, the high methoxylation aids gelation via strong hydrophobic interactions. Low methoxyl pectins (<40% esterified) are obtained from high methoxyl pectins (about 70% esterified) by demethylation with ammonia. Hydrogen bonding between the carboxylic acid groups and the hydroxyl groups displays a rigid gel. Thus, it has been shown that pectin gels with 40 to 60% methoxylation are stronger than those with 70 to 80% methoxylation. Low-methoxyl pectin gels are thermoreversible in the presence of calcium cations at pH 3 to 5. High-methoxyl pectin gels undergo a thermally irreversible process in the presence of sugar (65% by weight) at pH < 3.5.

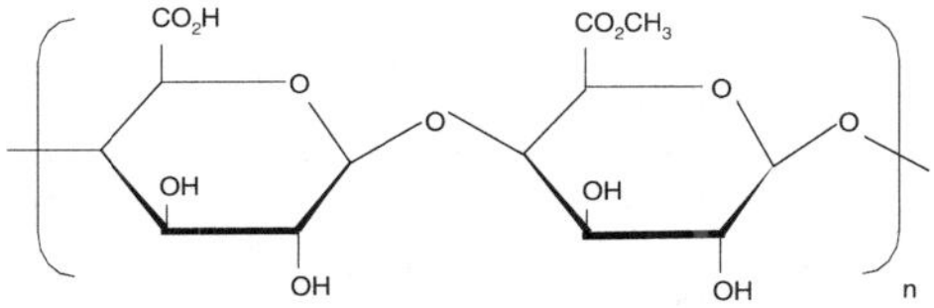

Pectin

Alginate is a linear polysaccharide (MW 47,000 to 370,000) extracted from brown seaweed (mainly *Laminaria*) consisting of D-mannuronic acid and L-guluronic acid residues. Sodium alginate forms a flexible, translucent gel upon contact with $CaCl_2$ solution (i.e., cross-linking) by replacing the hydrogen bonding and zipping guluronate chains together. The longer the cross-linked gel remains in the $CaCl_2$ solution, the more rigid the gel that will be obtained. The cross-links can be broken by placing them into brine. The rate of gelation of alginates is slower than that of pectins. Alginates with high L-guluronic acid content form a stronger gel. Like other polysaccharides, alginates precipitate in acidic conditions, but propylene glycol alginates are free of carboxylic acid in the macromolecular chains. Sodium alginates and propylene glycol alginate are used for a variety of applications such as cell immobilization (e.g., encapsulation of pancreas cells), wood dressings, antacids (e.g., Gaviscon), dental impression materials, pharmaceutical excipients, and drug delivery.

Sodium alginate

Carrageenan is a linear galactan with sulfate groups extracted from red seaweeds of the Furcellariaceae, Gigartinaceae, Phyllophorraceae, and Solieraceae families. They are composed of alternating 4-linked-α-D-galactopyranose and 3-linked-β-D-galactopyranose units. The three major types of carrageenans are κ-, ι-, and λ-carrageenan. They are different in the composition of repeating units and the degree of sulfation, which depend on algal sources. Unlike other polysaccharides comprised of carboxylic acid groups, carrageenan is not pH sensitive due to the sulfate groups. It strongly interacts with cationic compounds (i.e., complexation). It has been applied to deliver a variety of drugs from drug–carrageenan complexes without providing pH-dependent release. λ-Carrageenan, which has galactose repeating units, dissolves in water; the other carageenans, which have 3,6-anhydrogalactose units that allow for a helical structure, should be heated to about 80°C for complete solution. Carrageenans are used as suspending, thickening, and gelling agents.

Carrageenan (kappa)

7.5.5 GELATIN

Gelatin is obtained by the thermal denaturation or disintegration of collagen, a principal protein found in many animal skins and bones, including those of humans. It is composed of 18 different amino acids, including 4-hydroxyproline ($\approx$ 14%), proline ($\approx$ 16%), and glycine ($\approx$ 26%) groups, and with an extended left-handed helix conformation containing 300 to 4000 amino acid groups. However, it contains no tryptophan and is low in methionine.

There are two types of gelatin, depending on the source material and the preparation method. Type A is derived from an acid process, primarily of pigskin where the collagen is young. Type B is derived from alkaline or lime and acid processes, primarily of cattle or calf skins and bones where the collagen is older and densely cross-linked. Gelatin contains 84 to 90% protein, 1 to 2% mineral salts, and 5 to 15% water. In general, the two types of gelatin have the following properties:

Specification	Type A	Type B
Material	Pork skin	Cattle skin
pH	3.8 to 5.5	5.0 to 7.5
Isoelectric point	7.0 to 9.0	4.7 to 5.4
Gel strength (bloom)	50 to 300	50 to 280
Viscosity (mP)	15 to 75	20 to 75
Ash (%)	0.3 to 2.0	0.5 to 2.0

Gelatin is slightly soluble in water and completely soluble above 40°C. Its solution becomes a transparent thermoreversible gel upon cooling below 35°C (e.g., Jell-O®), and upon being spray dried from the solution, gelatin is readily soluble in cold water. Gelatin is very compatible with polyhydric alcohols such as sorbitol, propylene glycol, and glycerol, which are used to modify the hardness of gelatin films (e.g., soft gelatin capsules).

The film-forming property of gelatin finds many applications in pharmaceutical products (e.g., hard and soft capsules). Due to the shrinkage of gelatin films on drying, polyhydric alcohols are added to modify the properties of the dry gelatin film (e.g., adhesion and flexibility). High-molecular-weight gelatins are favored over low-molecular-weight gelatins for film forming.

Gelatin is amphoteric and amphiphilic and thus has limited emulsifying properties (HLB 9.8) (e.g., whipped cream) that can be used in water-in-oil emulsions such as low-fat margarine. Gelatin is also used as a foam stabilizer (e.g., mallow foam). It has mixed-film-forming properties with polysaccharides. At a pH where the gelatin and polysaccharide retain a positive charge and a negative charge, respectively, the opposite charges react to form an insoluble gelatin–polysaccharide complex around emulsified oil droplets (e.g., flavor oils) or particles (i.e., microencapsulation of carbon black). The formed films are hardened with glutaraldehyde or formaldehyde before recovering microcapsules. Due to the cross-linking ability with an oxidative group such as aldehyde or ketone, the rate of capsule dissolution may slow down.

Gelatin is also used for tablets, suppositories (e.g., glycerinated), hemostatics and others.

SUGGESTED READINGS

1. R. Baker, *Controlled Release of Biologically Active Agents,* Wiley Interscience, New York, 1987, Chapters 6–8.
2. N. C. Billingham, *Molar Mass Measurements in Polymer Science*, John Wiley and Sons, New York, 1977.
3. F. W. Billmeyer, Jr., *Textbook of Polymer Science*, 2nd Ed., Wiley Interscience, New York, 1971.
4. J. Brandrup, E. H. Immergut, E. A. Grulke (Eds.), *Polymer Handbook,* 4th Ed., John Wiley and Sons, New York, 1995.
5. R. O. Ebewele, *Polymer Science and Technology,* CRC Press, Boca Raton, FL, 2000.
6. A. E. Hamielec, *Polymer Reaction Engineering: An Intensive Short Course on Polymer Production Technology,* McMaster University, Hamilton, Ontario, 1980, Chapters 1 and 2.
7. R. A. A. Muzzarelli, *Chitin,* Pergamon Press, Oxford, 1977.
8. S. N. E. Omorodion, Size Exclusion Chromatography (SEC) in Aqueous Media, Ph.D. Dissertation, McMaster University, Hamilton, Ontario, 1980.
9. P. C. Painter and M. M. Coleman, *Fundamentals of Polymer Science: An Introductory Text,* Technomic Publishing Co., Lancaster, PA, 1997.
10. F. P. Rempp and E. W. Merrill, *Polymer Synthesis*, Huethig and Wepf, Basel, Switzerland, 1986.
11. F. Rodriguez, *Principles of Polymer Systems,* 2nd Ed., McGraw-Hill, New York, 1970.
12. K. E. Uhrich et al., Polymeric Systems for Controlled Drug Release, *Chem. Rev.,* 99, 3181 (1999).
13. R. L. Whistler and J. BeMiller, *Industrial Gums,* 3rd Ed., Academic Press, New York, 1993.

Index